Cancer Treatment and Research

Volume 160

Series Editor

Steven T. Rosen, Chicago, IL, USA

For further volumes:
http://www.springer.com/series/5808

Ritu Nayar
Editor

Cytopathology in Oncology

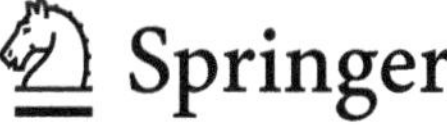 Springer

Editor
Ritu Nayar
Feinberg School of Medicine, Northwestern University
Chicago, IL
USA

ISSN 0927-3042
ISBN 978-3-642-38849-1   ISBN 978-3-642-38850-7   (eBook)
DOI 10.1007/978-3-642-38850-7
Springer Heidelberg New York Dordrecht London

Library of Congress Control Number: 2013947352

To my husband Rajeev—my inspiration and biggest support, my parents and many outstanding mentors

Preface

Cytopathology, a branch of pathology that studies and diagnoses diseases at the cellular level, was founded by Rudolf Virchow in 1858. The first cytopathology test, the Pap (anicolaou) test for screening and diagnosis of cervical cancer, was developed over 50 years ago and has proven to be not only the most successful screening test in medical history, but also the most effective global cancer reduction program. Since the development of the Pap test, the practice of cytopathology has expanded greatly to include samples from nearly all body sites which can be acquired during a range of procedures such as centesis, endoscopy, and fine needle aspiration. Cytologic sampling is minimally invasive, time efficient, and provides accurate, actionable information in the hands of qualified cytopathologists.

As expertise in cytopathology has developed and advances have occurred in medicine and oncology, the relationship between oncologist and cytopathologist has become exceedingly important for tumor diagnosis, prognostication, and targeted therapy selection. Cytopathologists are often the first physicians to make a diagnosis: adequacy assessment and triage for appropriate ancillary testing can be performed intraprocedurally by cytopathology in order to ensure that the specimen can provide the appropriate information required for the patient's management. In addition to fine needle aspiration, touch preparation assessment from thin-core biopsies has increasingly become a part of specimen acquisition.

To ensure a good working relationship between oncologist and cytopathologist and to maximize the value of cytopathology in patient care, each should have a basic understanding of one another's needs. In this text which is targeted toward our clinical colleagues, particularly those taking care of oncology patients, we aim to provide an overview of the basic principles of cytologic diagnosis at various body sites. We hope you will find it to be a useful reference for your practice.

Ritu Nayar, MD
Northwestern University,
Feinberg School of Medicine
and Robert H. Lurie Comprehensive Cancer Center

Contents

1 **Overview of Cytopathology Procedures and Techniques**   1
M. Ivanovic

2 **Ancillary Studies on Neoplastic Cytologic Specimens**   13
Y. Gong

3 **Head and Neck**.   31
Jose Dutra and Ajit Paintal

4 **Cytology of the Lung**   59
Sara Zydowicz, Anjana Yeldandi and Kirtee Raparia

5 **Liver Cytology**   83
Deborah J. Chute, Marc Sarti and Kristen A. Atkins

6 **Esophagus, Stomach, and Pancreas**. 111
Xiaoqi Lin and Srinadh Komanduri

7 **Genitourinary Cytopathology (Kidney and Urinary Tract)**. 149
Güliz A. Barkan and Eva M. Wojcik

8 **Body Cavity Fluids**. 185
Michael J. Thrall

9 **Cytopathology in the Diagnosis of Lymphoma**. 211
Yi-Hua Chen and Yun Gong

10 **Female Genital Tract** 241
Rosemary Tambouret

11 **Beyond the Standard of Care: The Role of Cytopathology
in Molecular Testing of Cancer**. 273
Peter Kulesza

Contributors

Kristen A. Atkins Department of Pathology, University of Virginia Medical System, 1215 Lee Street/Office 3034, Charlottesville, VA 22908, USA, e-mail: kaa2p@virginia.edu

Guliz A. Barkan Department of Pathology, Loyola University Medical Center, 2160 South First Avenue, Maywood, IL 60153, USA, e-mail: gbarkan@lumc.edu

Yi-Hua Chen Department of Pathology, Dean Northwestern University Feinberg School of Medicine, 251 E. Huron, Feinberg 7-209A, Chicago, IL 60611, USA, e-mail: y-chen5@northwestern.edu

Deborah J. Chute Department of Anatomic Pathology, Cleveland Clinic, 9500 Euclid Avenue L25, Cleveland, OH 44195, USA, e-mail: dchute1@gmail.com

Jose C. Dutra Department of Otolaryngology-Head and Neck Surgery, Northwestern Feinberg School of Medicine, 675 North Saint Clair, Galter Bldg 15-200, Chicago, IL 60611, USA, e-mail: jdutra@nmff.org

Yun Gong Department of Pathology, The University of Texas M. D. Anderson Cancer Center, Unit 53 1515 Holcombe Blvd, Houston, TX 77030, USA, e-mail: yungong@mdanderson.org

Marina Ivanovic Department of Pathology, University of Iowa, 200 Hawkins Drive, CRP 5243, Iowa City, IA 52242, USA, e-mail: marina-ivanovic@uiowa.edu

Srinadh Komanouri Department of Gastroenterology, Northwestern University, 676 N. St. Claire Street, 14th floor, Chicago, IL 60611, USA, e-mail: koman1973@gmail.com

Piotr Kulesa Department of Pathology, Northwestern University/Northwestern Memorial Hospital, 675 N St. Claire Street, Galter Pavillion 7-132-E, Chicago, IL 60611, USA, e-mail: p-kulesza@northwestern.edu

Xiaoqi Lin Department of Pathology, Northwestern University/Northwestern Memorial Hospital, 675 N St. Claire Street, Galter Pavillion 7-132F, Chicago, IL 60611, USA, e-mail: xlin@northwestern.edu

Kirtee Raparia Department of Pathology, Northwestern Memorial Hospital, 250 East Huron Street, Feinberg 7-335, Chicago, IL 60611, USA, e-mail: kraparia@northwestern.edu

Ajit Paintal Department of Pathology, Northwestern University/Northwestern Memorial Hospital, 251 East Huron Street, Galter 7-132G, Chicago, IL 60611, USA, e-mail: ajit.paintal@northwestern.edu

Marc Sarti Department of Radiology, Medical Director of Ultrasound and Cross-Sectional International Radiology, 1215 Lee Street, PO Box 800170, Charlottesville, VA 22908, USA, e-mail: marcsarti@gmail.com

Rosemary Tambouret Department of Pathology, Massachusetts General Hospital, Warren 105/55 Fruit Street, Boston, MA 02114, USA, e-mail: rtambouret@partners.org

Michael J. Thrall Department of Pathology, The Methodist Hospital, 6565 Fannin M227, Houston, TX 77030, USA, e-mail: mjthrall@tmhs.org

Eva M. Wojcik Department of Pathology, Loyola University Medical Center, 2160 South First Avenue, Maywood, IL 60153, USA, e-mail: ewojcik@lumc.edu

Anjana V. Yeldandi Department of Surgical Pathology, Northwestern Memorial Hospital, 251 E. Huron Street, Feinberg Pavilion 7-342, Chicago, IL 60612, USA, e-mail: a-yeldandi@northwestern.edu

Sara H. Zydowicz District Nine Medical Examiner's Office, 2350 E. Michigan Street, Orlando, FL 32806, USA, e-mail: sara.zydowicz@ocfl.net

Chapter 1
Overview of Cytopathology Procedures and Techniques

M. Ivanovic

1.1 General Specimen Labeling and Acceptance/Rejection Criteria Applicable to all Specimen Types

Each specimen (container/prepared glass slides) has to be labeled with two unique identifiers (patient name/medical record number/social security number/date of birth) and accompanied by an appropriate requisition form.

On the requisition form ordering physician should provide:

- Name of the patient
- Date of birth
- Medical record number
- Ordering physician's name and contact information
- Date of the procedure
- Type of the specimen (including procedure used to obtain it; for example urine-catheterized)
- Specimens obtained by fine needle aspiration should include:

  - Organ sampled
  - Laterality
  - Location of the lesion
  - Number of lesions
  - Size of the lesion and ultrasound characteristics (if available)
- Clinical history:

  - Reason for the procedure
  - Previous history of malignancy (if the prior malignancy was diagnosed in another institution, it is recommended to obtain patient written consent for the

M. Ivanovic (✉)
University of Iowa, Department of Pathology, 200 Hawkins Drive, CRP 5243, Iowa, IA 52242, USA
e-mail: marina-ivanovic@uiowa.edu

R. Nayar (ed.), *Cytopathology in Oncology*,
Cancer Treatment and Research 160, DOI: 10.1007/978-3-642-38850-7_1,
© Springer-Verlag Berlin Heidelberg 2014

release of the surgical report/slides if deemed necessary for comparison with current material).
– Besides the basic information about the patient, the requisition form accompanying the cervical sample (Pap test) should contain clinical information, date of last menstrual period, history of previous abnormal Pap tests or any gynecological surgeries, use of birth control pills, placement of IUD or any hormonal therapy [1].

Specimen will not be accepted for analysis by the cytology laboratory if[1]:

- The specimen is not labeled and accompanied by requisition form.
- The name of the patient written on the container is different than the name on the accompanying requisition form.
- The received slide(s) is broken and cannot be repaired.
- Contents of the container have leaked out of the container.

1.2 Fine Needle Aspiration

1.2.1 Superficial Fine Needle Aspiration

Superficial Fine Needle Aspiration (FNA) is a minimally invasive technique used to obtain diagnostic material from superficial, palpable lesions from organ sites such as thyroid, breast, lymph nodes, salivary glands, subcutaneous or adipose tissue [2]. Material is obtained either to determine the nature of the lesion (benign versus malignant) or to obtain material for further studies (microbiology, flow cytometry, or immunohistochemistry, molecular testing). It is usually performed by a cytopathologist or in a clinician's office with/or without the use of ultrasound.

Prior to beginning the procedure, clinical information/radiology findings are reviewed and the patient's identity and the procedure site/type are confirmed. The procedure, including potential risks and limitations, are described to the patient and a written consent is obtained.

The patient is put in a comfortable position and the size and location of the lesion are assessed. The skin is cleaned with alcohol or iodine and a small gauge needle (22–25G) is used for most procedures. Larger, 18G needles are used to obtain subcutaneous adipose tissue (fat pad) to determine the presence or the absence of amyloid by Congo red stain. The needle can be used alone or attached to the syringe placed in a metal holder (Fig. 1.1). If using a small gauge needle, no local anesthetic is necessary as injection of the anesthetic can cause more pain than the procedure itself, can make the lesion difficult to locate and may interfere with

---

[1] Each cytology laboratory has a specific acceptance/rejection policy and a written policy about informing the ordering physician of the rejected specimen.

the specimen quality [3]. Local anesthetic is given when using large 18G needle for fat pad aspiration. The lesion is localized and held in place by the operators thumb and index finger. The needle is introduced into the lesion and is moved in a cutting motion to ensure adequate material for analysis. Once the material is seen in the needle hub, the needle is withdrawn from the lesion. When using a needle alone, without an attached syringe, an empty syringe (10 ml) with the clip pulled half way is attached to the needle after it is withdrawn from the lesion to help expel the material on to the glass slide. If blood is noticed in the needle hub, the needle should be immediately withdrawn from the lesion to prevent clotting of the specimen.

Two slides are prepared from each pass, one that is immediately put in alcohol or spray fixed for Papanicolaou stain and another one that is air-dried and stained with Diff-Quick for immediate assessment of cellularity and triage based on morphological findings (Fig. 1.2). If an on site evaluation is being performed and the initial findings indicate infectious disease or hematological malignancy additional material can be obtained to triage for microbiology cultures or flow cytometry, respectively.

When using a syringe holder with needle attached to the syringe (usually 10–20-ml disposable plastic syringe), suction is applied after the needle is advanced into the lesion and is released before the needle is removed from the lesion to prevent dispersal of the specimen into the syringe. In some cases, multiple passes are required to obtain adequate diagnostic material.

After the needle is withdrawn from the lesion, pressure is applied to the procedure site with a sterile gauze for 2–3 min to ensure hemostasis [2]. When the procedure is completed, the procedure site is cleaned and a bandage is applied over the site. The patient is advised to monitor the procedure site for redness or any other changes and to contact his/her clinician if any complications related to the procedure are noticed.

At the time of the procedure, two slides, one air dried and the other alcohol fixed, are prepared from each pass. The air-dried smear is used for adequacy assessment and triage, as noted above, before termination of the procedure. The Papanicolaou stain has advantage over the Diff-Quick stain as it provides better nuclear detail; however, both types of stains are complimentary in assessment of

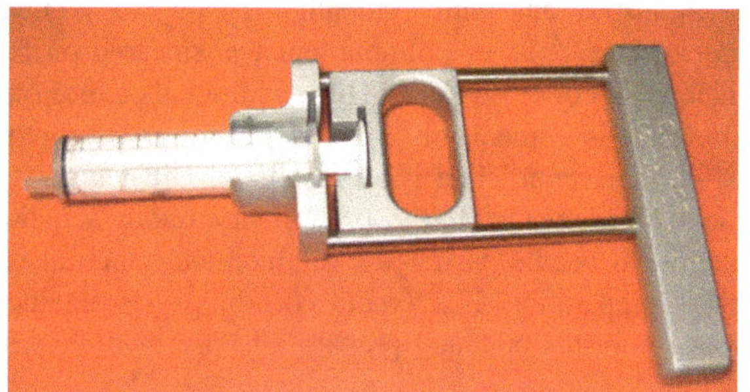

Fig. 1.1 Syringe placed in the metal syringe holder used for the fine needle aspiration. A variety of holders are available. Depicted here is the Cameco Holder

Fig. 1.2 Diff-Quick stain.
Air-dried smear prepared in
an ideal "tear drop" shape

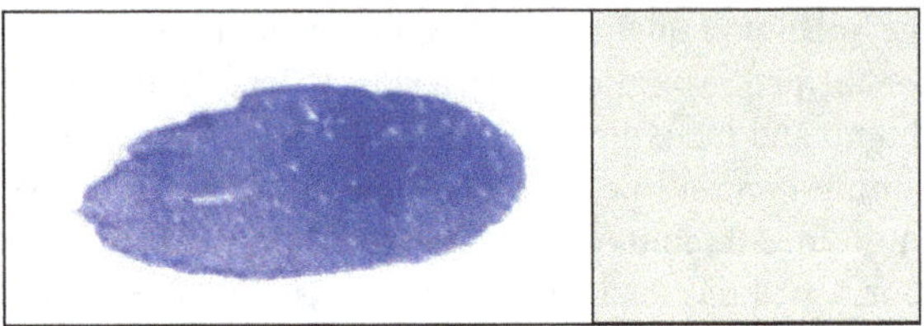

FNA biopsies. If indicated, needle rinsing and additional passes may be performed for making a cell block, which is processed in the histology laboratory.

The main limitation of FNA is lack of the tissue architecture. In very fibrotic and largely cystic lesions, it may be difficult to obtain adequate cellular material for diagnosis. Air drying artifact, bloody and thick smears are limiting factors in the interpretation of the FNA [2]. A cell block is useful if additional studies such as immunohistochemistry or if molecular studies need to be performed.

Complications are very rare (0.03 %) when using 22G needle and thinner. [4], and increase with increase in the diameter of the needle used [2]. Complications include bleeding (hematoma), infection [5] and pneumothorax [1] (when breast, axillary, and supraclavicular masses are aspirated). Rare cases of needle track seeding by tumor have been reported [5–7].

1.2.2 Endoscopic FNA

Endoscopic FNA is a sensitive method for assessing gastrointestinal or endobronchial lesions as well as organs/lesions adjacent to the gastrointestinal and endobronchial tracts. It can be used for obtaining primary diagnosis and for staging of the patients with unknown malignancy or for restaging patients with lung cancer after chemotherapy or chemoradiation [8].

The procedure is performed by gastroenterologists or pulmonologists with the patient under intravenous conscious sedation or general anesthesia [8, 9]. Target lesions are evaluated by using a radial or curvilinear echo endoscope. Usually a 22G needle is used for the obtaining tissue specimens by EUS-FNA [10]. If core biopsy material is required, a Trucut biopsy needle can be used in certain cases [11].

In institutions with cytopathology on site evaluation, material obtained by gastroenterologist or pulmonologist is smeared on two slides and all the excess material is collected in RPMI for additional studies (cell block or flow cytometry). One slide is immediately fixed in alcohol or is spray fixed for Papanicolaou stain, while the second slide is air-dried and Diff-Quick stained for immediate assessment of adequacy. If the preliminary findings indicate need for immunostains additional needle passes are obtained and material is collected in RPMI for cell block preparation. If a Trucut core biopsy is obtained during the procedure, the tissue imprints or touch preparations are made and slides are stained with Diff-

Quick for immediate assessment. The remaining tissue is put in formalin and sent to the histology laboratory for processing.

EUS-FNA is an operator-dependent technique and the accuracy of diagnosis depends on quality material obtained. Cystic lesions may yield insufficient material for diagnosis, as well as submucosal spindle cell lesions.

Complications of gastrointestinal EUS-FNA are rare. O'Toole found the overall incidence of complications to be 1.5 %, with high risk complications in cystic than solid lesions [8].

1.2.3 Image-Guided Percutaneous Fine Needle Aspiration

Image-guided percutaneous FNA is used for evaluation of non-palpable, deep-seated lesions of the lung, mediastinal, abdominal, and retroperitoneal organs.

Deep seated lesions are visualized either by US or CT scan and small (20–23G) needles are introduced into the lesion to obtain diagnostic material. The material obtained by FNA consists of a cell suspension and minute tissue fragments [12]. During the same procedure, a small tissue core biopsy maybe obtained to assess architecture of the lesion and to obtain tissue for immunohistochemical and/or molecular studies.

The radiologist puts a drop of the aspirated material on the glass slide (Fig. 1.3), and the rest of the material into RPMI for cell block preparation. The cytology staff prepares two slides, one slide that is immediately fixed in alcohol for Papanicolaou stain and second slide that is Diff-Quick stained for immediate adequacy assessment and specimen triage.

This procedure requires well trained interventional radiologists for accurate localization and sampling of the lesion. Location and fibrotic/cystic nature of the lesions can be limiting factors. Vascular lesions may produce bloody specimen with clotting artifact that limits cytologic evaluation. In such cases, a core biopsy is often helpful. On site evaluation and triage can be successfully done on touch preparations from core biopsies.

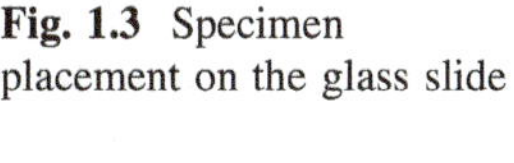

Fig. 1.3 Specimen placement on the glass slide

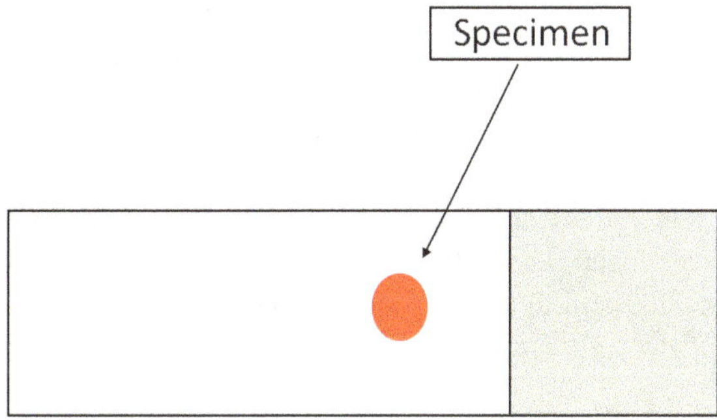

Complications of percutaneous FNA depend on the organ sampled. The most common complication is bleeding and is usually not of clinical significance. Rarely more serious bleeding requiring transfusion may occur. FNA biopsies of the lung or upper abdominal region can result in pneumothorax. The majority of these spontaneously reabsorb and do not require chest tube placement. When sampling abdominal organs, the needle may rarely perforate the gut but serious complications are rare due to the small needle diameter used for the procedure. Most common complications of pancreatic percutaneous FNA are hyperamylasemia, bile peritonitis, pancreatitis, and formation of pancreatic fistula [13]. Cases of the serious infections have been reported after FNA of the prostate in patients with acute prostatitis. Risk of the needle track seeding exists, but reported cases are very rare [2].

1.3 Exfoliative Cytology

1.3.1 Fluids (Peritoneal, Pleural, Pericardial, and Abdominal Washing)

Fluid accumulated in the body cavities may be symptomatic or asymptomatic and is removed either for therapeutic purposes or for diagnostic evaluation. The most common causes of pleural fluid accumulation in the United States are congestive heart disease, pneumonia, cancer, pulmonary embolism, viral disease, coronary artery bypass surgery, and cirrhosis [14]. The most common causes of abdominal fluid accumulation are cirrhosis, portal hypertension, cancer, heart failure, renal failure, tuberculosis, and pancreatic disease [15]. Causes of chronic pericardial effusions include congestive heart disease, other cardiac diseases, hypoalbuminemia, chronic renal disease, connective tissue diseases, neoplasms, and infections [16].

Pleural, peritoneal and pericardial fluid samples are obtained by inserting a wide-bore needle (under local anesthesia) through the body wall into the body cavity.

Abdominal washing specimen(s) are obtained by instilling saline solution into the abdominal cavity and withdrawing it for cytologic examination. It is mostly used for staging of patients with gynecologic malignancies.

The specimen is collected in a sterile container and sent to the cytology laboratory immediately after collecting it. If there is a delay in transportation the specimen is stored in the refrigerator at 4 °C [17]. It is not necessary to add fixative to the specimen.

The gross appearance of the specimen is evaluated. The specimen is mixed, centrifuged, and cytology slides are prepared either by direct smearing, cytospin method or a thin layer liquid-based preparation. The slides are stained with Papanicolaou stain and/or Diff-Quick and the remaining material is used for cell block preparation. The cell block is paraffin embedded and stained with H&E. Additional slides can be cut and used for special stains and/or immunohistochemistry.

Limitations are mostly encountered in small effusions when only a few milliliters of fluid can be obtained. The cytologic preparations may be hypocellular and suboptimal for evaluation. In addition, if small amounts of fluid are received, there will be insufficient material for cell block preparation. When available it is advised to send at least 20 ml of specimen to the cytology laboratory [18].

Complications of paracentesis include bleeding, bowel or bladder puncture, local infection or peritonitis, and a persistent leak at the site of the puncture [19]. Reported overall complication rate for ultrasound-guided thoracentesis in one study was 9.1 % with the two most common complications being pain (2.7 %) and pneumothorax (2.5 %). Other complications included shortness of breath, cough, vasovagal response, bleeding, hematoma and re-expansion pulmonary edema [20].

Rates of reported complications of echo-guided therapeutic pericardiocentesis were 1.2 % for major and 3.5 % for minor complications. Major complications were considered complications that required intervention and the minor complication ones that did not require intervention beside monitoring and follow-up. The major complications included chamber laceration, injury to an intercostal vessel, pneumothorax, ventricular tachycardia, and bacteriemia all of which required intervention. There was one case of death reported due to right ventricular puncture resulting in hemorrhagic tamponade. Minor complications included transient chamber entries, pneumothorax, vasovagal response, non-sustained supraventricular tachycardia, pericardial catheter occlusion, and possible pleuro-pericardial fistula [21].

1.3.2 Brushings

Endoscopic brushings are used to evaluate mucosal lesions or infections in bronchial, gastrointestinal and urinary tracts [18].

In esophageal and bronchial brushings, mucosal lesions/abnormalities are visualized by using the flexible fiberoptic endoscope. The endoscope possesses a channel through which the cytology brush is inserted [22]. Under visual guidance, the brush is moved back and forth over the lesion. Minimal bleeding can occurr during the procedure. If a tissue biopsy is taken at the same time, cytology washings and brushings should be obtained first [18].

Endoscopic retrograde cholangiopancreatography (ERCP) is used for evaluation of the pancreaticobilliary tract and for obtaining cytology material, bile/pancreatic duct brushing. It combines a radiologic and endoscopic approach and is performed under fluoroscopy. During the procedure, the stenotic area or the lesion are vigorously brushed to obtain diagnostic material [22].

Endoscopic brush cytology of the upper urinary tract (ureteral brushing) is performed by passing a small brush through the open-ended catheter [23]. Brush cytology is more sensitive than irrigation or catheterized urine in the detection of the upper urinary tract malignancies [24].

Material obtained by brush cytology is either directly smeared on to the slides at the time of the procedure or the tip of the brush is washed/or cut and submitted in fixative for cytologic processing/examination. If direct smearing is used, it is important to fix the slides immediately either in alcohol or by fixative spray to avoid air drying artifact which compromises specimen interpretation.

Biliary cytology (brushing and bile cytology) failed to provide tissue diagnosis in 25 % of cases either due to the sampling error or sclerotic nature of the lesion. Better diagnostic yield is reached if it is combined with FNA or tissue biopsy [25].

1.3.3 Sputum

Sputum is used for evaluation of the respiratory tract for inflammatory and malignant processes. Early morning sputum, produced by deep cough, is collected. Inhaling a heated solution of 15 % sodium chloride and 20 % propylene glycol for 20 min can be used to induce sputum production in patient who cannot produce sputum spontaneously [26].

The specimen is collected in a sterile container and immediately sent to the cytology laboratory. If there is a delay in transport, the specimen may be submitted in fixative. The specimen is examined grossly and all bloody portions or grossly visible tissue are smeared on the slides, fixed in 95 % alcohol and stained by the Papanicolaou method. The slides also can be prepared using the cytospin method or fix properly for one of the liquid-based preparations [18].

Sputum cytology is more successful in diagnosing centrally located tumors, that are more commonly squamous cell carcinomas, than peripherally located ones that are more likely to be adenocarcinomas. As we now have experienced a shift in the lung cancer type from squamous cell carcinoma to adenocarcinoma, and with the advent of targeted drug therapy in management of adenocarcinoma, the utility of the sputum cytology in lung cancer may decrease further [27].

1.3.4 Urine

Urine cytology is used in the evaluation of hematuria, follow-up of the patients with previously diagnosed urinary tract malignancies and in evaluation of patients with glomerular damage [18]. For evaluation of the urine specimen, it is very important to know by which method the urine sample was obtained.

Voided urine is the preferred specimen in male patients. Patient should be hydrated and the second voided morning urine, to avoid degeneration in the first voided specimen, should be collected for three consecutive days [28]. If voided specimens are collected in females, they should be instructed to clean the vulvar area before collection.

Obtaining catheterized urine is favored over the voided urine in female patients. It is obtained by inserting catheter in the urinary bladder [28].

Bladder and pelvic washing specimens are obtained during cystoscopy by injecting saline or Ringer's solution and collecting it in a sterile container [28]. Slides are either prepared using cytospins or thin layer liquid-based techniques. Certain types of lubricant used during procedure can interfere with the cytologic interpretation by obscuring the cells or interfering with cell transfer to the slide.

Urine cytology has a low sensitivity in diagnosing low grade papillary urothelial tumors and is very sensitive in diagnosing high-grade neoplasms [18].

1.3.5 Cerebrospinal Fluid

Examination of the cerebrospinal fluid (CSF) is used to exclude infections, to evaluate for lymphoma and for metastatic carcinoma, and for staging of primary central nervous system malignancies [18].

The specimen is obtained by lumbar puncture and fluid is collected into a sterile container. Occasionally fluid may be sent from a ventricular/Omaya shunt- if this is the case, the specimen source should be indicated on the requisition form accompanying the specimen.

The two most common methods for preparation of CSF specimens are membrane filtration and cytocentrifugation. Both of them have been developed to allow concentration of the cells in hypocellular specimens [29]. Hypocellular specimens and poor cell preservation may limit interpretation.

1.3.6 Cervical Cytology (Pap Tests)

The Pap test is a screening test for the detection of epithelial abnormalities of the uterine cervix and vagina.

Pap test can be obtained either by using an Ayre spatula (or similar device) together with endocervical brush or by using an endocevical broom. An ectocervical sample is obtained by a firm scrape of the cervix with a spatula. The spatula is rotated one full circle. The endocervix is sampled by insertion of the brush into the cervical os and rotation of the brush for 90–180°. When the specimen is collected by using a broom, the broom is inserted in the cervical os and rotated fully a few times [30].

The specimen is either smeared directly to the slide (conventional Pap) and fixed immediately or placed in a liquid-based cytology media (liquid-based Pap).

Two most commonly used methods in liquid-based gynecologic cytology are ThinPrep® and SurePath®. In the USA, the majority of clinicians/laboratories use liquid-based testing for cervical cytology.

For ThinPrep, cervical specimens are collected by a spatula and a brush or by a broom and the material is placed into vial containing a liquid medium (methanol-based). For SurePath, the head of the broom used to obtain the cervical sample is detached and submitted to the cytology laboratory in the ethanol-based liquid media [31].

For obtaining an optimal specimen, the cervix should be sampled from day 15 to 25. Before collecting a specimen for cervical cytology, women are advised not to douche, use vaginal medication/lubricants or vaginal contraceptives for 48 h and to abstain from sexual intercourse for 24 h prior to the collection, as all of these can interfere with a quality of the specimen or pose interpretation problems [30].

The Pap test is a screening test and can detect 50–90 % of the precursor lesions, however it also fails to detect 10–50 % of the lesions due to either a sampling error (no abnormal cells are present on the slide), or due to interpretation errors when cells are present on the slide but are not found or are not recognized as abnormal [32].

High risk HPV testing can be performed out of the vial sent for a liquid-based Pap test. It is approved by the FDA for both primary screening (as an adjunct to the Pap test) as well as for triage of abnormal cytology (ASCUS, post-menopausal LSIL), follow-up of patients post colposcopically when cytology is abnormal but a lesion has not been found, and post treatment for a high grade lesion. There is no role for testing for low risk HPV types in cervical cancer screening since they do not have oncologic potential. HPV genotyping for HPV16/18 is also approved for triage of patients with a positive HR-HPV test but as of 2010/2011 this has not penetrated significantly into practice. Updated guidelines for molecular testing in cervical cancer became available in 2012[33]. Further uptake of the HPV vaccine will also change the landscape of cervical cancer screening in the future.

References

1. Anderson G (1997) Cytologic screening programs. In: Bibbo M (ed) Comprehensive cytopathology, 2nd edn. W.B. Saunders Company, Philadelphia, pp 51–61
2. Wu M, Burstein DE (2004) Fine needle aspiration. Cancer Invest 22(4):620–628
3. Pitman MB et al (2008) Techniques for thyroid FNA: a synopsis of the national cancer institute thyroid fine-needle aspiration state of the science conference. Diagn Cytopathol 36(6):407–424
4. Frable W (1997) Fine needle biopsy techniques. In: Bibbo M (ed) Comprehensive cytopathology, 2nd edn. W.B. Saunders Company, Philadelphia, pp 623–642
5. Karwowski JK et al (2002) Needle track seeding of papillary thyroid carcinoma from fine needle aspiration biopsy-a case report. Acta Cytol 46(3):591–595
6. Shinohara S et al (2001) Implantation metastasis of head and neck cancer after fine needle aspiration biopsy. Auris Nasus Larynx 28(4):377–380
7. Agarwal G et al (2006) Implantation of parathyroid carcinoma along fine needle aspiration track. Langenbecks Arch Surg 391(6):623–626

8. O'Toole D et al (2001) Assessment of complications of EUS-guided fine-needle aspiration. Gastrointest Endosc 53(4):470–474

9. Keswani R, Azar R (2009) Role of endoscopic ultrasound in diagnosis and staging of pancreatic neoplasms. In: Heiken J (ed) Pancreatic cancer. Cambridge University Press, Cambridge, pp 152–171

10. Gines A et al (2003) Prospective study comparing endosonography-guided trucut (EUS-TCB) and endosonography-guided fine needle aspiration biopsy (EUS-FNAB). Gastrointestinal Endosc 57(5):Ab243

11. Cameron SEH, Andrade RS, Pambuccian SE (2010) Endobronchial ultrasound-guided transbronchial needle aspiration cytology: a state of the art review. Cytopathology 21(1):6–26

12. Tao LC et al (1980) Percutaneous fine-needle aspiration biopsy. I. Its value to clinical practice. Cancer 45(6):1480–1485

13. DeMay RM (1996) Fine needle aspiration biopsy. In: DeMay RM (ed) The art & science of cytopathology, 1st edn. American Society of Clinical Pathologists, Chicago, pp 463–492

14. Porcel JM, Light RW (2006) Diagnostic approach to pleural effusion in adults. Am Fam Physician 73(7):1211–1220

15. Zeller JL, Burke AE, Glass RM (2008) JAMA patient page. Abdom paracentesis. JAMA 299(10):1216

16. Karam N, Patel P, deFilippi C (2001) Diagnosis and management of chronic pericardial effusions. Am J Med Sci 322(2): 79–87

17. Naylor B (1997) Pleural, peritoneal, and pericardial fluids. In: Bibbo M (ed) Comprehensive cytopathology, 2nd edn. W.B. Saunders Company, Philadelphia, pp 551–621

18. Chandra A et al (2009) The BSCC code of practice-exfoliative cytopathology (excluding gynaecological cytopathology). Cytopathology 20(4):211–223

19. McGibbon A et al (2007) An evidence-based manual for abdominal paracentesis. Dig Dis Sci 52(12):3307–3315

20. Jones PW et al (2003) Ultrasound-guided thoracentesis: is it a safer method? Chest 123(2):418–423

21. Tsang TS et al (2002) Consecutive 1127 therapeutic echocardiographically guided pericardiocenteses: clinical profile, practice patterns, and outcomes spanning 21 years. Mayo Clin Proc 77(5):429–436

22. Geisinger KR (1997) Alimentary tract (esophagus, stomach, small intestine, colon, rectum, anus, billiary tract). In: Bibbo M (ed) Comprehensive cytopathology, 2nd edn. W.B. Saunders Company, Philadelphia, pp 413–444

23. Konety Badrinath R, Caroll Peter R (2011) Uothelial carcinoma: cancers of the bladder, ureter, & renal pelvis. In: Tanagho EA, McAninch JW (eds) Smith's general urology, 17th edn. McGraw-Hill, New York. http://www.accessmedicine.com/content.aspx?aID=3128012. Accessed 14 Oct 2011

24. Dodd LG et al (1997) Endoscopic brush cytology of the upper urinary tract. Evaluation of its efficacy and potential limitations in diagnosis. Acta Cytol 41(2):377–384

25. Kurzawinski TR et al (1993) A prospective study of biliary cytology in 100 patients with bile duct strictures. Hepatology 18(6):1399–1403

26. Johnston WW, Elson CE (1997) Respiratory tract. In: Bibbo M (ed) Comprehensive cytopathology, 2nd edn. W.B. Saunders Company, Philadelphia, pp 325–401

27. Bach PB, Niewoehner DE, Black WC (2003) Screening for lung cancer: the guidelines. Chest 123(1):83S–88S

28. Kern WH (1997) Urinary tract. In: Bibbo M (ed) Comprehensive cytopathology, 2nd edn. W.B. Saunders Company, Philadelphia, pp 445–476

29. Bigner SH (1997) Central nervous system. In: Bibbo M (ed) Comprehensive cytopathology, 2nd edn. W.B. Saunders Company, Philadelphia, pp 477–492

30. DeMay RM (2005) Clinical considerations. In: DeMay RM (ed) The pap test, 1st edn. American Society of Clinical Pathologists, Chicago, pp 195–202
31. DeMay RM (2005) Liquid-based cytology, death of the pap smear, and primary prevention. In: DeMay RM (ed) The pap test, 1st edn. American Society of Clinical Pathologists, Chicago, pp 213–233
32. DeMay RM (2005) Failure of the pap test. In: DeMay RM (ed) The pap test, 1st edn. American Society of Clinical Pathologists, Chicago, pp 203–212
33. Stewart ML, Einstein MH, Huh WK et al (2012) ASCCP consensus guidelines conference. Updated consensus guidelines for the management of abnormal cervical cancer screening tests and cancer precursors. J Low Genit Tract Dis 17(5):S1–S27

Chapter 2
Ancillary Studies on Neoplastic Cytologic Specimens

Y. Gong

2.1 Introduction

Fine-needle aspiration (FNA) is a safe, simple, rapid, and cost-effective procedure that is often used as an initial diagnostic modality to work up primary and metastatic tumors at almost any body site. FNA allows acquisition of samples not only from superficial and large lesions, but also from small- or deep-seated lesions, or from multiple lesions during the same biopsy procedure. It provides valuable information that enables oncologists to make optimal therapeutic decisions, including planning preoperative management for patients with operable tumors and choosing adequate medical therapy for patients with hematopoietic malignancies or nonresectable tumors. An informative cytologic diagnosis should address whether the lesion is neoplastic or nonneoplastic, benign or malignant, as well as the histogenesis of the tumor (e.g., epithelial, mesenchymal, melanocytic, or lymphoid), tumor type (e.g., adenocarcinoma, squamous carcinoma, or others), tumor origin (i.e., primary vs. metastatic and if possible the potential primary origin of a metastatic tumor) and information on prognostic and therapeutic markers. Frequently, this information needs to be obtained with the help of ancillary tests. Body cavity fluids may also be utilized for ancillary studies, when indicated.

This chapter outlines the utility of immunocytochemistry (ICC), flow cytometric (FCM), cytogenetic and molecular studies in the cytologic diagnosis of neoplastic lesions including the indications, sample requirements, reliability, and limitations.

Y. Gong (✉)
The University of Texas M.D. Anderson Cancer Center Department of Pathology,
Unit 53 1515 Holcombe Blvd, Houston, TX 77030, USA
e-mail: yungong@mail.mdanderson.org

R. Nayar (ed.), *Cytopathology in Oncology*,
Cancer Treatment and Research 160, DOI: 10.1007/978-3-642-38850-7_2,
© Springer-Verlag Berlin Heidelberg 2014

2.2 Immunocytochemistry

ICC combines cytologic, immunological and biochemical techniques for the identification of specific tissue/cell components by means of a specific antigen/ antibody reaction tagged with a visible label. Depending on characteristics of the cells, the ICC reaction can be seen in cytoplasm, nucleus or cell membrane, thus the ICC technique allows us to visualize the distribution and localization of specific biomarkers within a cell or tissue. The applications of ICC have increased in parallel with the discovery of novel markers in surgical pathology. It is important to emphasize that ICC should be considered only in the context of a proper differential diagnosis, and appropriate immunomarkers should be selected on the basis of the patient's medical history, current clinical and radiologic presentation, and cytolomorphologic features of the lesion. In general, if a lesion exhibits malignant features with poor differentiation and the patient has no known history of malignancy, the initial step in the workup is to identify the histogenesis of the tumor: epithelial (carcinoma), melanocytic (melanoma), hematopoietic (lymphoma), or mesenchymal (sarcoma). Accordingly, the basic markers should include at least keratin, melanoma markers, and leukocyte common antigen (CD45). If a carcinoma of unknown primary origin is encountered, the ICC panel usually starts with cytokeratin 7 (CK7) and CK20 to identify a likely primary site (Table 2.1) [1–3]. If a history of malignancy is known, corresponding markers relatively specific to an organ site (Table 2.2) and other markers that are relevant to cell differentiation may be added to the panel. Notably, the staining patterns and site-specific markers in Tables 2.1 and 2.2 are not absolute and may vary depending on variations in antibody sensitivity and specificity, staining conditions, and tumor differentiation. For example, TTF-1 is a tissue-specific transcription factor expressed in the thyroid and lung, and is one of the most frequently used markers to distinguish between pulmonary and extra pulmonary origin of an adenocaricnoma [4]. It can also be expressed in small-cell carcinomas (pulmonary and extra pulmonary) and in a small subset of squamous cell carcinomas, and carcinoid tumors of lung origin.

FNA specimens are usually prepared as direct smear(s) and cell block. Some laboratories may use liquid-based preparations (ThinPrep, SurePath) in parallel with or to replace direct smears. Air-dried smears are stained with Diff-Quik, and alcohol-fixed smears with Papanicolaou; the air-dried preparations are usually used for immediate on-site assessment for adequacy assessment and triage for ancillary studies. Cells obtained from the needle rinses or tissue fragments are collected in cell preservative medium to make a cell block or for cytospin preparation depending on the size of the pellet after centrifugation. For a cell block, the pellet is fixed in formalin, embedded in paraffin, then sectioned and stained with hematoxylin and eosin, a process virtually identical to that used for surgical tissue specimens. The cell block may partially retain the histologic architecture of a lesion. A cell block, or core biopsy if feasible, is the preferred sample type for ICC. Therefore, when an ICC workup is expected on the basis of immediate assessment,

Table 2.1 Common CK7 and CK20 staining patterns in tumors of various primary sites

CK7+/CK20+	Pancreas: pancreatic adenocarcinoma[a]
	Biliary duct: adenocarcinoma, including cholangiocarcinoma[a]
	Genitourinary tract: urothelial carcinoma[a]
	Stomach: gastric adenocarcinoma[a]
	Ovary: mucinous adenocarcinoma
CK7+/CK20-	Lung: non-small cell carcinoma, adenocarcinoma
	Breast: ductal carcinoma, lobular carcinoma
	Endometrium and uterine cervix: adenocarcinoma
	Ovary: adenocarcinoma other than mucinous type
	Thyroid: papillary carcinoma, follicular carcinoma, medullary carcinoma
	Salivary gland tumor
	Mesothelium: malignant mesothelioma
CK7-/CK20+	Colon and rectum: colorectal adenocarcinoma
	Skin: merkel cell carcinoma
CK7-/CK20-	Liver: hepatocellular carcinoma
	Kidney: renal cell carcinoma
	Adrenal gland: adrenal cortical tumor
	Prostate: prostatic adenocarcinoma
	Testis: germ cell tumor

[a] variable expression pattern

Table 2.2 Immunomarkers that are relatively site specific

TTF-1	Lung, thyroid
CDX2	Gastrointestinal organs, pancreas
Thyroglobulin	Thyroid
Calcitonin	Thyroid (medullary carcinoma)
Surfactant, napsin-A	Lung
HepPar-1	Liver (hepatocyte)
RCC	Kidney (renal cell)
PAX-8	Kidney (renal cell), gynecologic organs, thyroid
PSA, PAP	Prostate
PTH	Parathyroid
ER, PR	Breast, gynecologic organs
GCDFP-15, mammaglobin	Breast
Calretinin, mesothelin	Mesothelium
WT-1	Ovary (serous carcinoma), mesothelium
Mart-1, S-100, HMB-45, SOX-10, MITF	Skin (melanoma)
PLAP, AFP	Testis (germ cell tumor)

the on-site cytopathologist usually tries to obtain material for a cell block or core biopsy. Additional needle pass(es) might be obtained if deemed feasible by the aspirator. If a cell block is not available or contains insufficient cells, Papanicolaou-stained direct smear(s), cytospin preparation, and liquid-based preparation are also feasible for ICC as long as they have reasonable cellularity [5–7]. If the cells of interest are present on only a single or few smears without available cell block material when a panel of ICC is needed, a cell-transfer technique, in which the original smear material is divided into several pieces and then transferred onto multiple slides, may facilitate multiple ICC studies from the limited material [8–11]. This technique can avoid a repeat biopsy solely for immunophenotyping of tumors.

There are several disadvantages of ICC on the sample types other than cell block. (1) such sample types lack validated control tissue, which should be fixed in the same way as the test specimen at each run of ICC staining. (2) Certain stains such as S-100 cannot be reliably assessed on these preparations. (3) High background staining, often associated with crowding of cells in thick smear and poor cytoplasmic preservation, may be encountered occasionally, and prove problematic for interpretation. (4) A false-positive ICC interpretation may result from the lack of a histologic pattern in the aspirated material and mistaking entrapped benign cells at the biopsy site for tumor cells. For example, an aspirate of a carcinoma metastatic to the lung may contain entrapped benign and reactive bronchial cells that express TTF-1, which may lead to an erroneous conclusion that the tumor is focally TTF-1 positive and thus of lung origin. Last, a limitation that is intrinsic to all types of cytologic samples is scarcity of cells available for ICC due to sampling error, tumor necrosis, or tumor fibrosis. It is conceivable that ICC on a small sample may lead to a false-negative finding in tumors that express some markers only focally and heterogeneously. Therefore, caution should be exercised in the interpretation of ICC results.

The predictive factors commonly tested on cytologic specimens are estrogen receptor (ER), progesterone receptor (PR), HER2 status for breast cancer or gastric cancer, and epidermal growth factor receptor (EGFR), K-RAS and ALK mutations in lung cancer, K-RAS and thymidine synthetase in colorectal cancer. These tests are conducted to assess a patient's eligibility to receive anti-ER, anti-HER2, and anti-EGFR targeted therapies, or responsiveness to 5-FU-based regimens, respectively. Although testing for these biomarkers is usually performed on surgically resected or biopsy specimens of newly diagnosed primary carcinoma and requires standardized fixation conditions (i.e., fix in 10 % neutral buffered formalin for 6–48 h for ER, PR, and HER2), [12, 13] they are frequently determined on cytologic specimens, including aspirated metastatic carcinoma samples when the receptor status needs to be repeated in the relapsed disease, or on primary carcinoma when the cytologic samples are the only material available. ICC of ER and PR can be performed on cell blocks, direct smears, and liquid-based preparations; however, HER2 staining should be performed only on cell block section since ICC of HER2 on direct smears is not standardized and is associated with high variability in sample preparation, fixation, staining, and interpretation [14].

Sometimes, testing of ER, PR, and HER2 is requested by an oncologist after a cytologic diagnosis has been completed and extra slides for these markers are not available. In such case, the Papanicolaou-stained smears that have been used for routine morphologic diagnosis may be used for ER and PR staining [15]. Direct smears can be used for testing HER2 gene copy number via fluorescence in situ hybridization (FISH). The advantage of using archived slides is to enable the cytopathologist to visualize cytologic features and the amount of tumor cells on the smear prior to the tests, thereby allowing selection of the "most representative" slides for the tests. It is important to note that these markers should be assessed on the invasive component of the breast carcinoma. Since cytologic specimens cannot reliably discriminate invasive from in situ components, interpretation of ER, PR, and HER2 status in a primary setting should be done cautiously. Also, the reliability of ER, PR, and HER2 status determined on cytologic preparations needs to be validated according to the current guidelines [12]. In our experience, ER status in breast carcinoma is generally stable during progression to metastasis with a concordance rate between primary and paired metastatic breast carcinoma to be 92 % [16]. Detection of EGFR and K-RAS mutations is covered in the section on cytogenetic and molecular tests.

2.3 Flow Cytometry

FCM is a powerful tool for determining the phenotype and characteristics of cells. It uses the principles of light scattering, light excitation, and emission of fluorochrome molecules to generate specific multi-parameter data from particles and cells.

In the past decades, the applications of this technology have evolved substantially. With the wide use of FNA, FCM has become a main ancillary test to evaluate adenopathy and other lymphoid lesions, although the primary diagnosis of lymphoma is usually based on surgical biopsy specimens. However, an accurate cytologic diagnosis relies on correlation of cytologic features with immunophenotypic, genotypic, clinical, and radiologic information in view of the considerable overlap of cytologic features among some types of lymphomas and between low grade lymphomas and reactive lymphoid hyperplasia. FCM is the most commonly used ancillary test, especially in the setting of persistent or relapsed lymphoma. The role of FNA in rendering a primary diagnosis of lymphoma remains controversial.

2.3.1 Handling and Triaging of the FNA Specimen

At immediate on-site assessment, a cytopathologist evaluates the cell composition, features, and quantity of the aspirated material and ensures properly triaging of the specimen for ancillary studies. For example, if a lesion shows granulomas or abundant acute inflammatory cells, aspirates should be collected for microbiology culture(s) and special stains; if a lesion shows features of a nonhematopoietic tumor, an effort should be made to obtain a cell block for possible ICC workup; if cells show features suggestive of hematopoietic malignancy, collecting enough cells for FCM is the priority. Specifically, if a lesion is from a patient who has a history of non-Hodgkin lymphoma or has clinical and/or radiologic findings suggestive of non-Hodgkin lymphoma, even if it exhibits "reactive-like" cytologic appearance, a lymphoma workup by FCM should be performed. When a diagnosis of non-Hodgkin lymphoma is highly suspected in a patient without a history of lymphoma during immediate assessment, a concurrent core needle biopsy should be obtained for further histologic classification and grading. However, if a FNA sample exhibits cytologic features suggesting Hodgkin lymphoma, and/or the patient has a history of Hodgkin lymphoma, the sample should not be sent for FCM since FCM is not helpful in diagnosing Hodgkin lymphoma [17]. The same is true for anaplastic large-cell lymphoma. In such cases, a tissue biopsy is typically required for histologic confirmation and classification since the sensitivity of cytologic diagnosis for these types of lymphoma is relatively low.

At The University of Texas MD Anderson Cancer Center, we usually smear a portion of the aspirates from the first needle pass onto glass slides. If smears show a lymphoid population with features suspicious for non-Hodgkin lymphoma, cells from subsequent aspiration(s) should be collected directly into cell preservative medium (RPMI) and the cells quantified by using an automated counter (Coulter Electronics, Hialeah, FL) to determine if there is a sufficient number of cells for further workup. A minimum of 10 million cells from three or four needle passes is usually required for a standard lymphoma workup. We triage samples for lymphoma workup in the following steps:

A. Cytomorphologic evaluation on direct smears
B. Immunophenotyping by FCM (approximately 5 million cells)
C. Proliferation index (Ki67) assessment by immunostaining on a cytospin preparation; the result correlates strongly with the grade and outcome of lymphoma. To prepare the cytospin, cells in RPMI medium are processed over a Ficoll-Hypaque gradient to enrich mononucleated cells, which are then centrifuged onto glass slides (approximately 1×10^5 cells per slide) [18, 19].
D. When a specimen is hypercellular, an additional four to six cytospin slides will be kept in a tumor bank (-80 °C) for possible ICC or FISH. A panel of ICC including kappa, lambda, CD3, and Ki67 might be informative when FCM fails to demonstrate light chain restriction in a lesion that is clinically suspected for lymphoid neoplasm. FISH analysis may be needed to confirm characteristic chromosomal abnormalities in selected cases.
E. Aggregates of tissue in the RPMI medium will be salvaged to make a cell block, which can be used for ICC and FISH or in situ hybridization for Epstein-Barr virus infection.

2.3.2 Interpretation of Flow Cytometry

FCM is a highly sensitive technique that can quantify the expression of four or more markers on a single cell and therefore enables identification of aberrant cells within a complex cellular background. It is the preferred method of lineage determination of hematopoietic neoplasms and subclassification of B-cell lymphomas. The panels of antibodies should be selected on the basis of the cytologic features and clinical information; at first-time diagnosis, FCM should evaluate both B- and T-cell abnormalities.

Mature B-cell neoplasms account for more than 85 % of non-Hodgkin lymphomas, and are the most commonly encountered hematopoietic tumors in cytology practice. Therefore, evaluation of clonality by assessing immunoglobulin light chains (i.e., kappa and lambda light chains) together with CD19 and CD20 expression is important to establish a B-cell neoplastic nature. In non-neoplastic conditions, the specimen comprises a mixture of T- and B- cells. In addition to CD19, CD20, and CD22, mature non-neoplastic B cells typically express polyclonal surface immunoglobulin (i.e., the kappa to lambda light chain ratio is around 1.5:1). B-cell lymphomas, however, express a single clonal light chain (also called light chain restriction), so this ratio is either increased (greater than 3:1 in our experience) or decreased due to a significant lambda excess. B-cell lymphomas are often associated with aberrant expression of other antigens, some of which are of prognostic value. For example, CD38 expression in B-cell small lymphocytic lymphoma/chronic lymphocytic leukemia (SLL/CLL) is often associated with a more aggressive clinical course [20, 21]. Table 2.3 lists key immunophenotypic and molecular features of mature B-cell neoplasms commonly encountered in cytology practice.

Although the interpretation of FCM data in most cases is quite straightforward, potential pitfalls may be encountered and may lead to misinterpretation. A negative FCM result does not necessarily indicate a benign process [22]. Identical immunoprofiles may be seen in different types of lymphoma. It would be a mistake to attempt to interpret a case solely on the basis of FCM results. The common pitfalls include the following:

1. Immunoglobulin light chain may not be detectable due to too few neoplastic cells that may be masked by abundant benign lymphocytes in the background, a situation often seen in T-cell-rich B-cell lymphoma or a partially involved node. Gating on the large-cell population may separate neoplastic large cells from background reactive lymphocytes. In a case of partial involvement by follicular lymphoma, typically CD10-positive B cells demonstrate light chain restriction, whereas CD10-negative B cells express polyclonal light chain consistent with non-neoplastic nature.
2. Since FCM generally evaluates intact viable cells, poor cellular integrity, extensive fibrosis, and necrosis, which occur frequently in large-cell lymphoma, may lead to a false-negative FCM interpretation.
3. In some B-cell lymphomas, FCM shows negative light chain expression caused by aberrant loss of surface immunoglobulin expression. Using different antibodies for each light chain is important to verify true light chain loss or, in some cases, overcome false-negativity resulting from antibody issue. This is because a single pair of light chain antibodies may not successfully identify monotypic light chain expression in each lymphoma cases.

Table 2.3 Immunophenotypic and molecular features of mature B-cell neoplasms commonly encountered in cytology practice

	Immunophenotype	Molecular features
Follicular lymphoma	sIg, CD19+, CD20+, CD10+, BCL6+, BCL2+ CD5-, CD23±	Most common t(14;18)(q32;q21), rarely t(2;8)(p11;q21) and t(18;22)(q21;q11)
Marginal zone lymphoma	sIg, CD19+, CD20+ CD10-, CD5-, CD23-, BCL6-	t(11,18)(q21;q21), t(1;14)(p22;q32), t(14;18)(q32;q21), Trisomy 3, 7, 12, and 18
Mantle cell lymphoma	sIg, CD19+, CD20+, CD5+, FMC7+, CD79a+, cyclin D1+ CD10-, CD23-	t(11;14)(q13;q32)
Small lymphocytic lymphoma/ chronic lymphocytic leukemia (SLL/CLL)	sIg (dim), CD19±, CD20+(dim), CD22+(dim), CD5+, CD23+, CD38+(worse prognosis) CD10-, FMC7-	Trisomy 12, 13q14 deletion, 17p and 11q deletions
Lymphoplasmacytic lymphoma	sIg or cIg, CD19+, CD20+, CD38+, CD43± CD10−, CD5−, CD23−	
Burkitt/atypical Burkitt lymphoma	sIg, CD19+, CD20+, CD10+, BCL6+, Ki67 labeling index ≥ 99 % CD5−, CD23−	most common: t(8;14)(q24;q32), less common t(2;8) (p12;q24) or t(8;22)(q24;q11)
Large B-cell lymphoma	sIg, cIg or Ig undetectable, CD19+, CD20+, high Ki67 labeling index CD10∓, CD5∓, BCL6∓ (positive CD10 or BCL6 indicates follicular center cell origin)	t(14;18) (q32;q21)
Plasma cell neoplasm	cIg, CD45±, CD56+, CD38+, CD138+	

Ig immunoglobulin light chain, *sIg* surface Ig restriction, *cIg* cytoplasmic Ig restriction

4. Plasma cell neoplasms and some B-cell lymphomas are negative for surface light chain staining. In these cases, examination of cytoplasmic immunoglobulin light chains is the key to demonstrating clonality.
5. Marginal zone lymphoma, CD10-negative follicular lymphoma and lymphoplasmacytic lymphoma share similar immunophenotypes (i.e., CD5-negative, CD10-negative monoclonal B cells).
6. CD10-positive mature B-cell lymphomas include follicular lymphoma, Burkitt lymphoma, and some large B-cell lymphoma. Based on FCM alone, the distinction among the three may be difficult.
7. Some B-cell SLL/CLL may show an atypical phenotype with a brighter expression of pan-B cell markers and diminished CD23 expression, mimicking the phenotype of mantle cell lymphoma. Similarly, large B-cell lymphomas may show CD5 expression resembling the phenotype of mantle cell lymphoma. Because the prognosis and treatment of these lymphomas are significantly different from one another, it is critical to distinguish clearly among these lymphomas.
8. In some reactive conditions such as Hashimoto thyroiditis, a small population of monotypic B cells may be detected, caution is needed not to over interpret these as lymphoma [23].

Compared with B-cell lymphomas, T-cell lymphomas in general have less predictable patterns of immunophenotypic aberrancy. T-cell lymphomas often show deletion or loss of one or more pan-T-cell markers (i.e., CD2, CD3, CD5, CD7), which can be detected by FCM [24]. In addition, T-cell lymphomas often demonstrate aberrant CD4 and CD8 patterns. T-cell clonality may be detected by FCM using anti-T-cell receptor (TCR) V-beta antibodies, [25, 26] although this technique has not been used for FNA specimens. In difficult cases, polymerase chain reaction (PCR) can aid in the diagnosis by demonstrating *TCR* gene rearrangements that are present in most T-cell lymphomas [27, 28].

While FCM is a valuable adjunct for the diagnosis of lymphoma on cytologic specimens, it is important to view immunophenotyping results in conjunction with cytologic features, and to be alert to potential inconsistencies. When clinical features are not explained by FCM, repeating FNA or obtaining tissue biopsy, with addition of cytogenetic and molecular studies if possible is recommended.

2.4 Cytogenetic and Molecular Tests

Following the rapid advance in molecular and cytogenetic research, it has become clear that genomic alterations are involved in cancer initiation and progression. Two main genetic events are considered to trigger cancer initiation: activation of oncogenes as a consequence of point mutation, amplification, or chromosomal translocation; and/or inactivation of tumor suppressor genes due to chromosomal deletion, mutation, or epigenetic mechanisms.

Identification of specific cytogenetic and molecular abnormalities has several clinical implications.

1. They can help in more accurate diagnosis. As noted earlier, although cytologic features in conjunction with ICC or FCM are usually sufficient to make cytologic diagnosis, there are instances where identification of characteristic abnormalities at the chromosomal and/or molecular levels is necessary to arrive at a definitive cytologic diagnosis. For example, cytologic features of small-to-intermediate cell lymphomas (such as follicular lymphoma, marginal zone lymphoma or mantle cell lymphoma) can considerably overlap with one another as well as with those of reactive lymphoid hyperplasia. Some of these lymphomas, such as CD10-negative follicular lymphoma and marginal zone lymphoma, may share similar immunophenotypic features. A similar situation may be encountered in the cytologic diagnosis of small round blue cell tumors, a group of histogenetically different tumors that share some morphologic and immunophenotypic features. Since lymphomas and these solid tumors frequently carry nonrandom chromosomal aberrations (usually reciprocal chromosomal translocation) (Tables 2.3 and 2.4), a cytogenetic and/or molecular study would be a powerful adjunct for the diagnosis.

2. Demonstration of characteristic chromosomal abnormalities may help in prognostic assessment. For example, the presence of the t(2;5) translocation is associated with relatively good prognosis of anaplastic large-cell lymphoma. In SLL/CLL, trisomay 12, and 11q and 17p deletions are associated with poor prognosis, whereas 13q14 deletion is a marker of good prognosis.

3. Chromosomal abnormalities can be used to predict therapeutic response of some tumors. For example, marginal zone lymphoma of the MALT type with t(11;18) or t(1;14) is unlikely to respond to antibiotic therapy.

Table 2.4 Characteristic chromosomal translocations in some sarcomas

Tumor type	Translocation
Ewing sarcoma/peripheral primitive neuroectodermal tumor	t(11;22)(q24;q12)
	t(21;22)(q22;q12)
	t(7;22)(p22;q12)
	t(17;22)(q21;q12)
	t(2;22)(q33;q12)
Desmoplastic small round cell tumor	t(11;22)(p13;q12)
Synovial sarcoma	t(X;18)(p11;q11)
Myxoid liposarcoma	t(12;16)(q13;p11)
	t(12;22)(q13;q12)
Myxoid chondrosarcoma	t(9;22)(q22–31;q11–12)
	t(9;15)(q22;q21)
	t(9;17)(q22;q11)
Clear cell sarcoma	t(12;22)(q13;q12)
Alveolar rhabdomyosarcoma	t(2;13)(q35;q14)
	t(1;13)(p36;q14)
Alveolar soft part sarcoma	t(X;17)(p11;q25)

4. Identification of genetic abnormalities may also be used for identifying minimal residual disease in hematopoietic malignancies.

Cytogenetics is a branch of molecular genetics and is concerned with the study of the number and structure of the chromosomes such as translocations, amplification, deletions, inversions, duplications, or isochromosomes. It includes conventional cytogenetic analysis such as metaphase karyotyping using chromosome-banding techniques, and molecular cytogenetics such as FISH and comparative genomic hybridization. Conventional cytogenetic studies allow complete karyotype analysis and detect most chromosome anomalies; however it is a cumbersome and time-consuming procedure requiring adequate fresh tissue and special cell culture techniques in order to obtain adequate number of proliferating cells. In our experience, approximately 8 million tumor cells in sterile condition are needed for this procedure.

FISH is used widely as an easy and reliable technical substitute to search for well-documented specific chromosomal abnormalities. The method can be used on metaphase or on nondividing interphase cells, and allows the localization of specific genes and DNA segments on specific chromosomes, determines the position and orientation of adjacent genes along a specific chromosome, and can detect the presence of microdeletions or duplications that are not apparent by conventional cytogenetic studies. Furthermore, FISH test has a shorter turnaround time than conventional cytogenetic studies. The interphase FISH (I-FISH) method is particularly advantageous for FNA specimens because it requires only a few cells, and can facilitate a definitive diagnosis on some cases that otherwise fall into indeterminate (i.e., atypical or suspicious) diagnostic category due to scant cellularity [18]. The results of I-FISH are important integral part of cytologic diagnosis, especially for lymphoma and sarcoma. The most common abnormality of these tumors is reciprocal chromosomal translocation (Tables 2.3 and 2.4) [29]. However, in contrast to conventional cytogenetic studies, I-FISH is not informative to identify "unexpected" chromosome abnormalities that are not designed to detect. Cell block, direct smear (air-dried, alcohol-fixed or archived), cytospin preparation, or cellular touch imprint are all suitable for I-FISH. However, direct smear and cytospin preparation appear to be superior to cell block sections in that gene copy number can be enumerated on monolayered and entire tumor nuclei without tissue section-associated truncating artifacts, thereby yielding a more accurate score [30–33]. It is important to ensure that the scoring should be performed on cells of interest such as malignant cells. I-FISH on previously stained archival smears has the advantage of evaluating cytomorphologic features of cells on the same slides before the procedure.

HER2 status is a frequently tested on cytology specimens, using either ICC (on cell block) or FISH (on smear or cell block). Positive HER2 status (i.e., over expression of the HER2 protein with immunostaining or amplification of the HER2 gene with FISH) is associated with a poor clinical outcome, and more importantly, is a prerequisite for anti-HER2 (such as Trastuzumab/Herceptin) treatment. Dual-probe FISH is the preferred method over immunostaining [34].

This was based on the fact that FISH is less affected by preanalytic, analytic, and postanalytic variables and thus more stable and reproducible than immunostaining, as well as the fact that HER2 status determined with FISH is more strongly correlated with responsiveness to anti-HER2 therapy. HER2 status is highly concordant between primary carcinomas and paired metastatic tumors and is quite stable after chemotherapy, [35, 36] or trastuzumab treatment [37].

Bright-field chromogenic in situ hybridization (CISH) has shown potential to replace the I-FISH technique in detection of *HER2* gene amplification in tissue sections since it detects gene copy number using a conventional peroxidase reaction, and allows enumeration of the signals with simultaneous histologic examination by ordinary microscopy [38–41]. This technique is more straight-forward than FISH for scoring. The utility of CISH in cytologic specimens is still investigational [42–44].

Molecular tests have now become an important integral part of cytologic diagnosis. PCR is a technique to amplify a specific DNA sequence in an expo-nential manner. PCR and FISH are complementary for detecting predictable chromosomal abnormalities; however, the overall sensitivity of PCR is lower than that of I-FISH [18, 45–49]. For example, the detection rate of the t(14;18) trans-location in follicular lymphoma is less than 70 % with PCR, while it is around 90 % with FISH. This is mainly due to the presence of *BCL2* gene breakpoints outside the known major breakpoint region (*mbr*) and minor cluster region (*mcr*), that are unable to span with primers, whereas FISH circumvents this limitation by using a probe covering the entire *BCL2* region.

In contrast to detection of immunoglobulin heavy-chain (*IgH*) and *TCR* gene rearrangement that are encountered occasionally in cytology practice, detection of *EGFR* and *K-RAS* mutation in non-small cell lung cancer on cytologic specimens has been increasingly requested by oncologists to determine a patient's eligibility for anti-EGFR therapy (such as Gefitinib/Iressa or Erlotinib/Tarceva). Two classes of EGFR mutations, short deletions in exon 19 and the L858R point mutation in exon 21, are the most frequent mutations and account for approximately 90 % of EGFR mutations [50]. The presence of these mutations is associated with response to tyrosine kinase inhibitors. Mutations in *EGFR* and *K-RAS* appear to be mutually exclusive; tumors with a *K-RAS* mutation would not likely be affected by anti-EGFR therapy. Cell block material or cells scraped from direct smears are suitable for the mutation tests [51]. However, the efficacy of the tests is affected to a great extent by the amount of tumor cells available for analysis.

Another common application of molecular tests in cytology practice includes detection of human papillomavious (HPV) DNA in liquid-based cervical speci-mens using Hybrid Capture 2 or third Wave (Cervista) technology [52, 53], and diagnosis or surveillance of urothelial neoplasia using multi-probe FISH (UroVysion) [54]. These tests will be discussed in subsequent chapters.

Numerous other molecular tests have been investigated and some have shown substantial promise to aid cytologic diagnosis and optimize personalized man-agement. Gene expression profiling microarray has been used to identify sophis-ticated multigene prognostic and predictive factors of various tumors. Both core needle biopsy and FNA are feasible for procurement of fresh samples in the neoadjuvant setting [55–58]. Compared to core needle biopsy sample, FNA samples contain a higher proportion of neoplastic cells and fewer stromal components [59]. Gong et al. have assessed the reliability of testing ER and HER2 status via gene expression profiling and observed close correlation between mRNA levels of ER and HER2 and the routinely determined status via immunostaining and/or FISH, with overall accuracies ranging from 88 to 96 % [60]. In that study, mRNA cutoff values of ER and HER2 were defined using breast carcinomas sampled with FNA and the performance of each cutoff was validated in independent datasets of FNA specimens as well as surgical specimens obtained from seven institutions across 5 countries. These findings indicate that gene expression mircroarray not only generates large and comprehensive gene expression data from human cancers, this technique also reliably measure ER and HER2. Integration of the individual gene expression with multigene signatures generated from the same microarray data might improve predictive power of tumor response to targeted therapies and therefore optimize clinical decision-making and tailoring the therapeutic regimens on an individual basis.

Management of thyroid nodules largely depends on the FNA diagnosis. Approximately 15–25 % of thyroid FNA diagnoses are indeterminate for malignancy. *RET/PTC* gene rearrangements and mutational analysis of *BRAF* have shown promising potential to refine indeterminate cytologic diagnosis of thyroid lesions [61, 62].

Aberrant CpG methylation at the promoter region of tumor suppressor genes, a main epigenetic mechanism, is associated with transcriptional silencing and has a central role in tumorigenesis of different tissues. The application of promoter hypermethylation has been investigated in archival liquid-based cytologic specimens and showed potential to improve diagnostic certainty [63–65]. However, larger studies are required to validate these findings before clinical application.

2.5 Conclusion

With the rapid advent of sophisticated diagnostic technology and increased understanding of the molecular mechanisms of various tumors, the need to obtain diagnostic, prognostic, and predictive information from cytologic material continues to grow. In addition to adoption and incorporation of the new techniques into routine cytology practice, a major challenge is to standardize specimen processing and validation of testing procedures to ensure optimum results, especially for markers that predict response to targeted therapies. It is critical that ancillary test results be evaluated in concert with cytologic features and clinical and radiologic findings to avoid erroneous interpretation.

References

1. Chu P, Wu E, Weiss LM (2000) Cytokeratin 7 and cytokeratin 20 expression in epithelial neoplasms: a survey of 435 cases. Mod Pathol 13:962–972
2. Gyure KA, Morrison AL (2000) Cytokeratin 7 and 20 expression in choroid plexus tumors: utility in differentiating these neoplasms from metastatic carcinomas. Mod Pathol 13:638–643
3. Wang NP, Zee S, Zarbo RJ et al (1995) Coordinate expression of cytokeratins 7 and 20 defines unique subsets of carcinomas. Appl Immunohistochem 3:99–107
4. Moldvay J, Jackel M, Bogos K et al (2004) The role of TTF-1 in differentiating primary and metastatic lung adenocarcinomas. Pathol Oncol Res 10:85–88
5. Dabbs DJ, Abendroth CS, Grenko RT et al (1997) Immunocytochemistry on the Thinprep processor. Diagn Cytopathol 17:388–392
6. Guiter GE, Gatscha RM, Zakowski MF (1999) ThinPrep vs. conventional smears in fine-needle aspirations of sarcomas: a morphological and immunocytochemical study. Diagn Cytopathol 21:351–354
7. Leung SW, Bedard YC (1996) Immunocytochemical staining on ThinPrep processed smears. Mod Pathol 9:304–306
8. Mehta P, Battifora H 1993 How to do multiple immunostains when only one tissue slide is available. The "peel and stick" method. Appl Immunohistochem 1:297–298
9. Miller RT, Kubier P (2002) Immunohistochemistry on cytologic specimens and previously stained slides (when no paraffin block is available). J Histotechnology 25:251–257
10. Sherman ME, Jimenez-Joseph D, Gangi MD (1994) Immunostaining of small cytologic specimens. Facilitation with cell transfer. Acta Cytol 38:18–22
11. Gong Y, Joseph T, Sneige N (2005) Validation of commonly used immunostains on cell-transferred cytologic specimens. Cancer 105:158–164
12. Wolff AC, Hammond ME, Schwartz JN et al (2007) American society of clinical oncology/college of american pathologists guideline recommendations for human epidermal growth factor receptor 2 testing in breast cancer. J Clin Oncol 25:118–145
13. Goldstein NS, Ferkowicz M, Odish E et al (2003) Minimum formalin fixation time for consistent estrogen receptor immunohistochemical staining of invasive breast carcinoma. Am J Clin Pathol 120:86–92
14. Nizzoli R, Bozzetti C, Crafa P et al (2003) Immunocytochemical evaluation of HER-2/neu on fine-needle aspirates from primary breast carcinomas. Diagn Cytopathol 28:142–146
15. Gong Y, Symmans WF, Krishnamurthy S et al (2004) Optimal fixation conditions for immunocytochemical analysis of estrogen receptor in cytologic specimens of breast carcinoma. Cancer 102:34–40
16. Gong Y, Han E, Guo M et al (2010) Stability of estrogen receptor status in breast carcinoma: a comparison between primary and metastatic tumors with regard to disease course and intervening systemic therapy. Cancer 117(4):705–713
17. Jimenez-Heffernan JA, Vicandi B, Lopez-Ferrer P et al (2001) Value of fine needle aspiration cytology in the initial diagnosis of Hodgkin's disease. Analysis of 188 cases with an emphasis on diagnostic pitfalls. Acta Cytol 45:300–306
18. Gong Y, Caraway N, Gu J et al (2003) Evaluation of interphase fluorescence in situ hybridization for the t(14;18)(q32;q21) translocation in the diagnosis of follicular lymphoma on fine-needle aspirates: a comparison with flow cytometry immunophenotyping. Cancer 99:385–393
19. Katz RL (1991) Cytologic diagnosis of leukemia and lymphoma values and limitations. Clin Lab Med 11:469–499
20. Damle RN, Wasil T, Fais F et al (1999) Ig V gene mutation status and CD38 expression as novel prognostic indicators in chronic lymphocytic leukemia. Blood 94:1840–1847
21. Del Poeta G, Maurillo L, Venditti A et al (2001) Clinical significance of CD38 expression in chronic lymphocytic leukemia. Blood 98:2633–2639

22. Verstovsek G, Chakraborty S, Ramzy I et al (2002) Large B-cell lymphomas: fine-needle aspiration plays an important role in initial diagnosis of cases which are falsely negative by flow cytometry. Diagn Cytopathol 27:282–285
23. Chen HI, Akpolat I, Mody DR et al (2006) Restricted kappa/lambda light chain ratio by flow cytometry in germinal center B cells in hashimoto thyroiditis. Am J Clin Pathol 125:42–48
24. Jorgensen JL (2005) State of the art symposium: flow cytometry in the diagnosis of lymphoproliferative disorders by fine-needle aspiration. Cancer 105:443–451
25. Beck RC, Stahl S, O'Keefe CL et al (2003) Detection of mature T-cell leukemias by flow cytometry using anti-T-cell receptor V beta antibodies. Am J Clin Pathol 120:785–794
26. Morice WG, Kimlinger T, Katzmann JA et al (2004) Flow cytometric assessment of TCR-Vbeta expression in the evaluation of peripheral blood involvement by T-cell lymphoproliferative disorders: a comparison with conventional T-cell immunophenotyping and molecular genetic techniques. Am J Clin Pathol 121:373–383
27. Galindo LM, Garcia FU, Hanau CA et al (2000) Fine-needle aspiration biopsy in the evaluation of lymphadenopathy associated with cutaneous T-cell lymphoma (mycosis fungoides/sezary syndrome). Am J Clin Pathol 113:865–871
28. Katz RL, Hirsch-Ginsberg C, Childs C et al (1991) The role of gene rearrangements for antigen receptors in the diagnosis of lymphoma obtained by fine-needle aspiration. A study of 63 cases with concomitant immunophenotyping. Am J Clin Pathol 96:479–490
29. Barr FG (2004) Diagnostic applications of chromosomal translocations in bone and soft tissue sarcomas. Expert Rev Mol Diagn 4:579–582
30. Beatty BG, Bryant R, Wang W et al (2004) HER-2/neu detection in fine-needle aspirates of breast cancer: fluorescence in situ hybridization and immunocytochemical analysis. Am J Clin Pathol 122:246–255
31. Gu M, Ghafari S, Zhao M (2005) Fluorescence in situ hybridization for HER-2/neu amplification of breast carcinoma in archival fine needle aspiration biopsy specimens. Acta Cytol 49:471–476
32. Moore JG, To V, Patel SJ et al (2000) HER-2/neu gene amplification in breast imprint cytology analyzed by fluorescence in situ hybridization: direct comparison with companion tissue sections. Diagn Cytopathol 23:299–302
33. Tomas AR, Praca MJ, Fonseca R et al (2004) Assessing HER-2 status in fresh frozen and archival cytological samples obtained by fine needle aspiration cytology. Cytopathology 15:311–314
34. Sauter G, Lee J, Bartlett JM et al (2009) Guidelines for human epidermal growth factor receptor 2 testing: biologic and methodologic considerations. J Clin Oncol 27:1323–1333
35. Gong Y, Booser DJ, Sneige N (2005) Comparison of HER-2 status determined by fluorescence in situ hybridization in primary and metastatic breast carcinoma. Cancer 103:1763–1769
36. Tapia C, Savic S, Wagner U et al (2007) HER2 gene status in primary breast cancers and matched distant metastases. Breast Cancer Res 9:R31
37. Xiao C, Gong Y, Han EY et al (2011) Stability of HER2-positive status in breast carcinoma: a comparison between primary and paired metastatic tumors with regard to the possible impact of intervening trastuzumab treatment. Ann Oncol 22:1547–1553
38. Gong Y, Gilcrease M, Sneige N (2005) Reliability of chromogenic in situ hybridization for detecting HER-2 gene status in breast cancer: comparison with fluorescence in situ hybridization and assessment of interobserver reproducibility. Mod Pathol 18:1015–1021
39. Gong Y, Sweet W, Duh YJ et al (2009) Chromogenic in situ hybridization is a reliable method for detecting HER2 gene status in breast cancer: a multicenter study using conventional scoring criteria and the new ASCO/CAP recommendations. Am J Clin Pathol 131:490–497
40. Gong Y, Sweet W, Duh YJ et al (2009) Performance of chromogenic in situ hybridization on testing HER2 Status in breast carcinomas with chromosome 17 polysomy and equivocal (2+)

herceptest results: a study of two institutions using the conventional and new ASCO/CAP scoring criteria. Am J Clin Pathol 132:228–236

41. Tanner M, Gancberg D, Di Leo A et al (2000) Chromogenic in situ hybridization: a practical alternative for fluorescence in situ hybridization to detect HER-2/neu oncogene amplification in archival breast cancer samples. Am J Pathol 157:1467–1472

42. Kim GY, Oh YL (2004) Chromogenic in situ hybridization analysis of HER-2/neu status in cytological samples of breast carcinoma. Cytopathology 15:315–320

43. Lin F, Shen T, Prichard JW (2005) Detection of Her-2/neu oncogene in breast carcinoma by chromogenic in situ hybridization in cytologic specimens. Diagn Cytopathol 33:376–380

44. Vocaturo A, Novelli F, Benevolo M et al (2006) Chromogenic in situ hybridization to detect HER-2/neu gene amplification in histological and ThinPrep-processed breast cancer fine-needle aspirates: a sensitive and practical method in the trastuzumab era. Oncologist 11:878–886

45. Alkan S, Lehman C, Sarago C et al (1995) Polymerase chain reaction detection of immunoglobulin gene rearrangement and bcl-2 translocation in archival glass slides of cytologic material. Diagn Mol Pathol 4:25–31

46. Belaud-Rotureau MA, Parrens M, Carrere N et al (2007) Interphase fluorescence in situ hybridization is more sensitive than BIOMED-2 polymerase chain reaction protocol in detecting IGH-BCL2 rearrangement in both fixed and frozen lymph node with follicular lymphoma. Hum Pathol 38:365–372

47. Buno I, Nava P, Alvarez-Doval A et al (2005) Lymphoma associated chromosomal abnormalities can easily be detected by FISH on tissue imprints. An underused diagnostic alternative. J Clin Pathol 58:629–633

48. Kishimoto K, Kitamura T, Fujita K et al (2006) Cytologic differential diagnosis of follicular lymphoma grades 1 and 2 from reactive follicular hyperplasia: cytologic features of fine-needle aspiration smears with Pap stain and fluorescence in situ hybridization analysis to detect t(14;18)(q32;q21) chromosomal translocation. Diagn Cytopathol 34:11–17

49. Richmond J, Bryant R, Trotman W et al (2006) FISH detection of t(14;18) in follicular lymphoma on papanicolaou-stained archival cytology slides. Cancer 108:198–204

50. Ahmed SM, Salgia R (2006) Epidermal growth factor receptor mutations and susceptibility to targeted therapy in lung cancer. Respirology 11:687–692

51. Billah S, Stewart J, Staerkel G et al (2011) EGFR and KRAS mutations in lung carcinoma: molecular testing by using cytology specimens. Cancer cytopathol 119:111–117

52. Kulmala SM, Syrjanen S, Shabalova I et al (2004) Human papillomavirus testing with the hybrid capture 2 assay and PCR as screening tools. J Clin Microbiol 42:2470–2475

53. Day SP, Hudson A, Mast A et al (2009) Analytical performance of the investigational use only cervista HPV HR test as determined by a multi-center study. J Clin Virol 45(1):S63–S72

54. Arentsen HC, de la Rosette JJ, de Reijke TM et al (2007) Fluorescence in situ hybridization: a multitarget approach in diagnosis and management of urothelial cancer. Expert Rev Mol Diagn 7:11–19

55. Assersohn L, Gangi L, Zhao Y et al (2002) The feasibility of using fine needle aspiration from primary breast cancers for cDNA microarray analyses. Clin Cancer Res 8:794–801

56. Ayers M, Symmans WF, Stec J et al (2004) Gene expression profiles predict complete pathologic response to neoadjuvant paclitaxel and fluorouracil, doxorubicin, and cyclophosphamide chemotherapy in breast cancer. J Clin Oncol 22:2284–2293

57. Pusztai L, Ayers M, Stec J et al (2003) Gene expression profiles obtained from fine-needle aspirations of breast cancer reliably identify routine prognostic markers and reveal large-scale molecular differences between estrogen-negative and estrogen-positive tumors. Clin Cancer Res 9:2406–2415

58. Sotiriou C, Powles TJ, Dowsett M et al (2002) Gene expression profiles derived from fine needle aspiration correlate with response to systemic chemotherapy in breast cancer. Breast Cancer Res 4:R3

59. Symmans WF, Ayers M, Clark EA et al (2003) Total RNA yield and microarray gene expression profiles from fine-needle aspiration biopsy and core-needle biopsy samples of breast carcinoma. Cancer 97:2960–2971
60. Gong Y, Yan K, Lin F et al (2007) Determination of oestrogen-receptor status and ERBB2 status of breast carcinoma: a gene-expression profiling study. Lancet Oncol 8:203–211
61. Cheung CC, Carydis B, Ezzat S et al (2001) Analysis of ret/PTC gene rearrangements refines the fine needle aspiration diagnosis of thyroid cancer. J Clin Endocrinol Metab 86:2187–2190
62. Cohen Y, Rosenbaum E, Clark DP et al (2004) Mutational analysis of BRAF in fine needle aspiration biopsies of the thyroid: a potential application for the preoperative assessment of thyroid nodules. Clin Cancer Res 10:2761–2765
63. Gustafson KS, Furth EE, Heitjan DF et al (2004) DNA methylation profiling of cervical squamous intraepithelial lesions using liquid-based cytology specimens: an approach that utilizes receiver-operating characteristic analysis. Cancer 102:259–268
64. Pu RT, Laitala LE, Alli PM et al (2003) Methylation profiling of benign and malignant breast lesions and its application to cytopathology. Mod Pathol 16:1095–1101
65. Pu RT, Laitala LE, Clark DP (2006) Methylation profiling of urothelial carcinoma in bladder biopsy and urine. Acta Cytol 50:499–506

Chapter 3
Head and Neck

Jose Dutra and Ajit Paintal

3.1 Thyroid

3.1.1 Introduction

The American Cancer Society estimated that about 56,460 new cases of thyroid cancer were diagnosed in the U.S. in 2012 and 1,780 deaths could be attributed to thyroid cancer. Worldwide, the incidence of thyroid cancer varies from 0.5 to 10 per 100,000 individuals. Multiple studies have shown that since the 1980s the incidence of thyroid cancer has increased significantly. This is in large part attributable to the increase in incidentally discovered nodules during the workup of unrelated conditions. In many countries, thyroid cancer has become the most rapidly increasing tumor in regard to incidence and in the U.S, it is now the sixth most common cancer in women with an incidence of 14.9 cases per 100.000 women in 2005, up from 6.4 in 1988 [1–5]. Larger tumors have also increased in incidence and this does not appear to be related to access to medical care.

Thyroid nodules are very common in general clinical practice, with an estimated prevalence of palpable thyroid nodules between 4 and 7 % [6, 7]. When high resolution ultrasound is used as a screening tool in asymptomatic patients, nonpalpable thyroid nodules are present in about 30–50 % of the adult population [8, 9]. The incidence of cancer in thyroid nodules is reported to be between 5 and 10 %. Thyroid nodules are commonly reported by the patient or discovered during

J. Dutra
Northwestern Feinberg School of Medicine Department of Otolaryngology-Head and Neck,
Surgery 675 North Saint Clair, Galter Bldg 15-200, Chicago, IL 60611,
United States of America
e-mail: JDutra@nmff.org

A. Paintal (⊠)
Northwestern Memorial Hospital Feinberg School of Medicine Department of Pathology,
Galter 7-132G 251 East Huron Street, Chicago, IL 60611, United States of America
e-mail: ajit.paintal@northwestern.edu

R. Nayar (ed.), *Cytopathology in Oncology*,
Cancer Treatment and Research 160, DOI: 10.1007/978-3-642-38850-7_3,
© Springer-Verlag Berlin Heidelberg 2014

a routine physical examination. In an oncology clinic, thyroid nodules are also found on physical examination or incidentally during imaging studies for staging or follow-up of unrelated malignancies. More than 300,000 thyroid nodules are discovered yearly in the U.S. Because thyroid nodules are common and mostly benign, the clinician is left with the complex task of determining whether the discovered thyroid nodule can be safely followed or has a reasonable chance of being malignant and thus requires surgical removal.

3.1.2 Evaluation of Thyroid Nodules

The initial evaluation of a patient with a thyroid nodule includes a good history and careful physical examination. Hoarseness, dysphagia, and rapid progression of symptoms should alert the physician to the possibility of a malignancy. A history of head and neck irradiation, family history of thyroid malignancy in a first-degree relative, and hereditary syndromes such as familial adenomatous polyposis, Gardner syndrome, Cowden disease, Carney complex, and MEN are factors that increase the risk of malignancy. Extremes of age (younger than 20 or older than 65 years) also increase the risk for malignancy. Physical findings suggestive of malignancy include palpable lymphadenopathy, ipsilateral vocal cord paralysis or paresis, and a hard, fixed nodule. Measurement of serum TSH is obtained in every patient. Although 90–95 % of patients will have normal or elevated TSH, a suppressed TSH suggests a functional adenoma which is almost always benign [10]. Thyroid ultrasound should be performed in every patient with a palpable or incidentally discovered thyroid nodule. It accurately measures the size of the nodule and identifies features suspicious for malignancy. A 131 Iodine uptake scan is useful only if TSH is suppressed in order to identify a toxic adenoma or a cold nodule in a hyperfunctioning gland. Because of its cost-effectiveness, safety, and accuracy, fine-needle aspiration biopsy is usually the next step.

3.1.3 Thyroid Cytopathology

3.1.3.1 Overview

Thyroid fine needle aspiration cytology was first introduced in the early 1950 s in Scandinavia. It gained acceptance in the U.S. in the 1980s and has evolved to be widely utilized in the assessment of thyroid nodules. The effectiveness of this procedure has translated into a significant reduction in unnecessary thyroid operations and an increased yield of thyroid cancer in patients undergoing thyroidectomies with diagnostic intent [12–14, 16, 17]. Thyroid FNA is a safe and rapid procedure with very few complications [18]. Seeding of thyroid cancer along the needle tract is very rare and has been reported only once [19]. Belfiori et al. demonstrated that thyroid FNA decreases the overall cost of care by 25 % [20].

The use of thyroid ultrasound imaging coupled with cytology allows for effective triage of a patient with a thyroid nodule.

A cytopathologist should be familiar with all aspects of thyroid disease and their clinical intricacies. Knowledge of clinical history is often important in the diagnosis of thyroid lesions. The increasing number of practitioners relying on thyroid FNA attests to its important role in the critical decision making regarding thyroid patient management. The procedure is safe and accurate. Until recently, there was no standardized reporting system for FNA specimens [23, 24]. Consequently, an enormous variability in the reported incidence of the different cytologic categories exists in older published thyroid FNA studies. Physicians treating patients with thyroid nodules should consult with their cytopathologist and discuss cytologic reporting methodology so that there is clear communication.

Advantages of Thyroid FNA

1. reduces the number of patients referred for surgery by approximately 50 %
2. increases surgical yield of thyroid malignancy by approximately 30 %
3. reduce management costs, estimated at about 20 %
4. allows assessment of specimen adequacy during procedure, avoiding repeat visits/biopsy.

The criteria for thyroid FNA adequacy have been difficult to define. A practice followed by many cytopathologists is a requirement of at least 6 groups of follicular cells with a minimum of 10 cells in each group. Other factors that influence adequacy and consequently interpretation include smear thickness, clot and obscuring blood, the number of passes, and preparatory artifacts. Overall the specimen should be appropriately collected, fixed, and stained. It must contain a minimum amount of cellular material allowing for identification and quantification of the cellular elements and colloid.

3.1.3.2 Noncellular Components Seen in Thyroid Fine-Needle Aspiration

Colloid Colloid is a characteristic, proteinaceous material containing thyroglobulin and thyroid hormone produced by the thyroid gland. It is a distinctive component of thyroid FNA's. The presence of large quantities of colloid in an aspirate smear generally indicates a benign thyroid nodule. A particularly thick and viscous form ("bubble gum colloid") is present in some cases of papillary thyroid carcinoma.

Amyloid The presence of amyloid on thyroid smears is frequently associated with medullary carcinoma. It is characterized by a dense "cracked" appearance, oftentimes with entrapped fibroblasts. In systemic amyloidosis, clumps of amyloid may be found in the absence of neoplastic C cells.

Calcium and psammoma bodies While in isolation psammoma bodies are not diagnostic of papillary thyroid carcinoma (PTC), their presence is strongly suggestive of the diagnosis and they are seen as "microcalcifications" on thyroid ultrasound. Psammoma bodies can also be seen in hyalinizing trabecular adenoma and oxyphilic tumors. Conversely, nonspecific calcifications, are associated with degeneration secondary to hemorrhage, cystic degeneration, and fibrosis and are a common occurrence. These calcifications should be distinguished from true psammoma bodies which are concentrically lamellated calcospherites of calcium phosphate, non-birefringent and have a glassy appearance.

Crystals Cholesterol crystals and birefringent calcium-oxalate crystals are a common degenerative change in benign thyroid nodules. They account for the majority of "macrocalcifications" on thyroid ultrasound.

Pigment Hemosiderin can be seen within macrophages in association with benign degenerative changes and hemorrhage of adenomatous nodules but rarely in association with PTC.

3.1.3.3 Cellular Components of a Thyroid Smear

Follicular cells Thyroid follicular epithelial cells are generally the most numerous cellular element in thyroid FNA specimens. Normal follicular cells are small and display indistinct cell borders and uniform round nuclei with granular chromatin. The arrangement of follicular cells in relationship to one another (architecture) is important in the assessment of thyroid FNA specimens. The presence of flat sheets of follicular cells is associated with benign thyroid nodules, while three-dimensional clusters of follicular cells and microfollicles (less than 12 cells in diameter) are associated with follicular neoplasms.

Hurthle cells Hurthle cells are a variant of follicular epithelial cells that contain abundant granular eosinophilic cytoplasm and numerous mitochondria. Hurthle cells are often found admixed with normal follicular cells in benign thyroid nodules. Hurthle cell change is also a hallmark of Hashimoto's thyroiditis. In an aspirate specimen comprised exclusively of Hurthle cells, the possibility of a Hurthle cell neoplasm should be considered.

C cells Normal C cells are not specifically recognized in thyroid aspirate specimens. In medullary carcinoma, neoplastic C cells can assume a variety of morphologies including spindle cell, epithelioid (round), and giant cell forms.

Macrophages Numerous macrophages in FNA specimens of the thyroid, and from other sites, generally indicate a cystic component within the lesion being sampled. The most frequent cystic lesions that occur in the thyroid are degenerating benign thyroid nodules and papillary thyroid carcinoma. The distinction of these two entities requires that the epithelial/solid portion of the lesion be sampled.

Lymphocytes A significant lymphoid component within a thyroid aspirate specimen is usually associated with chronic lymphocytic thyroiditis. When the lymphoid component is scant, it can be difficult to distinguish from circulating lymphocytes from the peripheral blood.

3.1.3.4 Reporting Thyroid Smears and Diagnostic Categories

Several reporting schemes have been recommended by several clinical organizations including the Papanicolaou Society for Cytopathology, American Association of Clinical Endocrinologists, and American Thyroid Association [15]. The classification used in this publication is the result of the National Cancer Institute (NCI) sponsored NCI Thyroid Fine-needle Aspiration (FNA) State of the Science Conference in October 22 and 23, 2007 in Bethesda, MD. It contains six diagnostic categories: Nondiagnostic/unsatisfactory, benign, follicular lesion of undetermined significance/atypia of undetermined significance, follicular/Hurthle neoplasm, suspicious for malignancy, and malignant.

Nondiagnostic FNA (Unsatisfactory/Insufficient) Numerous publications have reported FNA's sensitivity and specificity rates to be 65–98 % and 72–100 %, respectively [15]. Despite growing expertise in thyroid aspirate interpretation among cytopathologists, there is still a significant proportion of specimens, from 8 to 25 %, for which a nondiagnostic result is rendered. Aspiration of cystic lesions often produces a specimen comprised of granular cystic debris and macrophages ("cyst contents"). Specimens comprised entirely of "cyst contents" are considered nondiagnostic as without an epithelial component, papillary thyroid carcinoma (which is often at least partially cystic in nature) cannot be excluded. A nondiagnostic interpretation is also rendered when there is lack of follicular cells, excessive blood, or other technical issue that ultimately obscures the cellular features and renders the specimen uninterpretable. A repeat biopsy should be recomended and is successful in about 50-60% of cases [25]. Malignancy can be found in about 5 % of the initially nondiagnostic cases and thus correlation with ultrasound findings is always important [26, 27]. If initially done by palpation alone, an ultrasound guided FNA should be performed in subsequent biopsies [28, 29]. On site cytologic assessment of the specimen at the time of the repeat procedure will generate, in most cases, a satisfactory specimen. If repeated FNA yields a "nondiagnostic" aspirate, correlation with clinical and family history, and close follow-up should be performed [30]. In the case of cystic or complex nodules, many authors would consider surgical resection due to the low but real incidence of cystic papillary carcinoma. If the nodule is solid and repeated aspirates remain nondiagnostic, surgery should be strongly considered [11, 30–32]. Nodules greater than 1 cm with ultrasound findings suspicious for malignancy (microcalcifications, irregular borders, hypoechoic solid nodules) should also be referred for surgery.

Benign The benign category includes multinodular goiter, hyperplastic/adenomatoid nodule, and Hashimoto's thyroiditis. Other terms frequently used to describe benign aspirates are "negative for malignancy" or "nonneoplastic". In large series, hyperplastic nodules represent about 90 % of all benign aspirates (Fig. 3.1). The other 10 % are chronic inflammatory or subacute thyroiditis (Fig. 3.2). [20, 33] The false-negative rate associated with a "benign" cytologic diagnosis is low and varies from 1.3 to 11.5 % in different series [21, 34, 35].

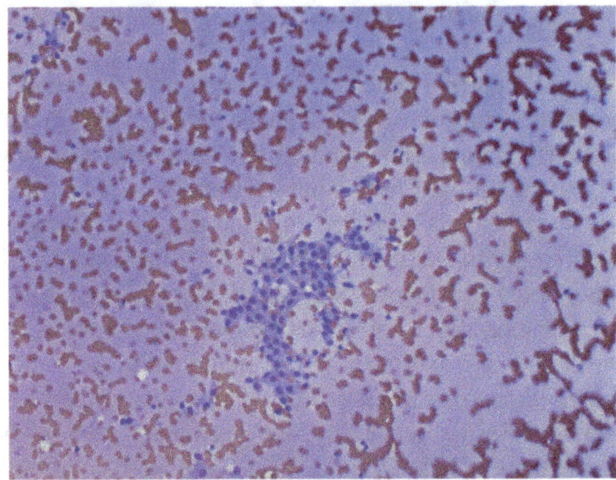

Fig. 3.1 Benign thyroid nodule (Diff-Quick, 20x). Abundant blue-staining colloid is present in the background. Follicular cells may be numerous but are arranged as flat sheets and contain bland round nuclei

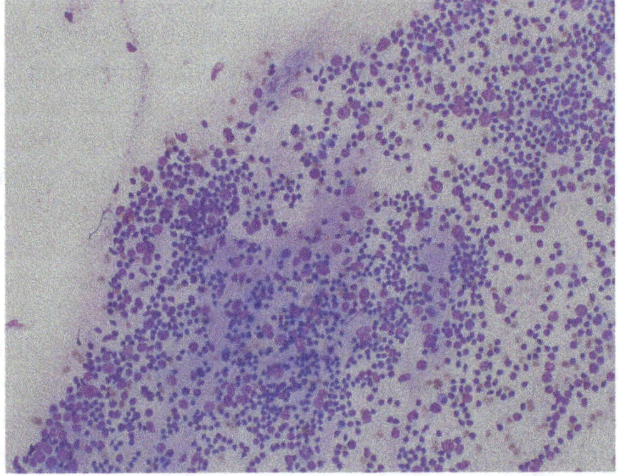

Fig. 3.2 Chronic lymphocytic thyroiditis (Diff-Quick, 20x). Numerous lymphocytes of varying sizes are present admixed with larger Hurthle cells (a variant of normal follicular cells). The Hurthle cells contain abundant granular cytoplasm, even chromatin, and prominent nucleoli. In the context of chronic lymphocytic thyroiditis, a moderate degree of nuclear atypia and enlargement are often seen

Although probably not cost-effective, a repeat FNA in benign aspirates would reduce the false-negative rate by 50 % [35–37].

A solitary thyroid nodule is a discrete mass in an otherwise normal thyroid gland. Most of these nodules are benign hyperplastic nodules. The nodules are composed of irregularly enlarged follicles with large amounts of colloid and bland follicular cells. The follicular epithelium is heterogeneous and generally is present in flat sheets, consistent with large follicle ("macrofollicle") formation. The cytoplasm is scant and may contain degenerative paravacuolar granules containing hemosiderin and lipofuscin pigment. Macrophages are seen in nodules with cystic degeneration. A variable number of admixed Hurthle cells can be observed.

Clinical follow-up is recommended for all patients with benign diagnoses due to the approximately 5 % false-negative rate. The ultrasonographic appearance of the nodules should also be considered when deciding the appropriate follow-up schedule. In patients with nodules with suspicious features such as microcalcifications or irregular borders in a solid hypoechoic nodule, a repeat biopsy in 6 months should be performed. Patients with risk factors for thyroid cancer such as a family history of thyroid malignancy or radiation therapy to the head and neck would also benefit from more frequent follow-up and repeat biopsy.

For most benign, palpable lesions in reliable patients, clinical follow-up with thyroid ultrasound after a 6–18 month interval is recommended. For patients with nonpalpable nodules, thyroid ultrasound examination should be performed at a similar interval. Nonpalpable thyroid nodules have a similar risk of malignancy as palpable nodules. Changes in nodule size or appearance, such as more prominent microcalcifications or an increase in the solid component of a complex nodule will require further cytologic evaluation. Changes in patient symptoms also may require reevaluation of the nodule. Benign nodules may require surgery if associated with significant neck discomfort or pressure, difficulty swallowing, cosmetic deformity of the neck, and if the lesion is substernal. Surgery is also indicated if the nodule repeatedly hemorrhages causing pain and neck swelling. Cystic lesions that reaccumulate fluid after aspiration and cause symptoms should also be given consideration for surgery. Thyroid lobectomy is usually indicated in the case of single or multiple nodules with a normal contralateral lobe. Total thyroidectomy should be considered in patients with a history of radiation therapy to avoid reoperation and to eradicate the risk of subsequent malignancy.

A multinodular goiter may be defined as a structurally and functionally heterogeneous thyroid enlargement [38]. Patients with multiple nodules have the same risk of malignancy as those with a single thyroid nodule. Therefore, careful follow-up is recommended in a similar fashion described for solitary nodules. Periodic ultrasonography of the gland at 6–18 months should be performed, the nodules measured systematically, and the gland thoroughly evaluated for changes in the appearance of the nodules and the occurrence of new nodules. Reaspiration or surgical removal should be performed if significant changes occur [11].

According to the American Thyroid Association Guidelines, hormone suppressive therapy should not be employed as a diagnostic maneuver for confirmation of benignancy [11]. Hormone suppressive therapy was widely used as a treatment for euthyroid patients with multinodular thyroids or single thyroid nodules and to confirm the benign nature of the nodule. The basic assumption underlying this treatment was that the growth of thyroid nodules is dependent on thyrotropin. Consequently, thyrotropin suppression would result in a decrease in nodule size and prevent the development of new nodules. Studies, however, have shown that this treatment seems to be beneficial only in a subgroup of patients with small thyroid nodules. Less than 20 % of solitary nodules will regress significantly by more than 50 % of initial size, but regrowth is common after discontinuation of therapy. Gharib and Mazzaferi, after extensive review of the literature, have also concluded that benign solitary nodules are best followed without suppression. Suppressive therapy results in subclinical hyperthyroidism which may have adverse effects including an increased risk of atrial fibrillation, accelerated osteoporosis, and other cardiac effects. Elderly and postmenopausal women are especially at risk.

Ethanol ablation can be used with caution on recurrent cystic lesions. As with all sclerosing agents, treatment may be complicated by severe and chronic pain, and recurrent laryngeal nerve palsy has been reported.

Follicular lesion or Atypia of undetermined significance (AUS/FLUS) This category includes lesions that cannot be classified as benign due to the absence of compelling and incontestable features of benignity, but lack the degree of cellular or architectural atypia necessary for classification as a "follicular neoplasm" or "suspicious for malignancy" [23]. The diagnostic heading of AUS/FLUS encompasses a broad range of diagnostic scenarios including cases with (1) cytologic atypia insufficient for surgical triage but too concerning to dismiss as benign (2) architectural atypia insufficient for a diagnosis of follicular neoplasm (3) a scant aspirate with a worrisome degree of atypia, but limited cellularity (4) an aspirate with mild atypia where a definitive assessment is precluded by excess blood or various preparatory artifacts. (5) In addition, a diagnosis of AUS/FLUS may be rendered in smears that would otherwise be considered as follicular neoplasms or Hurthle cell neoplasms if there is a clinical background of a multinodular goiter or Hashimoto's thyroiditis, respectively. This is owing to the decreased risk of malignancy that these patterns convey in those settings. Given that the AUS/FLUS category is heterogeneous and its application requires subjective assessment of mild degrees of atypia, interobserver variability among cytopathologists for this diagnosis is high. The risk of malignancy in this group varies, but is generally reported to be between 5 and 10 %. Repeated FNA, within 3–6 months, is usually performed. In these cases, a benign diagnosis will be rendered in approximately 50 % [22]. If the repeat FNA is again indeterminate, surgery should be considered. Clinical and radiological correlation is also advised. If the patient reports a family history of thyroid cancer or radiation therapy to the head and neck region, surgical consultation should be recommended. In addition, if ultrasound features suspicious for malignancy are present, surgery should also be considered. If a conservative approach is taken, a repeat FNA and ultrasound should be performed. More recently triage of these cases by molecular testing has become a viable option and both "rule in" and "rule out" malignancy tests are commercially available [39]

Follicular neoplasm or suspicious for follicular neoplasm This group of lesions refers to nonpapillary follicular patterned lesions and Hurthle cell neoplasms. The aspirates are generally quite cellular with a paucity of colloid. The follicular cells are bland but, in contrast to benign thyroid aspirates, are predominantly present in either three-dimensional clusters or microfollicles (Fig. 3.3). Microfollicles are defined as small rings of often overlapping cells comprised of up to 15 follicular cells. Hurthle cell neoplasms are similar, but comprised of Hurthle cells (Fig. 3.4). Of note, a predominantly microfollicular aspirate may be seen in follicular/Hurthle cell carcinoma, follicular adenoma, and in cellular adenomatoid nodules. As capsular and lymphovascular invasion, the diagnostic hallmarks of follicular carcinoma, cannot be assessed in FNA biopsies, follicular adenoma/carcinoma are

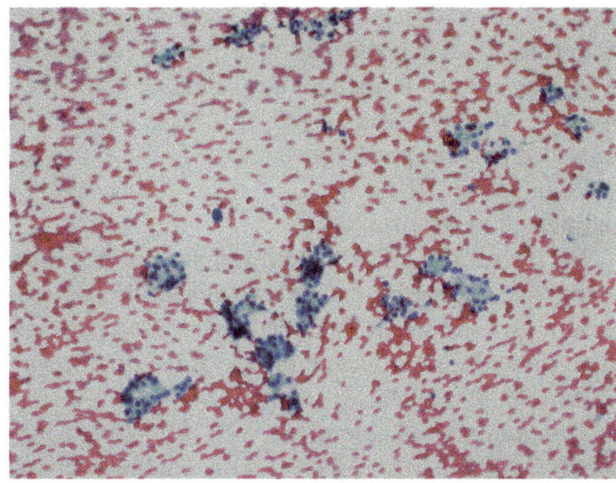

Fig. 3.3 Follicular neoplasm (Pap stain, 20x). Colloid is absent, The follicular cells, while bland and without atypia, are almost exclusively arranged in small, round, two-dimensional formations (microfollicles)

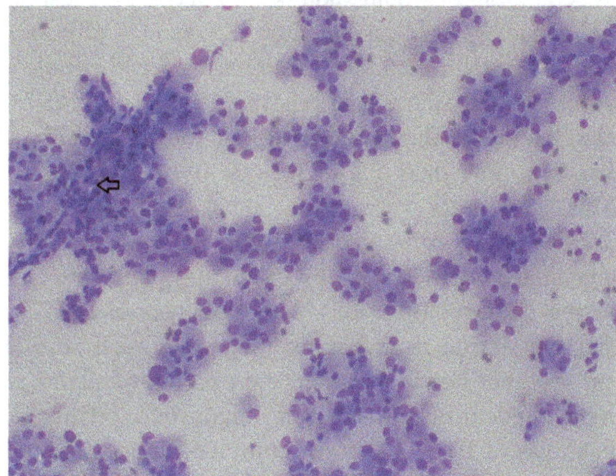

Fig. 3.4 Hurthle cell neoplasm (Diff Quick, 20x). The aspirate is almost exclusively comprised of Hurthle cells with no colloid. The Hurthle cells are arranged in three dimensional clusters and microfollicles. Occasional blood vessels are seen transgressing the cell clusters (*arrow*)

impossible to distinguish in FNA specimens and require surgical excision of the nodule for definitive diagnosis.

The risk of malignancy in this category is reported to be between 20 and 30 %. This percentage can be even higher if the lesion is larger than 4 cm and of the Hurthle cell type. The high incidence of carcinoma in these lesions mandates surgical treatment. Usually a thyroid lobectomy is indicated; total thyroidectomy may be performed if subsequent histologic examination reveals vascular and/or capsular invasion.

Some factors may favor a total thyroidectomy at the time of the initial surgery—the presence of contralateral nodules, documented hypothyroidism, patient's age and the presence of co-morbidities, and patient's unwillingness to accept the risk of a second thyroid operation.

Suspicious for malignancy This diagnostic category conveys the presence of cellularity and cytologic characteristics that are suggestive of malignancy (usually papillary thyroid carcinoma) but lacking all features necessary for a definitive diagnosis. This may be due to a paucity of abnormal cells or diffuse mild to moderate atypia. Resection ultimately reveals the presence of malignancy in 50–75 % of these lesions [28, 40]. The surgical approach, total versus partial thyroidectomy, depends on bilaterality of the lesions, patient's age, history of radiation therapy to the head and neck, strong family history of thyroid carcinoma, and patient preference.

Malignant Malignant thyroid lesions reported in this category include papillary carcinoma, medullary carcinoma, anaplastic carcinoma, lymphomas, poorly differentiated carcinomas, and metastases. Thyroid malignancy is found on 5–10 % of all thyroid FNAs. The predictive value of a "malignant" diagnosis in a thyroid FNA is 95–99 % in most series.

Papillary thyroid carcinoma Well-differentiated thyroid carcinoma accounts for 80–90 % of all malignancies, with papillary thyroid carcinoma (PTC) and its variants being the most common (about 85 % [4, 41, 42] of cases). These tumors are common in young adults and have the best prognosis among all thyroid malignancies. Women are more frequently affected, nearly three to four times more often than men. The National Cancer Institute's SEER database shows that among women, the 5-year relative survival rate is 97.4 %. According to the SEER data, the rate of distant metastasis in men at the time of the diagnosis is more than two-fold more than that of women (9 % vs 4 %) in data collected from 1974 to 2003.

PTC arises from thyroid follicular cells, and, typically, has a microscopic appearance characterized by branching papillae or follicles/sheets and distinctive nuclear features (Fig. 3.5). The diagnosis of PTC is based predominantly on its characteristic nuclear features that, when well developed, are extremely sensitive and specific. For this reason, the excellent cellular preservation in aspirate specimens renders FNA a superior diagnostic modality relative to core biopsy for the diagnosis of PTC. The most common diagnostic features include:

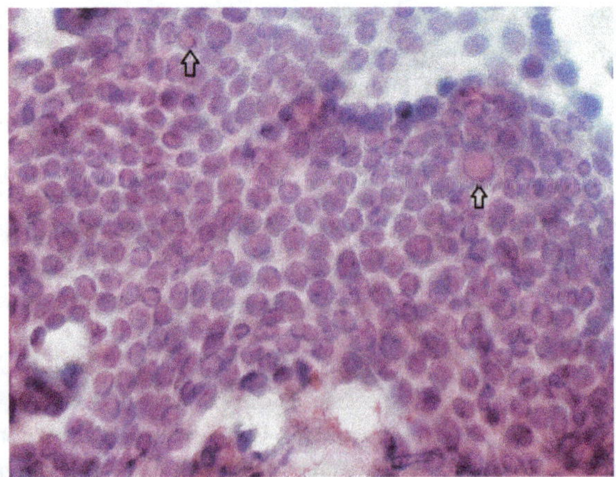

Fig. 3.5 Papillary thyroid carcinoma (Pap stain, 60x). Aspirates commonly contain predominantly flat sheets of cells with markedly enlarged, overlapping nuclei. The chromatin pattern is pale and cleared out and nuclei are frequently ovoid in shape. Nuclear grooves are common and scattered intranuclear pseudoinclusions are seen (*arrows*)

1. Enlarged nuclei with grooves and pseudoinclusions (invaginations of cytoplasm within the nucleus) and cleared chromatin.
2. Change in shape of the nucleus to oval.
3. Dense, "squamoid" cytoplasm.
4. Psammoma bodies (up to 50 % of the cases).
5. Dense bubble gum-like colloid.
6. Multinucleated giant cells.

Encapsulated cases of PTC demonstrating a pure follicular growth pattern without papillae formation are termed follicular variant of PTC (FVPTC). They comprise about 20–40 % of all cases of PTC. The nuclear features in FVPTC are often less fully developed than in conventional cases of PTC. As a result, the degree of inter-observer variability by pathologists in both FNA cytology and resections is high. Recent molecular data suggests that FVPTC, when strictly defined, may be more similar to follicular lesions than PTC in regard to behavior and genetics [43].

Some histologic variants of PTC such as the tall-cell variant and the rarer columnar-cell variant are more aggressive and have a more reserved prognosis.

The treatment of PTC is complex and its discussion is beyond the scope of this chapter. In general, a risk-stratification approach is recommended. This combines clinical factors present during the initial work-up and surgical findings to predict risk of death, recurrence, and risk of failing initial therapy. Postoperative radio-iodine ablation, the extent of surgical resection, the degree of thyrotropin suppression and the follow-up strategy is then individualized [44].

Total thyroidectomy or near total thyroidectomy, with or without central neck dissection is usually performed for most localized lesions [11]. For patients with bulky thyroid tumors or nodal disease, preoperative cross-sectional imaging should be obtained to assess the extent of disease. Lateral neck dissection is performed if positive nodes are present in the lateral compartment of the neck. Prognostic factors in PTC have been extensively studied.

Measurement of thyroglobulin (TG) on FNA specimens is a useful ancillary test in the work up of postsurgical recurrence in lymph nodes, especially those that are cystic and may thus not yield a definitive diagnosis on FNA biopsy [45].

Medullary thyroid carcinoma (MTC) is seen in about 2–5 % of thyroid FNAs. MTC originates from parafollicular C cells of neuroectodermal origin, contrasting with the epithelial nature of other thyroid tumors. About 15–25 % of MTC cases are familial. They occur in association with three familial syndromes: multiple endocrine neoplasia (MEN) type 2A or 2B, and familial MTC (FMTC). The other 75–85 % are sporadic. Germline mutations of the RET proto-oncogene have been demonstrated to be the causative genetic factor in familial cases of MTC. C-cell hyperplasia (CCH) is recognized as the precursor lesion of MTC. The progression of CCH to MTC occurs at different rates which appear to be related to the particular mutation of the RET proto-oncogene [46]. Mutations in different codons are associated with different phenotypic expressions of the disease. Although patients with MTC may present at any age, sporadic MTC has a mean presentation age of

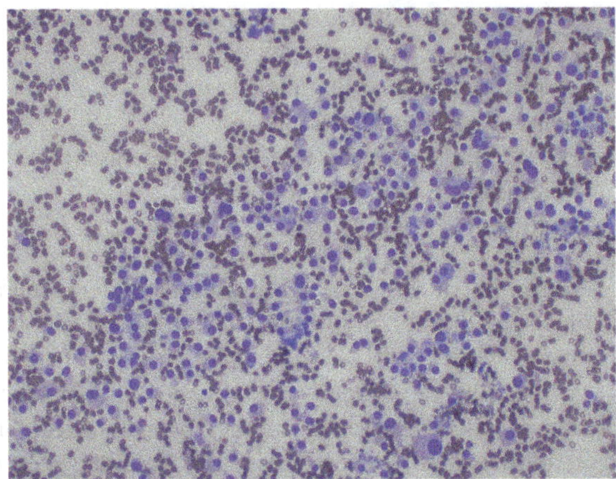

Fig. 3.6 Medullary carcinoma (Diff Quick, 20x). The aspirate is cellular and contains numerous single cells. The cells are polygonal and contain round uniform nuclei that are placed along one the edge of the cell (plasmacytoid). The chromatin pattern is granular and evenly dispersed

49 years in contrast with 30 years for the familial type [47]. Almost all patients with MTC will be present with elevated serum calcitonin, a peptide hormone composed of 32 amino acids which is secreted by C cells. An elevated calcitonin level confirms the presence of MTC, but a normal level does not exclude the diagnosis [48]. Carcinoembryonic antigen (CEA) is also frequently elevated.

Aspirates of medullary carcinoma are typically cellular. The neoplastic cells may take many forms, but are frequently spindled or round with eccentrically placed nuclei (plasmacytoid). The nuclei may be hyperchromatic but typically have dispersed, finely granular "salt and pepper" chromatin (Fig. 3.6). Nuclear pseudoinclusions may be seen creating the potential for confusion with PTC. Amyloid is found in variable amounts as an acellular material associated with tumor cells or in isolation. Immunohistochemistry performed on a cell block/core biopsy or correlation with serum calcitonin measurements is extremely useful for confirmation. Immunohistochemical stains for calcitonin, CEA, synaptophysin, and chromogranin are positive in the vast majority of MTC.

It is estimated that 14 % of all thyroid cancer associated with deaths are related to MTC [49, 50]. The MTC cancer specific mortality rate is approximately 25 % at 10 years [50]. The average 5-year survival rate is 78–98 %. Surgery is the only effective treatment and should be performed after careful evaluation of the extent of the disease and the presence of pheochromocytoma. Because MTC frequently metastasizes to regional neck lymph nodes, even at early stages of the disease, surgical dissection of the central neck, lateral lymph nodal chains, and upper mediastinum is usually recommended in addition to total thyroidectomy. When a RET mutation is found in an index case all first-degree relatives must be screened for identification of carriers. Theoretically, half of first-degree relatives will not carry the mutated gene. The risk of developing MTC in this group is the same as the general population [51]. The timing and extent of prophylactic thyroidectomy in RET mutation positive asymptomatic patients should be individualized-based predominantly on the results of a RET mutation analysis [46, 52, 53]. Prognostic factors to predict biochemical cure are pre-operative calcitonin levels and regional lymph node metastases [54]. The mortality rate tends to be worse in sporadic tumors and/or when metastases are found at the time of the diagnosis. Patients above 50 years and with MEN-2 phenotype also have worse prognosis [55].

Anaplastic thyroid carcinoma (ATC), the most aggressive of all thyroid malignancies, is seen in 1–3 % of cases of thyroid carcinoma [50]. These tumors occur in the elderly population with a greater incidence in the seventh decade, women representing 55–75 % of the cases. ATC has a dismal prognosis with survival measured in months [56]. ATC may arise "de novo" but in many cases develops from a preexisting well-differentiated thyroid carcinoma (follicular carcinoma or PTC) [56–59] In most cases ATC presents as a progressively enlarging thyroid mass, infiltrating adjacent structures in over 70 % of all patients and causing respiratory symptoms in at least a third of them [56, 58]. Hoarseness and cough are frequently present. Tumors are greater than 5 cm in 80 % of the patients and a third present with vocal cord paralysis [60]. A third of patients have distant metastases at the time of the diagnosis, lungs being the most common site [60]. Aspirates of ATC are typically extremely poorly differentiated and classically comprised of overtly malignant spindled and epithelioid (round) cells. The nuclei are extremely pleomorphic and morphologically, it is often difficult to recognize these tumors as carcinomas or as primary thyroid tumors (Fig. 3.7). The most important differential diagnostic consideration is metastasis from another site. Oftentimes this is difficult to resolve as many patients present with lung lesions as well. Exclusion of a metastatic lesion is impossible based on morphology alone and requires clinicopathologic correlation as well as the application of immunohistochemistry. If ATC is suspected clinically or during on site pathologic assessment, a cell block/core biopsy should be obtained for immunohistochemical studies. While ATC, by definition, loses expression of most thyroid-specific markers (TTF1, thyroglobulin), expression of the transcription factor, Pax8, is retained in most cases and is relatively specific for thyroid origin in this context.

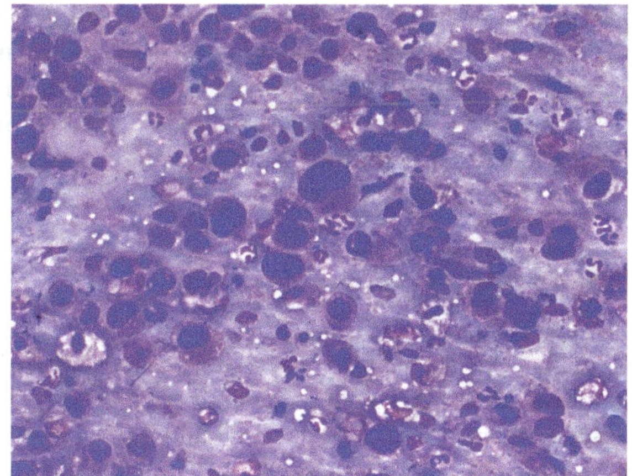

Fig. 3.7 Anaplastic thyroid carcinoma (Diff Quick 40x). Markedly enlarged cells with striking variation in cell and nuclear size and shape. Multinucleated forms are frequent. This morphologic pattern is not specific and may be seen in metastatic poorly different carcinomas from a variety of sites. Correlation with clinical and radiographic data is imperative in the diagnosis of this entity

ATC is rarely cured. The best results are obtained with combined surgery, hyperfractionated external beam radiation therapy and chemotherapy [61, 62]. Total thyroidectomy with clear margins of resection is almost never feasible and may have little impact on outcomes.

Lymphomas Can be difficult to diagnose and accurately subtype in cytology specimens. Triage of biopsy material for flow cytometry is often invaluable for both diagnosis and subtyping. An open biopsy is often recommended if the cytologic diagnosis is suspicious or positive for lymphoma.

Patients with a history of Hashimoto's thyroiditis are at increased risk for non-Hodgkin lymphoma. The clinician should exercise caution and clinical judgment when assessing hypothyroid patients with rapidly enlarging thyroid nodules. Thyroid lymphoma may present with a solitary or multiple nodules. False negatives may occur in low-grade lymphomas. Low-grade lymphomas are extremely difficult to distinguish from lymphocytic thyroiditis on the basis of morphology alone. If the thyroid mass is relatively large or has rapidly increased in size, on site evaluation with flow cytometry triage and/or open biopsy should be considered.

Metastasis to the Thyroid Metastatic lesions to the thyroid are infrequently seen, but are reliably diagnosed by FNA in the proper clinicopathologic context. Renal cell carcinoma is the most common metastatic tumor followed by lung and breast carcinoma, and occasionally melanoma. If no other metastases are found after complete metastatic work-up, total thyroidectomy may be recommended to avoid local complications. The appearance of metastasis to the thyroid gland frequent portends a poor prognosis.

3.2 Parathyroid

Fine-needle aspiration is rarely performed in the context of a known parathyroid lesion. Parathyroid tissue is extremely difficult to distinguish from thyroid tissue in aspirate specimens and mischaracterization of parathyroid tissue as a thyroid follicular neoplasm is a well-described pitfall, particularly in the case of an intrathyroidal parathyroid gland. Clinicopathologic correlation and triage of aspirate material for PTH measurements is vital in the accurate diagnosis of suspected parathyroid lesions. There is no general agreement on the cytopathologic criteria for parathyroid adenoma, hyperplasia, or parathyroid cyst [63, 64]. Suspected parathyroid lesions identified on neck ultrasound following unsuccessful parathyroid exploration may be aspirated and PTH levels assayed [65].

3.3 Salivary Glands

Neoplasms of the salivary glands account for about 5–7 % of all head and neck neoplasms in adults. The parotid, submandibular, and sublingual glands are commonly described as major salivary glands. Minor salivary glands are aggregates of salivary gland tissue located in the submucosa of the aerodigestive tract. Approximately 2,500 new cases are diagnosed yearly in the U.S. Because of their rarity and varied histology (over 40 subtypes) salivary gland neoplasms represent a unique category of head and neck tumors and one of the most challenging areas of cytopathology.

3.3.1 Clinical Presentation

Salivary gland tumors occur in all age groups with a peak of incidence in the sixth to seventh decades. Although demographics may differ according to tumor type, most salivary gland tumors occur more frequently in women. In children, mesenchymal tumors are more common and mucoepidermoid carcinoma is the most common malignancy.

Most salivary gland tumors occur in the parotid gland (85 %), and the vast majority of them (80 %) are benign. Tumors of the submandibular gland are less common and account for about 10–15 % of all salivary gland neoplasms with an incidence of malignancy up to 50 %. Tumors of the sublingual gland are extremely rare (less than 1 %) with an incidence of malignancy exceeding 90 %. Neoplasms of the minor salivary glands account for 5 % of all salivary gland tumors. Most tumors occur in the oral cavity with the palate being the most common site. Malignant neoplasms represent the greater proportion of tumors (80 %). Rarely, salivary gland tumors may develop in heterotopic salivary gland tissue present in the sinuses, lacrimal gland, skin, ear, bones and lymph nodes of the head and neck.

The most common benign tumor is pleomorphic adenoma, 85 % of which occur in the parotid gland. A rare but well-recognized subtype, metastasizing pleomorphic adenoma, behaves as a malignancy, with 50 % of patients ultimately dying from metastases to lungs, bones, and others organs. Warthin's tumor (benign cystadenoma lymphomatosum) is the second most common benign salivary gland tumor comprising about 10 % of all benign tumors. These tumors are commonly seen in the parotid glands but rarely in other glands. They can be bilateral in 10 % of cases. The most common salivary gland malignancies are adenoid cystic carcinoma, mucoepidermoid carcinoma, adenocarcinoma, not otherwise specified, and acinic cell carcinoma

Risk factors associated with the development of salivary gland neoplasms include radiation exposure, particularly radiation treatment to the head and neck. There is no clear relationship between use of tobacco or ethanol and the development of salivary gland malignancy. However, smoking has been associated with the development of Warthin's tumors. Familial or genetic predisposition has not been identified except for patients with Brooke-Spiegler syndrome who present with an increased risk for salivary gland basal cell tumors. Epstein-Barr virus has been linked to the development of lymphoepithelial carcinoma. Also, exposure to industrial chemicals such as nickel alloy, chromium, asbestos, woodworking, and silica dust has been linked to salivary gland tumors.

3.3.2 Clinical Evaluation

The majority of patients with salivary gland tumors present with a slow growing, asymptomatic mass palpated by the patient or discovered incidentally during a head and neck imaging study for an unrelated condition. A complete history and physical examination can usually distinguish inflammatory conditions from tumors. Both benign and malignant tumors can have a protracted history. Rapid enlargement of a longstanding mass or development of a cervical lymphadenopathy should raise the possibility of malignant transformation of a pleomorphic adenoma. Persistent pain, facial nerve dysfunction, trismus, adenopathy, a fixed mass, and tumor extension to the skin are suggestive of malignancy. Facial nerve involvement is associated with increased morbidity and mortality.

In patients with Sjogren's syndrome, an asymmetric enlargement of the parotid gland should raise the suspicion of lymphoma. This may occur in 15 % of patients with typical Sjogren's lymphoepithelial lesions. Primary lymphoma of the major salivary glands represents 2 % of all salivary gland tumors and approximately 5 % of all extranodal lymphomas with the parotid gland affected in 80 % of the cases. Among primary non-Hodgkin's lymphomas of the salivary glands, 35 % are large B-cell lymphoma, 35 % are follicular lymphoma, and extranodal marginal lymphoma accounts for the remaining 30 %.

There is strong evidence that exposure to ionizing radiation may raise the risk of developing neoplasms, both benign and malignant, in the salivary glands. In patients with a history of head and neck irradiation, the development of a mass in the salivary gland should prompt a clinical investigation to rule out a primary neoplasm of the affected gland or the presence of metastatic disease. Metastatic masses to the parotid region may be the initial presentation of cutaneous malignancies of the scalp, forehead, and temporal region such as melanoma or squamous cell. Melanoma and squamous cell carcinoma account for about 90 % of these metastatic lesions. Head and neck Merkel's cell carcinoma can also metastasize to the parotid glands. Kidney, lungs, and breast are the most frequent nonhead and neck cancer metastasizing to the parotid glands. In contrast, 85 % of metastases to the submandibular gland originate from infraclavicular primary tumors such as breast, lungs, and kidney.

3.3.3 Imaging Studies

A number of imaging studies are available for the evaluation of salivary gland neoplasms and include ultrasonography, computed tomography, magnetic resonance imaging, and PET scan.

Ultrasonography (US) is inexpensive, easy to perform and can be completed during the initial clinical consultation in the surgeon's office. US is used to distinguish between solid and cystic masses. It is also used in the evaluation of superficial mass to distinguish extrinsic from parenchymal lesions. It can demonstrate deep-lobe extension of superficial lesions and identify cervical lymphadenopathy. Also, the use of US guidance increases the accuracy of fine-needle aspiration biopsy particularly in deep-lobe or nonpalpable tumors and complex cystic lesions.

Computed tomography (CT) and magnetic resonance imaging (MRI) are frequently used in evaluating patients with tumors of the major salivary glands. Both CT and MRI help elucidate the tumor's relationship to vital structures of the neck and parapharyngeal space, to assess cervical lymphadenopathy, and to demonstrate whether a mass is intra or extraglandular. CT is superior to MRI for detection of bone erosions in the mastoid bone and mandible. CT can also be used to guide needle biopsies of deep-seated salivary gland tumors. There are instances where tumors are not visualized on CT scans but clearly demonstrated on MRI. Contrasted MRI is more widely used and is currently the method of choice in evaluating salivary gland masses. In the assessment of parapharyngeal space masses MRI has better contrast resolution helping discriminate between a deep lobe parotid tumor and other primary tumors of the parapharyngeal space such as Schwannoma or glomus tumor. MRI is also superior for the assessment of ductal architecture and parenchymal disease.

CT and MRI provide useful information in regard to the anatomic extent of the tumors but neither provides information regarding the specific histologic diagnosis. New MRI technologies (dynamic contrast-enhanced MRI, proton MRI spectroscopy, diffusion-weighted MRI) are being developed and show encouraging results in the differentiation of benign and malignant neoplasms.

PET scans are not commonly used in the initial assessment of salivary gland masses. Salivary gland tumors have demonstrated high variability and inconsistency in the uptake of F-18 fluorodeoxyglucose (FDG). PET also cannot consistently separate benign from malignant tumors. Normal salivary gland tissue, Warthin's tumor, and pleomorphic adenomas often show metabolic uptake of FDG.

3.3.4 Fine-Needle Aspiration Biopsy

3.3.4.1 Advantages and Disadvantages

Fine-needle aspiration biopsy (FNAB) has become an important tool in the clinical investigation of salivary gland lesions, particularly in the parotid and submandibular glands. The procedure is safe, simple to perform, minimally invasive, and relatively inexpensive. The morbidity is very low with hematomas and infection being the most common complications. Material from FNABs can be easily utilized for ancillary studies such as cultures, immunophenotyping, and molecular analysis in the case of a suspected lymphoma.

Although discredited by several studies, fear of seeding malignant tumor cells in the needle tract has always being a point of contention. Some authors claim that FNAB of pleomorphic adenomas may increase the incidence of local recurrence. A large study by Engzell and colleagues has demonstrated no support for such a claim [66]. Because the vast majority of salivary gland tumors are ultimately surgically removed, critics of preoperative FNAB argue that its use does not significantly change management in most cases [67, 68]. One study, however, showed that the results of FNAB in a series of 101 patients changed the clinical approach in 35 % of cases [69].

Some authors argue that salivary gland tumors are not suitable for FNAB due to their rarity, heterogeneous morphology, and the significant cytologic overlap between benign and malignant lesions. FNAB can be quite accurate in distinguishing common benign and malignant tumors, but accuracy breaks down in the case of less common, more obscure lesions. Some tumors are characterized by a combination of morphologies; in these tumors limited sampling will not provide a complete representation of the overall morphologic pattern [70] Another limitation of FNAB is its inability to recognize an infiltrative growth pattern, an important, and definitive feature of malignancy. Conversely, FNAB can also cause histologic changes such as pseudo-capsular invasion or extensive squamous metaplasia which could be erroneously interpreted as true invasion or squamous cell carcinoma, respectively, at the time of resection. Complete tumor necrosis after FNAB, a rather rare complication, has also been described and could preclude an accurate histopathologic interpretation in a resected specimen.

Despite these potential shortcomings, review of the literature shows that, overall, FNAB is accurate and useful in the initial work-up of salivary gland tumors. Published accuracy rates have ranged from 74 to 100 % [71–82]. In the Postema et al. study of 388 salivary gland tumors, the sensitivity, specificity, and accuracy of FNAB in distinguishing benign from malignant lesions were 88, 99, and 96 %, respectively. In this study the overall accuracy rate was 96 % [83].

Preoperative FNAB can be beneficial in many circumstances. Complications are minimal when compared with core or open biopsies. Damage to the facial nerve, bleeding, and infection are rare. FNAB improves patient selection for surgery. FNAB can identify conditions such as inflammatory or reactive lymphadenopathies, benign cysts, and granulomatous processes that can mimic neoplasms clinically. The information obtained by FNAB is useful for patient counseling and guides additional preoperative work-up. A benign diagnosis on FNAB relieves the patient's anxiety and helps in the decision making process; the surgery can be postponed or the patient can be followed if clinical conditions pose a significant surgical risk [84].

In clinically suspicious cases, it is useful to obtain a diagnosis of malignancy prior to surgery. A positive result facilitates preoperative planning and expedites treatment. It mandates an open discussion about the extent of the surgery to obtain clear margins of resection, management of the neck lymph nodes, surgical scar, and the likelihood of facial nerve resection. Imaging studies, a contrasted CT scan or MRI, should be acquired. Metastatic lesions to intraparotid lymph nodes are a frequent occurrence. Melanomas and squamous cell carcinomas of the temporal and forehead areas are the most common causes. Distant metastasis from kidney, breast, and other primary sites are less commonly encountered. FNAB in these cases is of utmost importance in establishing the correct course of management.

3.3.4.2 Diagnostic Entities

Most salivary gland lesions undergoing aspiration biopsy are benign pleomorphic adenomas. Warthin's tumors and chronic sialadenitis are also common. Adenoid cystic carcinoma, mucoepidermoid carcinoma, and acinic cell carcinoma are the most common salivary gland malignancies. Interpretation of FNAB is usually performed in combination with radiologic and clinical findings along with an accurate medical history. Image guidance improves the quality of the specimen and its accuracy. Immediate on-site screening of the aspirate specimen using a Diff-Quick stain also improves the diagnostic yield. The cytologist, when present during the procedure, will examine the patient, obtain important additional history, and communicate his initial impression to the surgeon. If there are sampling issues or if ancillary tests are necessary, such as microbiologic cultures if infection is suspected or flow cytometry for predominantly lymphoid smears, additional material can be immediately obtained. Benign lesions that are most often mis-diagnosed as malignant are monomorphic adenoma, intraparotid lymph node, Warthin tumor, and granulomatous sialadenitis. Malignant lesions most often misdiagnosed as benign includes lymphoma, acinic cell carcinoma, low-grade mucoepidermoid carcinoma, and adenoid cystic carcinoma [85].

Pleomorphic adenoma Aspirates from pleomorphic adenomas classically display an admixture of stroma, epithelial cells, and myoepithelial cells (Fig. 3.8). The epithelial component can show a wide range of morphologies and be comprised of either glandular or squamous cells. The myoepithelial cells are typically

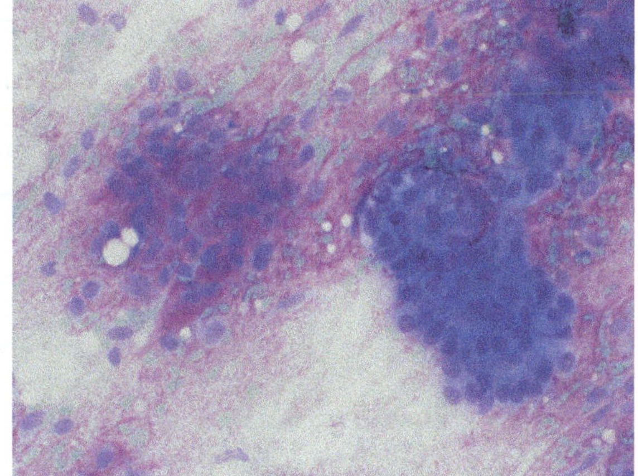

Fig. 3.8 Pleomorphic adenoma (Diff Quick 60x). A typical aspirate from a pleomorphic adenoma contains three components as seen here. (1) Magenta fibrillary stroma (2) Single myoepithelial cells dispersed throughout the stroma (*left*) (3) Epithelial cells forming clusters (*right*)

plasmacytoid (round with eccentric nuclei), but may also be spindled. Myoepithelial cells are typically intermixed with fibrillary metachromatic (pink in the Diff Quik stain) stroma which is the diagnostic hallmark of this tumor.

The main differential diagnostic consideration is adenoid cystic carcinoma which also shows a combination of metachromatic stroma, myoepithelial cells, and epithelium. The character of the stroma as well as its relationship to the myoepithelial cells generally allows the accurate morphologic distinction of these two entities. Knowledge of the clinical and radiographic findings is also useful in this setting.

Chronic sialadenitis Aspirates from chronic sialadenitis generally contain a lymphoid component, ductal epithelium, and fragments of dense fibrosis. The lack of acinar cells (generally the most common cellular element in normal salivary gland) as well as the prominence of the ductal cells may prompt consideration of a neoplasm, particularly mucoepidermoid carcinoma. If the lymphoid component is florid and predominates, it may be difficult to distinguish chronic sialadenitis from lymphoma or an intraparotid lymph node. Flow cytometry may be useful for diagnosis or exclusion of the former.

Warthin's tumor Papillary cystadenoma lymphomatosum (Warthin's tumor) occurs almost exclusively in the parotid glands. This tumor has a striking male predominance and is frequently multiple and cystic. Warthin's tumors are characterized by three distinct components: (1) uniform flat sheets of onococytes with abundant granular cytoplasm, round nuclei, even chromatin, and prominent nucleoli, (2) a lymphoid component, (3) cyst contents comprised of granular debris and macrophages (Fig. 3.9). When all three components are present, the diagnosis is generally straightforward. If only the epithelial component is seen, the differential diagnosis will include a spectrum of oncocytic neoplasms. When only the lymphoid portion is sampled, a lymphoma may be considered. If only the cystic component is present in the biopsy, it is impossible to definitively exclude a low-grade mucoepidermoid carcinoma or other cystic neoplasm. Warthin's tumor can

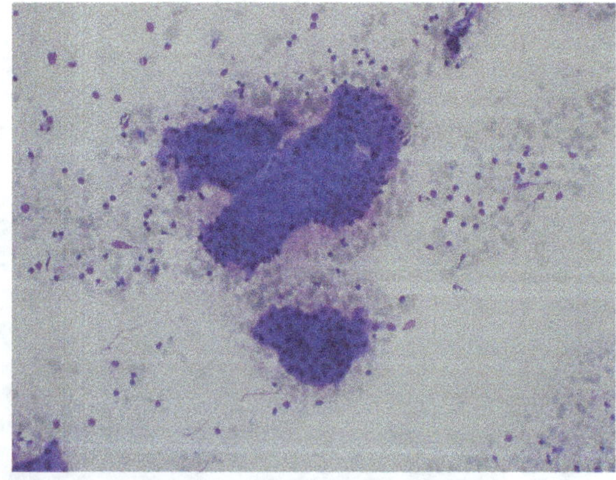

Fig. 3.9 Warthin tumor (Diff Quick 40x). The three typical components of a Warthin tumor are seen here: (1) Flat sheets of uniform cells with abundant granular cytoplasm (2) Lymphocytes (3) Granular debris (cyst contents)

Fig. 3.10 Adenoid cystic carcinoma (Diff Quick 40x). The most notable feature is well defined magenta stroma forming rounded structures ("gumballs"). The cells are uniform and contain relatively small bland nuclei and little cytoplasm. In contrast to pleomorphic adenoma, a range of cell types is typically not seen and cells are not present within the stroma

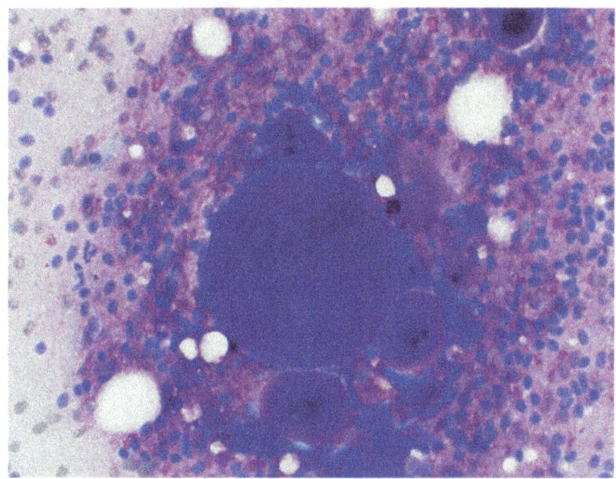

undergo infarction causing atypical squamous metaplasia and necrosis which should be distinguished from squamous cell carcinoma.

Adenoid cystic carcinoma Adenoid cystic carcinoma is the second most common malignant tumor of the salivary glands and the most common malignant tumor of the minor salivary glands. It is generally a low-grade tumor with indolent behavior although more virulent high grade and dedifferentiated forms exist. Perineural spread is particularly common. Adenoid cystic carcinoma is generally comprised of basaloid (bland uniform cells high nuclear:cytoplasmic ratios) epithelial and myoepithelial cells. Round, well-demarcated globules of metachromatic (pink) stroma are the classic diagnostic finding in these tumors and generally allow distinction from a pleomorphic adenoma (Fig. 3.10). In some cases, areas of a pleomorphic adenoma may almost precisely mimic an adenoid cystic carcinoma resulting in misdiagnosis in a small biopsy or aspirate.

Mucoepidermoid carcinoma Although relatively common among malignant salivary gland tumors, mucoepidermoid carcinoma is difficult to accurately diagnose. Aspirates from mucoepidermoid carcinomas contain a combination of cell types including epidermoid (nonkeratinizing squamous cells), intermediate, and mucin producing cells (Fig. 3.11). Low-grade mucoepidermoid carcinomas are more indolent with predominantly mucin producing cells and a cystic component. In the absence of a sampled epithelial component, it is impossible to distinguish low-grade mucoepidermoid carcinoma from a mucocele. High-grade mucoepidermoid carcinoma is generally solid and composed of more squamoid cells with only a paucity of glandular elements. In aspirates, high-grade mucoepidermoid carcinoma is very difficult to distinguish from other high-grade neoplasms particularly ductal carcinoma, carcinoma ex pleomorphic adenoma, and metastatic squamous cell carcinoma.

Acinic cell carcinoma Acinic cell carcinoma represents 2–5 % of all parotid neoplasms. It is bilateral in 3 % of the cases. It is generally classified as a low-grade carcinoma. The dedifferentiated form can be very aggressive. Aspirates of

Fig. 3.11 Mucoepidermoid carcinoma (Diff Quik 40x). A cluster of vacuolated mucin producing cells (*right*) is seen juxtaposed to a group of squamoid/intermediate cells with more dense cytoplasm (*left*). The background contains numerous inflammatory cells and thin blue mucin

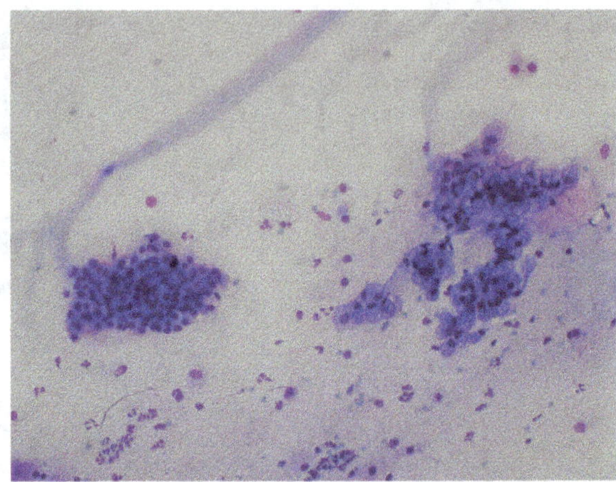

Fig. 3.12 Acinic cell carcinoma (Diff Quik 60x). Irregular clusters of cells are present amidst a background of naked, stripped nuclei. The cells contain abundant granular and vacuolated cytoplasm. The nuclei are oriented along one edge of the cell and are large with prominent nucleoli

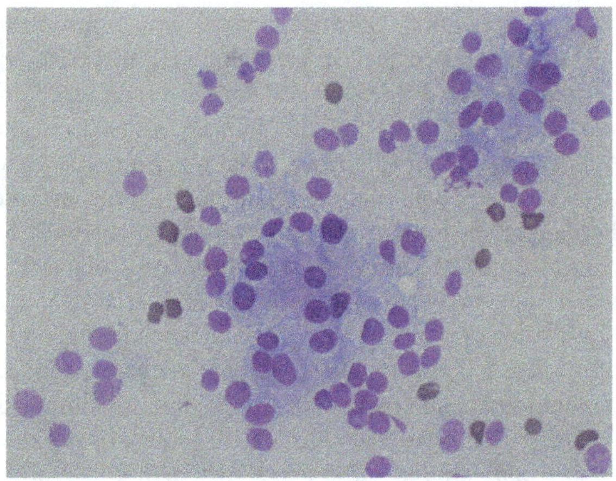

acinic cell carcinoma are typically cellular with numerous stripped ("naked") nuclei and haphazard three-dimensional clusters of acinic cells (Fig. 3.12). The cells typically have abundant delicate, coarsely granular cytoplasm and eccentric nuclei containing prominent nucleoli. Cytoplasmic vacuolization may be prominent. In contrast to normal salivary gland parenchyma, the acinic cells in acinic cell carcinoma display more atypia and lack an organized lobulated configuration. Misinterpretation of an aspirate of normal salivary gland parenchyma is a potential source of false positives.

Carcinoma ex-pleomorphic adenoma This rare entity develops in association with recurrent pleomorphic adenomas. It is usually a high-grade carcinoma and represents the malignant transformation of the epithelial component within a preexisting pleomorphic adenoma. Accurate diagnosis in an FNA specimen is difficult without recognition of the prior pleomorphic adenoma. These tumors are extremely aggressive with a 5-year survival rate of 0 % [86].

3.3.5 *Conclusions*

There is widespread acceptance of the use of fine-needle aspiration biopsy in the work-up of salivary gland tumors. The procedure is very reliable, safe, and inexpensive. This modality is very reliable in distinguishing benign from malignant tumors, and neoplastic from nonneoplastic lesions. However, because of their rarity and varied histology, subclassification of more obscure salivary gland neoplasms remains difficult. Nevertheless, FNAB is a powerful and cost-effective initial approach in the management of salivary gland tumors.

References

1. Lubina A, Cohen O, Barchana M et al (2006) Time trends of incidence rates of thyroid cancer in Israel: what might explain the sharp increase. Thyroid 16:1033–1040
2. Colonna M, Grosclaude P, Remontet L et al (2002) Incidence of thyroid cancer in adults recorded by French cancer registries (1978–1997). Eur J Cancer 38:1762–1768
3. Leenhardt L, Grosclaude P, Cherie-Challine L (2004) Increased incidence of thyroid carcinoma in france: a true epidemic or thyroid nodule management effects? Report from the French Thyroid Cancer Committee. Thyroid 14:1056–1060
4. Davies L, Welch HG, Davies L, Welch HG (2006) Increasing incidence of thyroid cancer in the United States, 1973–2002.[see comment]. JAMA 295:2164–2167
5. Liu S, Semenciw R, Ugnat AM, Mao Y (2001) Increasing thyroid cancer incidence in Canada, 1970–1996: time trends and age-period-cohort effects. Br J Cancer 85:1335–1339
6. Gharib H, Papini E, Gharib H, Papini E () Thyroid nodules: clinical importance, assessment, and treatment. Endocrinol Metab Clin N Am 36:707–735
7. Tunbridge WM, Evered DC, Hall R et al (1977) The spectrum of thyroid disease in a community: the Whickham survey. Clin Endocrinol 7:481–493
8. Brander A, Viikinkoski P, Nickels J, Kivisaari L (1991) Thyroid gland: US screening in a random adult population. Radiology 181:683–687
9. Tan GH, Gharib H (1997) Thyroid incidentalomas: management approaches to nonpalpable nodules discovered incidentally on thyroid imaging. Ann Intern Med 126:226–231
10. Alexander EK (2008) Approach to the patient with a cytologically indeterminate thyroid nodule. J Clin Endocrinol Metab 93:4175–4182
11. Cooper DS, Doherty GM, Haugen BR et al (2006) Management guidelines for patients with thyroid nodules and differentiated thyroid cancer.[see comment]. Thyroid 16:109–142
12. Castro MR, Gharib H, Castro MR, Gharib H (2003) Thyroid fine-needle aspiration biopsy: progress, practice, and pitfalls. Endocrine Practice 9:128–136
13. Hegedus L, Hegedus L (2004) Clinical practice. The thyroid nodule. N Engl J Med 351:1764–1771
14. Yang J, Schnadig V, Logrono R et al (2007) Fine-needle aspiration of thyroid nodules: a study of 4703 patients with histologic and clinical correlations. Cancer 111:306–315
15. Gharib H, Papini E, Valcavi R et al (2006) American Association of Clinical Endocrinologists and Associazione Medici Endocrinologi medical guidelines for clinical practice for the diagnosis and management of thyroid nodules.[see comment][erratum appears in Endocr Pract. 2008 Sep, 14(6), pp. 802–3 Note: multiple author names added]. Endocrine Pract 12:63–102

16. Sidawy MK, Del Vecchio DM, Knoll SM (1997) Fine-needle aspiration of thyroid nodules: correlation between cytology and histology and evaluation of discrepant cases. Cancer 81:253–259
17. Garcia-Mayor RV (1997) Perez Mendez LF, Paramo C, et al. Fine-needle aspiration biopsy of thyroid nodules: impact on clinical practice. J Endocrinol Invest 20:482–487
18. Seiberling KA, Dutra JC, Gunn J, Seiberling KA, Dutra JC, Gunn J (2008) Ultrasound-guided fine needle aspiration biopsy of thyroid nodules performed in the office. Laryngoscope 118:228–231
19. Hales MS, Hsu FS (1990) Needle tract implantation of papillary carcinoma of the thyroid following aspiration biopsy. Acta Cytol 34:801–804
20. Belfiore A, La Rosa GL (2001) Fine-needle aspiration biopsy of the thyroid. Endocrinol Metab Clin North Am 30:361–400
21. Gharib H, Goellner JR (1993) Fine-needle aspiration biopsy of the thyroid: an appraisal.[see comment]. Ann Intern Med 118:282–289
22. Yassa L, Cibas ES, Benson CB et al (2007) Long-term assessment of a multidisciplinary approach to thyroid nodule diagnostic evaluation. Cancer 111:508–516
23. Baloch ZW, LiVolsi VA, Asa SL et al (2008) Diagnostic terminology and morphologic criteria for cytologic diagnosis of thyroid lesions: a synopsis of the National Cancer Institute Thyroid Fine-Needle Aspiration State of the Science Conference. Diagn Cytopathol 36:425–437
24. Wang HH (2006) Reporting thyroid fine-needle aspiration: literature review and a proposal. Diagn Cytopathol 34:67–76
25. Grant CS, Hay ID, Gough IR, McCarthy PM, Goellner JR (1989) Long-term follow-up of patients with benign thyroid fine-needle aspiration cytologic diagnoses. Surgery 106:980–985; discussion 5–6
26. Alexander EK, Heering JP, Benson CB et al (2002) Assessment of nondiagnostic ultrasound-guided fine needle aspirations of thyroid nodules. J Clin Endocrinol Metab 87:4924–4927
27. de los Santos ET, Keyhani-Rofagha S, Cunningham JJ, Mazzaferri EL (1990) Cystic thyroid nodules. The dilemma of malignant lesions.[see comment]. Archives of Internal Medicine 150:1422–7
28. Layfield LJ, Cibas ES, Gharib H, Mandel SJ (2009) Thyroid aspiration cytology: current status. CA Cancer J Clin 59:99–110
29. Izquierdo R, Arekat MR, Knudson PE et al (2006) Comparison of palpation-guided versus ultrasound-guided fine-needle aspiration biopsies of thyroid nodules in an outpatient endocrinology practice. Endo Pract 12:609–614
30. Layfield LJ, Abrams J, Cochand-Priollet B et al (2008) Post-thyroid FNA testing and treatment options: a synopsis of the National Cancer Institute Thyroid Fine Needle Aspiration State of the Science Conference. Diagn Cytopathol 36:442–448
31. MacDonald L, Yazdi HM (1996) Nondiagnostic fine needle aspiration biopsy of the thyroid gland: a diagnostic dilemma. Acta Cytol 40:423–428
32. Hall TL, Layfield LJ, Philippe A, Rosenthal DL (1989) Sources of diagnostic error in fine needle aspiration of the thyroid. Cancer 63:718–725
33. Amrikachi M, Ramzy I, Rubenfeld S, Wheeler TM (2001) Accuracy of fine-needle aspiration of thyroid. Arch Pathol Lab Med 125:484–488
34. Danese D, Sciacchitano S, Farsetti A, Andreoli M, Pontecorvi A (1998) Diagnostic accuracy of conventional versus sonography-guided fine-needle aspiration biopsy of thyroid nodules. Thyroid 8:15–21
35. Erdogan MF, Kamel N, Aras D, Akdogan A, Baskal N, Erdogan G (1998) Value of re-aspirations in benign nodular thyroid disease. Thyroid 8:1087–1090
36. Chehade JM, Silverberg AB, Kim J, Case C, Mooradian AD (2001) Role of repeated fine-needle aspiration of thyroid nodules with benign cytologic feature [see comment]. Endocr Pract 7:237–243
37. Mittendorf EA, McHenry CR. Follow-up evaluation and clinical course of patients with benign nodular thyroid disease. American Surgeon 1999;65:653–7; discussion 7–8

38. Hermus AR, Huysmans DA (1998) Treatment of benign nodular thyroid disease. N Engl J Med 338:1438–1447
39. Kim MI, Alexander EK (2012) Diagnostic use of molecular markers in the evaluation of thyroid nodules. Endocr Pract18(5):796–802
40. Layfield LJ, Skripenova S, Bentz J, Smock C (2008) Cytologic fine needle aspiration findings by vegetant intravascular hemangioendothelioma. Acta Cytol 52:273–275
41. Hundahl SA (1998) Perspective: National Cancer Institute summary report about estimated exposures and thyroid doses received from iodine 131 in fallout after Nevada atmospheric nuclear bomb tests. CA Cancer J Clinicians 48:285–298
42. Hayat MJ, Howlader N, Reichman ME et al (2007) Cancer statistics, trends, and multiple primary cancer analyses from the Surveillance, Epidemiology, and End Results (SEER) Program. Oncologist 12:20–37
43. Rivera M, Ricarte-Filho J, Knauf J, Shaha A, Tuttle M, Fagin JA, Ghossein RA (2010) Molecular genotyping of papillary thyroid carcinoma follicular variant according to its histological subtypes (encapsulated vs infiltrative) reveals distinct BRAF and RAS mutation patterns. Mod Pathol 23:1191–1200
44. Tuttle RM (2008) Risk-adapted management of thyroid cancer. Endocr Pract 14:764–774
45. Baloch ZW, Buretta JE, Gupta PK et al (2008) Thyroglobulin measurement in fine-needle aspiration biopsy specimens of lymph nodes in the diagnosis of recurrent thyroid carcinoma. Cytojournal 5:1
46. Machens A, Dralle H (2007) Genotype-phenotype based surgical concept of hereditary medullary thyroid carcinoma. World J Surg 31:957–968
47. Raue F (1998) German medullary thyroid carcinoma/multiple endocrine neoplasia registry. German MTC/MEN study group. medullary thyroid carcinoma/multiple endocrine neoplasia type 2. Langenbecks Arch Surg 383:334–336
48. Redding AH, Levine SN, Fowler MR (2000) Normal preoperative calcitonin levels do not always exclude medullary thyroid carcinoma in patients with large palpable thyroid masses. Thyroid 10:919–922
49. Gilliland FD, Hunt WC, Morris DM, Key CR (1997) Prognostic factors for thyroid carcinoma. A population-based study of 15,698 cases from the Surveillance, Epidemiology and End Results (SEER) program 1973–1991. Cancer 79:564–573
50. Hundahl SA, Fleming ID, Fremgen AM, Menck HR (1998) A National Cancer Data Base report on 53,856 cases of thyroid carcinoma treated in the U.S., 1985–1995 [see commetns]. Cancer 83:2638–2648
51. Dionigi G, Tanda ML, Piantanida E (2008) Medullary thyroid carcinoma: surgical treatment advances. Curr Opin Otolaryngol Head Neck Surg 16:158–162
52. Brandi ML, Gagel RF, Angeli A et al (2001) Guidelines for diagnosis and therapy of MEN type 1 and type 2. J Clin Endocrinol Metab 86:5658–5671
53. Al-Rawi M, Wheeler MH (2006) Medullary thyroid carcinoma–update and present management controversies. Ann R Coll Surg Engl 88:433–438
54. Machens A, Schneyer U, Holzhausen HJ, Dralle H (2005) Prospects of remission in medullary thyroid carcinoma according to basal calcitonin level. J Clin Endocrinol Metab 90:2029–2034
55. Sipos J, Mazzaferri E (2008) Medullary Thyroid Carcinoma, Anaplastic Thyroid Carcinoma, and Thyroid Lymphoma. In: Cooper DS (ed.) Medical management of thyroid disease. 2nd ed. New York: Informa Healthcare, p. 448
56. Venkatesh YS, Ordonez NG, Schultz PN, Hickey RC, Goepfert H, Samaan NA (1990) Anaplastic carcinoma of the thyroid. A clinicopathologic study of 121 cases. Cancer 66:321–330
57. Demeter JG, De Jong SA, Lawrence AM, Paloyan E (1991) Anaplastic thyroid carcinoma: risk factors and outcome. Surgery 110:956–961; discussion 61–3
58. Chiacchio S, Lorenzoni A, Boni G, Rubello D, Elisei R, Mariani G (2008) Anaplastic thyroid cancer: prevalence, diagnosis and treatment. Minerva Endocrinol 33:341–357

59. Carcangiu ML, Steeper T, Zampi G, Rosai J (1985) Anaplastic thyroid carcinoma. A study of 70 cases. Am J Clin Pathol 83:135–158
60. Nel CJ, van Heerden JA, Goellner JR et al (1985) Anaplastic carcinoma of the thyroid: a clinicopathologic study of 82 cases. Mayo Clin Proc 60:51–58
61. Tennvall J, Lundell G, Wahlberg P et al (2002) Anaplastic thyroid carcinoma: three protocols combining doxorubicin, hyperfractionated radiotherapy and surgery. Br J Cancer 86:1848–1853
62. Kebebew E, Greenspan FS, Clark OH et al (2005) Anaplastic thyroid carcinoma. Treatment outcome and prognostic factors. Cancer 103:1330–1335
63. Davey DD, Glant MD, Berger EK (1986) Parathyroid cytopathology. Diagn Cytopathol 2:76–80
64. Abati A, Skarulis MC, Shawker T, Solomon D (1995) Ultrasound-guided fine-needle aspiration of parathyroid lesions: a morphological and immunocytochemical approach. Hum Pathol 26:338–343
65. Pacini F, Antonelli A, Lari R, Gasperini L, Baschieri L, Pinchera A (1985) Unsuspected parathyroid cysts diagnosed by measurement of thyroglobulin and parathyroid hormone concentrations in fluid aspirates. Ann Intern Med 102:793–794
66. Engzell U, Esposti PL, Rubio C, Sigurdson A, Zajicek J (1971) Investigation on tumour spread in connection with aspiration biopsy. Acta Radiol Ther Phys Biol 10:385–398
67. Que Hee CG, Perry CF (2001) Fine-needle aspiration cytology of parotid tumours: is it useful? ANZ J Surg 71:345–348
68. Olsen KD (1987) The parotid lump–don't biopsy it! An approach to avoiding misadventure. Postgrad Med 81:225–229, 32–34
69. Heller KS, Dubner S, Chess Q, Attie JN (1992) Value of fine needle aspiration biopsy of salivary gland masses in clinical decision-making. Am J Surg 164:667–670
70. Westra WH (1999) The surgical pathology of salivary gland neoplasms. Otolaryngol Clin North Am 32:919–943
71. Zhang S, Bao R, Bagby J et al (2009) Fine needle aspiration of salivary glands: 5-year experience from a single academic center. Acta Cytol 53:375–382
72. Daneshbod Y, Daneshbod K, Khademi B, Daneshbod Y, Daneshbod K, Khademi B (2009) Diagnostic difficulties in the interpretation of fine needle aspirate samples in salivary lesions: diagnostic pitfalls revisited. Acta Cytol 53:53–70
73. Goncalves AJ, Menezes MB, Kavabata NK et al (2007) Fine needle aspiration in salivary gland tumors: specificity and sensitivity. Rev Assoc Med Bras 53:267–271
74. Elagoz S, Gulluoglu M, Yilmazbayhan D, Ozer H, Arslan I (2007) The value of fine-needle aspiration cytology in salivary gland lesions, 1994–2004. J Otorhinolaryngol Relat Spec 69:51–56
75. Tan LG, Khoo ML, Tan LGL, Khoo MLC (2006) Accuracy of fine needle aspiration cytology and frozen section histopathology for lesions of the major salivary glands. Ann Acad Med Singapore 35:242–248
76. Seethala RR, LiVolsi VA, Baloch ZW, Seethala RR, LiVolsi VA, Baloch ZW (2005) Relative accuracy of fine-needle aspiration and frozen section in the diagnosis of lesions of the parotid gland. Head Neck 27:217–223
77. Mukunyadzi P, Mukunyadzi P (2002) Review of fine-needle aspiration cytology of salivary gland neoplasms, with emphasis on differential diagnosis. Am J Clin Pathol 118(Suppl):S100–S115
78. Stewart CJ, MacKenzie K, McGarry GW, Mowat A (2000) Fine-needle aspiration cytology of salivary gland: a review of 341 cases. Diagn Cytopathol 22:139–146
79. Zbaren P, Nuyens M, Loosli H et al (2004) Diagnostic accuracy of fine-needle aspiration cytology and frozen section in primary parotid carcinoma. Cancer 100:1876–1883
80. Schindler S, Nayar R, Dutra J, Bedrossian CW (2001) Diagnostic challenges in aspiration cytology of the salivary glands. Semin Diagn Pathol 18:124–146

81. Cajulis RS, Gokaslan ST, Yu GH, Frias-Hidvegi D (1997) Fine needle aspiration biopsy of the salivary glands. A five-year experience with emphasis on diagnostic pitfalls. Acta Cytol 41:1412–1420
82. Orell SR (1995) Diagnostic difficulties in the interpretation of fine needle aspirates of salivary gland lesions: the problem revisited.[see comment]. Cytopathology 6:285–300
83. Postema RJ, van Velthuysen ML, van den Brekel MW et al (2004) Accuracy of fine-needle aspiration cytology of salivary gland lesions in the netherlands cancer institute. Head Neck 26:418–424
84. Hughes JH, Volk EE, Wilbur DC et al (2005) Pitfalls in salivary gland fine-needle aspiration cytology: lessons from the College of American Pathologists Interlaboratory Comparison Program in Nongynecologic Cytology.[see comment]. Arch Pathol Lab Med 129:26–31
85. Layfield LJ, Tan P, Glasgow BJ (1987) Fine-needle aspiration of salivary gland lesions. Comparison with frozen sections and histologic findings. Arch Pathol Lab Med 111:346–353
86. Orell SR, Nettle WJ (1988) Fine needle aspiration biopsy of salivary gland tumours. Problems and pitfalls. Pathology 20:332–337

Chapter 4
Cytology of the Lung

Sara Zydowicz, Anjana Yeldandi and Kirtee Raparia

4.1 Introduction

Use of cytologic methods in the diagnosis of pulmonary malignancies dates back to the mid-1800s when sputum was examined for exfoliated neoplastic cells. Hamplen recorded the first series in the early 1900s in which 13–25 patients were effectively diagnosed with pulmonary malignancies via examination of sputum [1]. With the advent of fine needle aspiration (FNA) as a less invasive alternative to open or transbronchial biopsy, there was a renewed interest in pulmonary cytology in the 1970s and 1980s. The techniques were further refined by advances in imaging, allowing for detection and localization of smaller lesions as well mechanical improvements in bronchoscopes themselves resulting in improved sample yield and reduced numbers of unsatisfactory specimens. With increasing demand for less invasive procedures and more precise sub classification of neoplasms for molecular-targeted therapy, cytologic methods are increasingly employed for both diagnosis and prognosis [2].

S. Zydowicz
Office of the Medical Examiner, District 9, 2350 E. Michigan St, Orlando, FL 32806, USA

A. Yeldandi
Department of Surgical Pathology, Northwestern Memorial Hospital, 251 E. Huron St., Feinberg Pavilion 7-342, Chicago, IL 60611, USA
e-mail: a-yeldandi@northwestern.edu

K. Raparia (✉)
Department of Pathology, Northwestern Memorial Hospital, 250 East Huron Street Feinberg 7-335, Chicago, IL 60611, USA
e-mail: kraparia@northwestern.edu

R. Nayar (ed.), *Cytopathology in Oncology*,
Cancer Treatment and Research 160, DOI: 10.1007/978-3-642-38850-7_4,
© Springer-Verlag Berlin Heidelberg 2014

Lung Cytology

4.2 Reporting/Diagnostic Categories

There is variability in reporting terminology by the individual pathologist as well as institution. Commonly used words and phrases to convey the diagnostic impression in the cytology report are described below.

4.2.1 Negative for Malignancy

Benign cellular components are present in the specimen including bronchial epithelial cells, reserve cells, goblet cells and any other indigenous cells expected depending on the route of procurement, i.e., squamous cells seen as oral contamination during bronchoscopy, or mesothelial cells from transthoracic needle biopsy.

4.2.2 Atypical

The atypical category encompasses cellular changes favoring a reactive process in which there is no evidence of an underlying lesion or when the cellular material is degenerated to the point where reliable morphologic features are distorted. In such cases, neoplasia cannot be excluded with certainty.

4.2.3 Suspicious for Malignancy

The suspicious category is employed when a rare highly atypical cells are seen yet are too few or qualitative suboptimal for a definitive diagnosis.

4.2.4 Positive for Malignancy

The positive for malignancy category is used when there is presence of cells in sufficient quantities fulfilling morphologic criteria, which establish an undisputable diagnosis of malignancy.

4.3 Approaches to Respiratory Cytology

There are five basic cytologic modalities available to assess pulmonary lesions ranging from non-invasive to invasive techniques requiring sedation: sputum analysis, bronchial washings, brushings and bronchoalveolar lavage (BAL) are minimally invasive procedures performed during bronchoscopy. FNA can be performed percutaneously for peripheral lesions; although transbronchial FNA, especially with ultrasound guidance, is increasingly being utilized for both diagnostic and staging purposes. The choice of procedure depends on a number of factors including the nature of the disease process (i.e., localized or diffuse), anatomic location, status of the patient, and comfort level and/or familiarity of the physician with a particular procedure.

Exfoliative cytology encompasses commonly used techniques such as bronchial aspirations, washings, and BAL to sample central lung lesions or in the assessment of pneumonic processes where infectious etiology is suspected. The advent of flexible bronchoscopy has significantly improved sampling and virtually any part of the respiratory tract is amenable to this technique. Complications from bronchoscopy are rare and include bronchospams, laryngospasm, seizure, hypoxia, cardiac conduction disturbances, and sepsis [3, 4].

4.3.1 Bronchial Aspirations and Washings

Direct aspiration of bronchial secretions can be obtained via flexible bronchoscopy. More commonly, a small volume (up to 10 mL) of sterile saline is instilled directly into the airways via a flexible bronchoscope. The fluid is then aspirated and the 'washing' is placed directly into a ThinPrep® or sterile vial. A cytospin of the aspirated fluid is prepared by centrifuging a fixed volume of the washing to concentrate the cells. Centrifugation must not be too vigorous in order to preserve cellular structure. A monolayer of cells is placed on a glass slide and subsequently stained with the Papanicolaou stain. This method yields variable amounts of cells depending on the cellular concentration of the specimen. Alternatively, the fluid can be centrifuged, treated with a coagulant and processed as if it were a solid tissue specimen, offering the advantage of material amenable to ancillary testing.

4.3.2 Bronchial Brushings

During bronchoscopy, a brush can be introduced through the flexible bronchoscope, swiped over the respiratory mucosa and directly smeared onto slides or the brush can be placed in Cytolyt® solution and a cytospin (as described above) can be prepared. This method allows for sampling of a larger surface area and the mechanical force of the brush 'coaxes' the most superficial cells away from the underlying mucosa. Ideally, brushings should be done prior to transbronchial biopsies in order to avoid the field becoming bloody, which will compromise the quality of the brushing.

4.3.3 Bronchoalveolar Lavage

Similar to bronchial aspirations and washings, sterile fluid is introduced into the airways and then aspirated. The intention in a BAL is to sample the most distal airways; therefore the bronchoscope is advanced as far as possible. Sterile saline is then injected and aspirated. There will be representative cells from the larger airways as well as the more distal alveolar spaces. This method is especially useful for suspected infectious processes and material from the BAL can be sent directly to the microbiology laboratory. "Reticulo-nodular" or infiltrative lung disease that is diagnosed on BAL includes pneumocystis, alveolar proteinosis, intra-alveolar hemorrhage, pneumonia, and adenocarcinoma with a lepidic growth pattern.

4.3.4 Sputum

Sputum collection was the first cytologic method employed in the diagnosis of pulmonary neoplasms, is relatively easy to obtain and well tolerated by patients. This method has fallen out of favor for a number of reasons, most notably a low sensitivity unless multiple consecutive specimens are collected and an overall low specificity for tumor classification [5]. Additionally, sputum historically has had the highest number of unsatisfactory specimens usually related to low cellularity, oral contamination and inability to collect a "true" sputum sample containing alveolar macrophages versus saliva.

4.3.5 Transbronchial FNA

Performed via flexible bronchoscope, transbronchial FNA is useful for centrally located lesions, particularly those lying in the submucosa. This technique can be used in conjunction with exfoliative cytology (BAL, brushing, etc.) to increase the diagnostic yield. Typically, the exfoliated samples are collected first to avoid contamination by blood or other obscuring elements. Aspirated material is expelled onto a glass slide then a second glass slide is placed on top of the material and gently 'dragged' along, dispersing the specimen on both slides. One slide is immediately placed into alcohol for staining with the Papanicolaou stain while the other slide is air dried and stained with the Diff Quik stain for immediate assessment. It is advantageous to have on-site assessment by the cytopathology staff to ensure adequate lesional material is collected [6].

Transbronchial ultrasound guided (EBUS), FNA is now commonly performed in most large centers. EBUS allows staging of non-small cell lung cancer, diagnostic evaluation of endobronchial lesions, peripheral pulmonary nodules, mediastinal abnormalities (e.g., lymphadenopathy), as well as endobronchial therapy. (6) For the pathologist, contamination by reactive bronchial epithelium can be a pitfall. It is also important to mention if lymphoid cells are present or not, if the target is a lymph node, since this is important for adequacy of the sample.

4.3.6 Transthoracic FNA

Transthoracic biopsy is preferred for peripherally located, discrete mass lesions which would otherwise not be attainable via transbronchial collection. Lesions are sampled under contrast tomography (CT), fluoroscopic or ultrasound guidance. On-site evaluation of collected material by cytopathology staff improves the diagnostic yield of tissue as well as prevents unnecessary needle passes. The complication rate is low and includes pneumothorax (most common), in which at least 5 % of patients will require a chest tube [3, 7]. Additional complications include hemorrhage and hematoma. Tumor seeding via needle tract is exceedingly rare; indeed only a few case report studies are available in the literature. Relative contraindications to transthoracic biopsy include pulmonary hypertension, bleeding diathesis, and emphysematous bullae.

4.4 Diagnostic Accuracy of Exfoliative Cytology and FNA

The diagnostic accuracy of exfoliative cytology is influenced by many factors including location of the lesion (peripheral lesions are difficult to detect), tumor type, operator experience and status of the patient to name a few. In general, bronchial brushings have the highest diagnostic yield of the exfoliative modalities with sensitivities ranging from 35 to 70 % with an overall specificity of 80 %, comparable to transbronchial biopsy [4, 8, 9].

Compared to exfoliative cytology, FNA biopsy is superior in accurate diagnosis of pulmonary neoplasms with an overall sensitivity ranging from 75 to 95 % and specificity from 95 to 100 %. False negative results occur in about 0.8 % of specimens and most times are due to sampling errors such as fibrous or necrotic tissue surrounding the neoplasm or simply a geographic miss. The false positive rate is reported to be near 8 % and in most cases is attributed to reactive cellular changes mimicking carcinoma [4, 8, 10]. Fewer complications, diagnostic accuracy and the cost of FNA biopsies make it an appealing diagnostic tool.

4.5 Cytology

4.5.1 Normal Respiratory Components

Knowledge of method of specimen collection and preparation is imperative in respiratory cytology as different cell types are represented in different portions of the respiratory tract. The upper respiratory tract defined as nasal, oral, and large conducting airways is comprised of predominantly ciliated columnar cells and squamous cells. The presence of squamous cells often represents oral contamination of a specimen. Furthermore, squamous cells from the oral cavity may have atypical features which can be misinterpreted as dysplasia or carcinoma [11]. Lower respiratory constituents from the trachea and bronchi include ciliated columnar cells, goblet cells, reserve cells (also called basal cells), and neuroendocrine cells (Kulchitsky cells). Collections from the terminal bronchioles will yield flat, thin type I pneumocytes and full, round type II pneumocytes with characteristic vacuolated cytoplasm. Alveolar macrophages are common in lower respiratory samples and are variable in their morphology due to phagocytosed material ('dust' pigment or hemosiderin), usually with one or two nuclei and abundant foamy cytoplasm.

In addition to the normal cellular elements, various non-cellular components produced or inhaled and ambient contaminants are commonly encountered. Charcot-Leyden crystals are associated with allergic disorders such as asthma and are the by-product of degenerating eosinophils. The crystals are orange-pink and rhomboid-shaped. Curshmann's spirals are helical structures composed of inspissated mucous and are non-specific. Ferruginous bodies are a significant finding in patients with a history of asbestos exposure, although they are occasionally seen in individuals without documented exposure. Ferroproteins precipitate on a mineral fiber to give rise to the characteristic dumbbell shaped ferruginous bodies [12]. Specimens may become contaminated with vegetable matter (endogenous to the host) and various pollens and molds from the environment.

4.5.2 Infections

4.5.2.1 Bacteria

Exfoliative cytology is not useful for the identification of specific bacteria. Definitive microbial identification should be carried out by the microbiology laboratory.

4.5.2.2 Fungi

Detection of fungal organisms can be readily appreciated in both exfoliative and aspirated cytologic specimens and are especially useful in evaluation of the immunocompromised patient. Concurrent collection of material for microbiologic studies is recommended when clinical suspicion for an infectious process is high. Identification of fungal organisms on cytologic preparations is often of great clinical value in sick patients, since they are turned around within 1 or 2 days whereas cultures can take days to weeks to grow. Of note, the inflammatory cellular response, and therefore the cellular milieu, can be altered and/or decreased in the immunocompromised patient. The most commonly encountered fungi will be addressed in this chapter.

Infection with members of *Aspergillus* species is commonly encountered and can present as a vast array of clinical manifestations, each with corresponding cytologic change. The diffuse pneumonic presentation of bronchopulmonary aspergillosis is best sampled via exfoliative methods and is recognized in washings and/or BAL by fungal organisms (usually), mucus plugs, eosinophils and occasionally Charcot-Leyden crystals. In the setting of invasive pulmonary aspergillosis and aspergilloma (fungus ball), a discrete mass or enlarged lymph node is amenable to FNA. FNA smears show fungal hyphae, some of which undergo sporulation, seen amid a 'grungy' background due to the hemorrhagic necrosis inflicted by the angioinvasive nature of the fungus. Additionally the lining of the mycetomal cavity may undergo squamous metaplasia, mimicking squamous cell carcinoma. The *Aspergillus* species are recognized by the presence of true septate hyphae of uniform width (5–10 µm) and dichotomous branching at 45° angle. (Fig. 4.1) Rarely, the conidiophores, reminiscent of a hand-held fan, may be seen, typically in a cavitary lesion. The two most common Aspergillus species, *A. fumigatus* and *A. niger*, cannot be distinguished by morphology alone and require culture for definitive speciation. Importantly, morphologic features are used to distinguish *Aspergillus* from the zygomycetes (*Mucor, Rhizopus*), which lack true hyphae and have irregular, broad, ribbon-like appearance with 90° angle branching [3, 4].

The dimorphic fungus *Blastomyces dermatidis* a mid-to-large size yeast (ranging from 8 to 20 µm) and is the etiologic agent responsible for the varied presentation of blastomycoses. While pulmonary involvement is most commonly

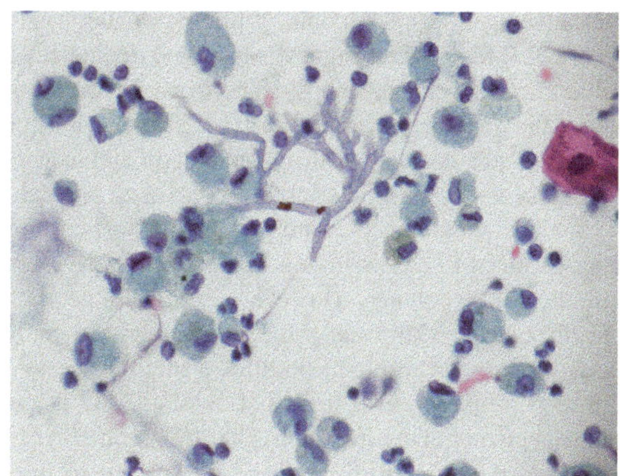

Fig. 4.1 BAL, 60X, Papaniculaou stain. Fungus morphologically consistent with *Aspergillus*. True septate hyphae with branching at 45°. Alveolar macrophages, inflammatory cells and a single squamous cell in the background

encountered, dissemination to bone, skin and urinary tract is not unusual. Involvement of the lungs characteristically presents as isolated densities, consolidation or mass-like infiltrates owing to the suppurative granulomas associated with the disease, and as such is best sampled via aspiration. Smears of the aspirates show a non-specific inflammatory background of acute inflammation, necrotic debris, macrophages, histiocytes, and occasionally multi-nucleated giant cells. The organism can be seen amid the non-descript background, but is easily overlooked as they are often out of the plane of focus due to the thick cellular wall. *Blastomyces* is a rigid, round organism with distinctive broad-based budding as well as a 'double contour', a hazy clearing surrounding the entire organism, seen in routine stains. Due to its slow growth, cultures can take several weeks [3, 4].

Histoplasmosis occurs as a primary infection from inhalation of the dimorphic yeast *Histoplasma capsulatum*. Up to 80 % of individuals exposed/infected to *H. capsulatum* in low/ambient levels will be asymptomatic or have vague symptoms at most, unless there is prolonged or high-level exposure in which case up to 75 % of those exposed will develop symptoms. Alternatively, clinically apparent histoplasmosis can result from reactivation of latent infection secondary to compromised immunity in previously exposed individuals. The spectrum of disease includes acute, chronic, disseminated, and much less commonly granulomatous and fibrosing mediastinitis. *Histoplasma capsulatum* is the smallest dimorphic fungus (3–5 μm) and is seen, for the most part, intracellularly. Macrophages engulf the organisms where they appear as vacuolated oval or foamy structures within the cytoplasm when stained with Diff-Quik®. Papanicolaou staining is not helpful. Confirmation is established with the Gomori-methanamine silver stain, although caution must be exercised as other organisms such as *Blastomyces*, *Cryptococcus*, Candida, *Pneumocystis* and *Toxoplasma* or even contaminating debris can be misinterpreted as *H. capulatum* [3].

Taxonomic classification of *Pneumocystis jirovecii* (formerly *Pneumocystic carinii*) has vacillated over time; once considered a protozoan, currently Pneumocystis is classified as a fungus based on biochemical and nucleic acid studies [13, 14]. Problematic in the immunocompromised individuals, Pneumocystis is a causative agent of pneumonia. While bronchial washings and induced sputum can be used, BAL has the highest sensitivity for detection of Pneumocystis, comparable to transbronchial biopsy. The trophozoite forms are visible with Diff-Quik® where the tiny organisms (1.5 μm) are seen as blue dots lying within the cysts [15]. The cysts are not visible in Papaniculaou stained preparations, rather spheres of foamy proteinaceous material (alveolar casts) are a clue to the diagnosis (Fig. 4.2).

While Candida species are part of the normal flora of the gastrointestinal and genitourinary tract, disruption of host immunity opens the door to opportunistic infection in the lungs. However, candidal pneumonia is exceedingly rare and usually occurs within the setting of known disseminated disease, via hematogenous spread with resultant multifocal microabscess formation. Candidal elements are seen frequently in exfoliative cytology and are indicative of oral contamination. Typically, both pseudohyphae (elongated yeast forms with budding) and yeast forms are seen together and the overall picture is sometimes referred to as

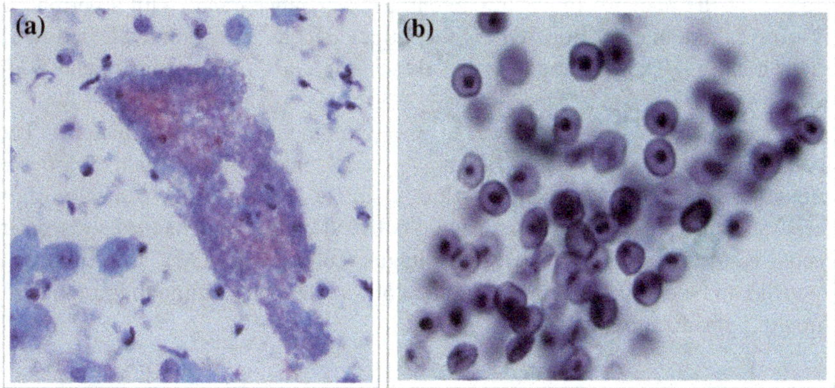

Fig. 4.2 BAL, **a** 60X, Papanicolaou stain. **b** GMS stain highlights the cysts *Pneumocystis* in a BAL can be easily dismissed as debris. A fluffy, proteinaceous mass with dot-like trophozoites

'spaghetti and meatballs' or 'sticks and stones' (Fig. 4.3). In the instance where a true infectious etiology is suspected, the distinction between contamination and infection can be problematic; however, the presence of pseudohyphae seen in a background of inflammatory cells and debris should raise the suspicion for an infectious process [3, 16].

4.5.2.3 Viral

Herpes simplex virus causing pneumonitis and tracheobronchitis is most often caused by HSV-1. Washings, brushings, or BAL demonstrate the characteristic virally induced cytopathologic changes. Notably, the respiratory epithelial cells show intranuclear accumulation of viral particles forcing the chromatin to the

Fig. 4.3 BAL, 40X, Papaniculaou stain. *Candida Albicans* with pseudohyphae with numerous macrophages in the background

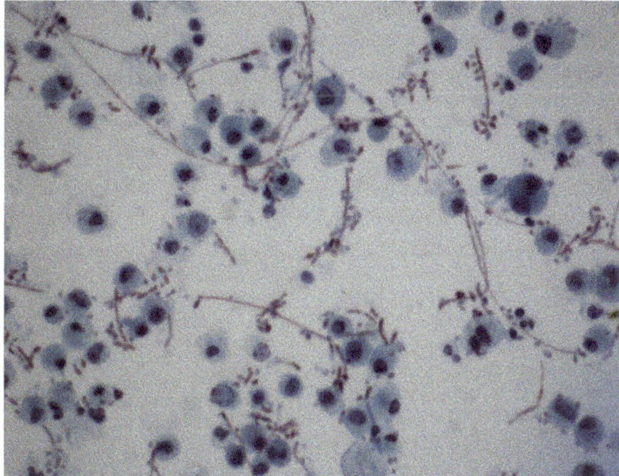

periphery of the nucleus, imparting a central glassy appearance with a peripheral dark rim called margination. Often the infected cells are multinucleated with nuclear molding. These changes are easily seen in washings, brushings and BAL [4] (Fig. 4.4).

Cytomegalovirus is often seen in the immunocompromised patient. The infected respiratory epithelial cells show overall enlargement and a prominent nucleus with a solitary basophilic nuclear inclusion and a perinuclear halo, often referred to as 'owl's eye' (Fig. 4.5). Identical viral cytopathic changes are seen in infected epithelial cells elsewhere (esophagus, colon) with CMV infection. The diagnosis can be confirmed with immunocytohistochemistry, immunoflourescence, or in situ hybridization [17].

4.6 Non-Infectious/Non-Neoplastic

4.6.1 Sarcoidosis

Sarcoidosis is a systemic, granulomatous disease of unknown etiology and is predominantly a diagnosis of exclusion, requiring clinic-radiologic features, tissue diagnosis, and exclusion of similar diseases. Although the disease is widespread, the lungs are the most common site of involvement, with variable involvement of the lung parenchyma and hilar lymph nodes. Either lymph nodes or parenchyma can be sampled via FNA. Transbronchial biopsy is non-diagnostic in up to 30 %, however improved sensitivity and specificity (up to 95 %) is attained with endoscopic ultrasound guided FNA of hilar lymph nodes [3]. The characteristic granulomas of sarcoidosis are compact, non-caseating and comprised of epithelioid histiocytes. The histiocyte is a large cell with vague cell borders and a gently curved nucleus, likened to a 'footprint.' Special stains should be utilized whenever granulomas are encountered in order to exclude infectious etiologies.

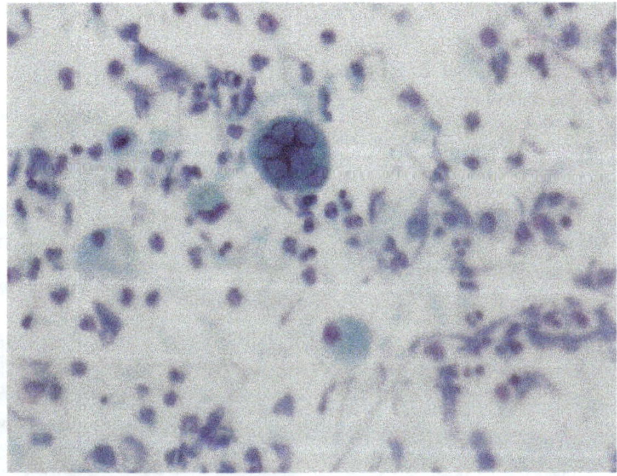

Fig. 4.4 BAL, 60X, Diff Quik stain. Viral cytopathlogic change in an epithelial cell due to *Herpes Simplex* virus with classic "three M's": multinucleationi, nuclear molding, and margination of the nuclear chromatin

Fig. 4.5 BAL, 60X, Papaniculaou stain. Brick red intranuclear viral inclusion of *cytomegalovirus*, sometimes referred to as 'owl's eye' inclusion

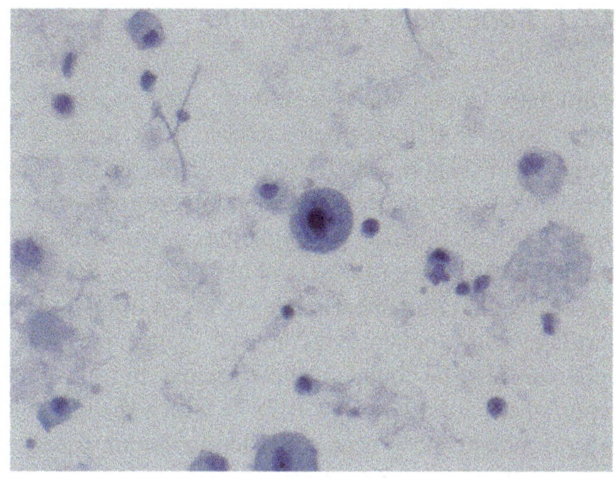

4.6.2 Wegener's Granulomatosis

The necrotizing vasculitis of Wegener's granulomatosis can present as a mass-like lesion in the lungs. Aspirations are non-specific and yield variable amounts of neutrophils, necrotic collagen, granular debris, giant cells, and epithelioid histiocytes. Correlation with serologic studies and clinical criteria is warranted for a definitive diagnosis.

4.6.3 Non-Infectious Inflammatory

The most commonly encountered non-infectious inflammatory conditions seen in cytology include resolving pneumonia, transplant rejection, diffuse alveolar damage, and cryptogenic organizing pneumonia (COP), formerly called bronchiolitis obliterans organizing pneumonia (BOOP). The cytologic features show considerable overlap and consist of variable amounts of inflammatory cells and reactive pneumocytes.

4.7 Benign Neoplasms (Epithelial and Mesenchymal)

Benign neoplasms of the lung are reasonably rare, especially in comparison to the prevalence of their malignant counterparts. Nevertheless, a mass lesion in the lung is an alarming finding and requires a pathologic diagnosis to determine the true nature of the lesion.

4.7.1 Pulmonary Hamartoma

Pulmonary hamartoma is seen most often as solitary, asymptomatic nodule and is often discovered incidentally. Chest films show a subpleural, well demarcated, round 'coin' lesion, which may have delicate calcifications. These lesions are not detectable by exfoliative cytology, but are readily sampled by FNA. Cytologically there is a combination of epithelial and mesenchymal elements (Fig. 4.6). The epithelial cells are uniform, oval to round benign-looking epithelial cells, while the mesenchymal component ranges from an immature fibromyxoid matrix to mature cartilage with chondrocytes housed in lacunae. Adipocytes and bland glandular cells can also be found in these lesions but are not required for diagnosis. The reported sensitivity of FNA is 78 % with a specificity of nearly 100 % [18]. Clonal rearrangements have been consistently demonstrated in these lesions, supporting a true neoplastic rather than reactive origin [19].

4.7.2 Other Benign Mass Lesions

Inflammatory myofibroblastic tumor, also known as inflammatory pseudotumor is seen younger patients and is the most common lung tumor seen in children less than 16 years of age. Chest films show a solitary, peripheral nodule. Cytologically, there is a population of bland spindle cells in a storiform (cartwheeling) pattern with a prominent mixed inflammatory infiltrate and necrotic debris. The behavior of inflammatory myofibroblastic tumor ranges from essentially benign to locally aggressive and destructive lesions.

Localized or solitary fibrous tumors are rare tumors, seen commonly in the pleura but also reported to involve the lung. Fine needle aspirates show scant to variable cellularity, fragments of ropy collagen, and oval to spindle cells.

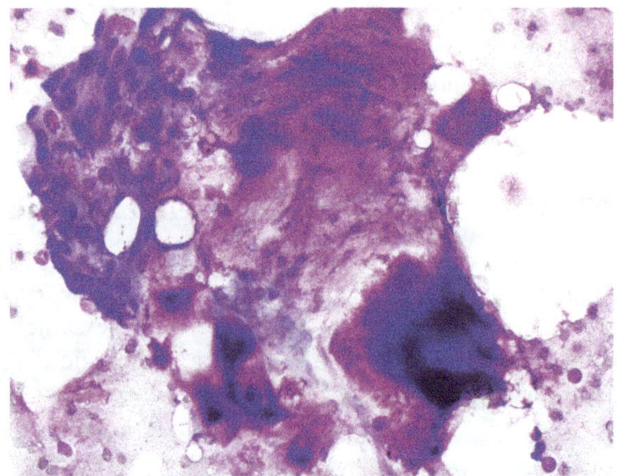

Fig. 4.6 Fine needle aspiration biopsy, 40X, Diff Quik® stain,Hamartoma. Cytologic preparation showing deeply basophilic purplish blue chondroid mesenchymal material containing chondrocytes mixed with bland spindle-shaped cells, oval to round epithelial cells and fat deposit

Endobronchial granular cell tumors are, as the name implies, are found centrally in the bronchial tree. Due to their submucosal location, the cells do not exfoliate, but may be collected by brushings or endobronchial ultrasound (EBUS). The neoplastic cells are typically in small groups or singly and have a small, round, dark, regular nuclei and abundant granular cytoplasm.

Other rare benign neoplasms include, neoplasms derived from the seromucimous glands of the airway such as pleomorphic adenoma with mixed epithelial and mesenchymal components. Typically, a fibrillar chondromyxoid matrix background is seen in these tumors, which shows a characteristic metachromasia on DiffQuik stain.

4.8 Carcinoma: Clinical and Cytopathologic Overview

Lung cancer remains the leading cause of cancer deaths in the United States and worldwide. It is estimated that in the USA 226,160 new cases of lung cancer (116,470 men and 109, 690 women) will be diagnosed and 160,340 will die from lung cancer in 2012, accounting for about 28 % of all cancer deaths [20]. With the undisputable link to cigarette smoking, considering that an estimated 45 million individuals in the USA alone are smokers it is not surprising that death from lung cancer ranks first above breast and colorectal carcinomas. In addition to the increasing incidence of pulmonary malignancies, there has been an as of yet unexplained shift in prevalence of histologic subtypes. Currently, adenocarcinoma has replaced squamous cell carcinoma as the most common malignant pulmonary neoplasm.

Histologic classification and tumor stage are critical to the diagnosis and treatment of lung cancer. Cytopathologists play a vital role in the diagnosis as most lung cancers are diagnosed by small biopsies or cytology specimens. Traditionally, the diagnosis of non-small cell lung carcinoma (NSCLC) was reflective of the relative lack of distinct therapeutic options available for pulmonary malignancies other than small cell lung cancer (SCLC); therefore a cytologic diagnosis of NSCLC was sufficient. NSCLCs include three major cell types (adenocarcinoma, squamous cell carcinoma, and large cell carcinoma). In addition to SCLCs, there are other less common neuroendocrine carcinomas of the lung.

In recent years, there has been a significant increase in research about lung cancer with new insights into histologic classification, pathological-clinical correlations, imaging, molecular pathology and therapy protocols. Correlation of certain molecular mutations with particular histologic subtypes has been well documented. As a result, the International Association of the study of lung cancer, American Thoracic Society and European Respiratory Society have proposed revisions to the traditional classification, of lung adenocarcinomas [21].

Recent understanding of the biology of pulmonary neoplasms at the molecular level, particularly the activating mutations of the epidermal growth factor receptor (EGFR) has changed the approach to diagnosis of these lesions. Briefly, the EGFR is a tyrosine kinase receptor, which when activated by appropriate ligand binding signals the intracellular pathways PI3 K/AKT and RAS/RAF/MAPK which regulate cellular activities such as cellular proliferation and apoptosis [12, 22]. Specific mutations in the EGFR gene have been demonstrated in well differentiated adenocarcinoma (non mucinous bronchioalveolar carcinoma) in specific populations. More importantly, the lesions harboring these mutations respond to the tyrosine kinase inhibitors erlotinib and geftininib. Because targeted therapy is available for this subset of neoplasms there is a need for the pathologist to report the histologic subtype so appropriate ancillary testing can be performed and expedite treatment [23–25]. Other potential targets of molecular therapy with specific histologic association includes K-ras mutations in mucinous adenocarcinomas.

Histologic subclassification presents specific challenges for the pathologist. First, there is frequently more than one histologic subtype within the same tumor underscoring the significance of sampling. Additionally, in poorly differentiated lesions it may not be possible to determine the histologic subtypes, although this may be less of an issue in regards to targeted therapy as EGFR mutations are not seen in poorly differentiated lesions (as mentioned above). In such situations, a diagnosis of "non-small cell carcinoma" may occasionally be unavoidable, although with the use of ancillary studies suggestion of cell type should be provided if possible.

It should be stated that one of the most daunting aspects of respiratory cytology is that any portion of the normal respiratory constituents, when reactive or degenerate, can mimic carcinoma. Degenerating squamous cells from oral contamination can mimic squamous cell carcinoma. Reactive bronchial epithelial cells and goblet cell hyperplasia can mimic adenocarcinoma. Reserve cell hyperplasia can mimic small cell carcinoma. Therapy related changes are notorious for appearing especially sinister. Clinical history is an integral component of the interpretation of respiratory cytologic specimens and the primary diagnosis of malignancy in the absence of supporting clinical data should be cautiously interpreted [4, 11].

4.8.1 Adenocarcinoma

Adenocarcinoma, as previously mentioned, is the most common primary lung malignancy has a slight predilection for women and is the most common histologic subtype of carcinoma found in non-smokers. According to the 2004 World Health Organization (WHO) classification, there are five subtypes of adenocarcinoma based on histologic features: acinar, papillary, bronchioloalveolar carcinoma (BAC), solid with mucin production and mixed subtypes. There has been considerable debate over the definition, diagnosis and biologic implications of BAC, and in practice 'pure' BAC is rarely diagnosed, and instead is usually seen as a component of adenocarcinoma. Similar to small transbronchial biopsies, it is not possible to distinguish between bronchogenic adenocarcinoma and BAC in cytologic preparations as evidence of invasion into pulmonary parenchyma, pleura or vascular invasion (or lack thereof) is required for diagnosis [26, 27]. The recent classification recommends that the term BAC should not be used for the diagnosis of lung adenocarcinoma in both resections and cytology specimens.

Morphologically, FNA smears are usually cellular with cohesive groups of cell in sheets with acinar/glandular formations and three-dimensional clusters. The neoplastic cells are variably pleomorphic with increased nuclear cytoplasmic ratios, scant, vacuolated cytoplasm eccentrically placed nuclei and large nucleoli. Well-differentiated adenocarcinoma with BAC can be deceptively 'normal' in cytologic preparations. A diagnosis of adenocarcinoma with BAC features is considered when the smear is cellular with cells in papillary clusters and sheets. Psammoma bodies and intranuclear inclusions are soft findings of BAC and are helpful in support of the diagnosis. The differential diagnosis of adenocarcinoma includes metastatic adenocarcinoma, reactive pneumocytes, reparative changes, and granulomatous inflammation (Figs. 4.7 and 4.8).

Thyroid transcription factor-1 (TTF-1) shows nuclear immunopoisitivity in 75–85 % of pulmonary adenocarcinomas and is routinely used to support the pulmonary origin of the adenocarcinomas. More recently, Napsin-A has been noted to be expressed in 80 % of lung adenocarcinomas with characteristic cytoplasmic immunostaining. In some situations, where the differential diagnosis between solid pattern of adenocarcinoma and squamous cell carcinoma is difficult, however, the distinction is important to make for the treatment purposes, an immunohistochemistry panel consisting of p63 and CK5/6 (frequently immuno-positive in squamous cell carcinoma) and TTF-1 and Napsin-A (positive in adenocarcinoma) has been proposed [28]. Once the diagnosis of adenocarcinoma is rendered, the cytology specimen (cell block or the biopsy) is sent to molecular pathology for mutation analysis. Recent studies strongly support the suitability of cytologic specimens for the new therapeutic paradigms in non small cell carcinoma [29].

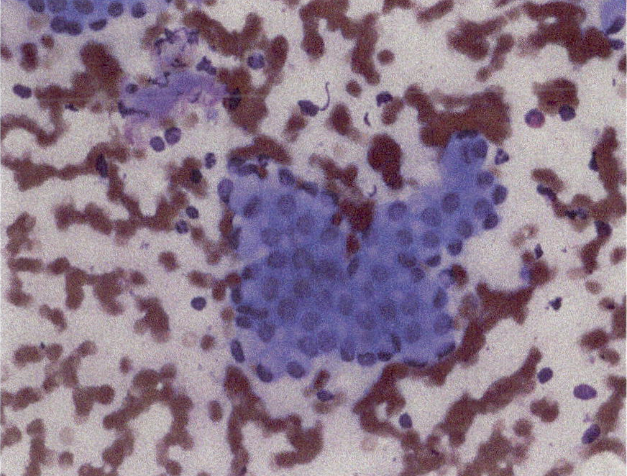

Fig. 4.7 Fine needle aspiration biopsy, 40X, Diff Quik® stain. Adenocarcinoma, mucinous type. Three dimensional cluster of neoplastic cells which are deceptively bland. The cells are polarized (nuclei pushed to one side) and there is visible cytoplasmic mucin, resembling goblet cells. In normal lung tissue, only 1 in 5 epithelial cells are goblet (contain mucin)

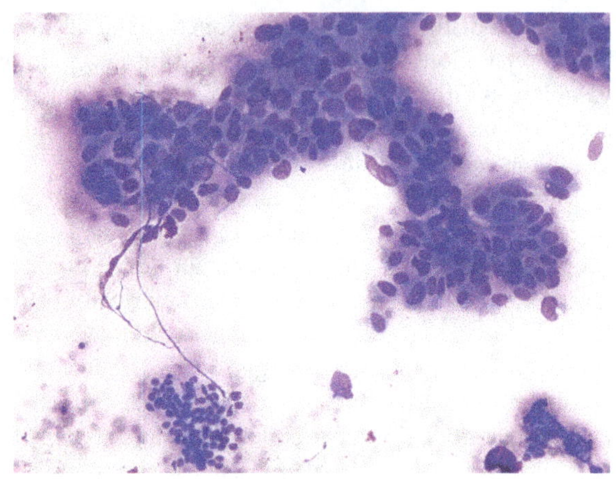

Fig. 4.8 Fine needle aspiration biopsy, 40X, Diff Quik® stain. Primary lung adenocarcinoma. Cohesive sheets of large, polygonal cells with pleomorphic nuclei and visible nucleoli. Compare to the small group of normal respiratory cells are in the lower middle field

4.8.2 Squamous Cell Carcinoma

Squamous cell carcinoma is the second most prevalent primary lung malignancy after adenocarcinoma, accounting for nearly 30 % of pulmonary malignancies and is most strongly associated with cigarette smoking. There is a significant predilection for males with a male to female ratio between 6 and 15:1 [3]. Rates of primary squamous cell carcinoma of the lung are decreasing and may reflect changes in smoking habits. A majority of squamous cell carcinomas arise centrally from a main or segmental bronchus, with growth extending along the endobronchial channels and invading into parenchyma with significant necrosis and resultant cavitation. Due to the compressive nature of these tumors, portions of lung distal to the mass are vulnerable and prone to develop atelectasis, bronchopneumonia and lipid pneumonia.

Whether material is collected via exfoliative methods or needle biopsy, the morphologic features of squamous cell carcinoma are similar. The preparations are cellular with very little cellular cohesion, usually seen amid a background of necrotic debris. The neoplastic cells can be round, oval or elongated into 'tadpole' or 'fiber' cells with characteristic dense cytoplasm (Figs. 4.9 and 4.10). Although some cells will stain a vibrant orange (orangeophilia) with Papanicolaou stain due to the large amount of keratin, it is the quality of the cytoplasm (dense, hard), which defines squamous differentiation. The nuclei are dark to pyknotic, to the extent that chromatin detail is obscured and irregular nuclear membranes. Ancillary testing can be performed on smears, cell block or core biopsy material to support the diagnosis if warranted. Squamous cell carcinomas are positive for CK5/6 and p63 and negative for TTF-1 [30] The differential diagnosis includes reactive or infectious etiologies, pulmonary infarct metastatic squamous cell carcinoma from a head and neck primary, urothelial carcinoma and adenocarcinoma (in poorly differentiated lesions).

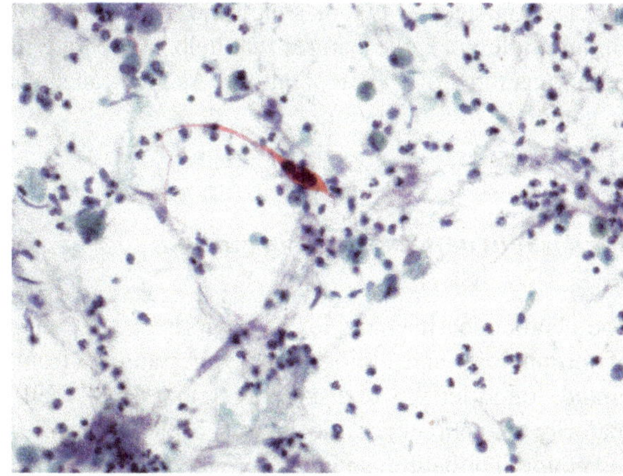

Fig. 4.9 BAL 40X, Papanicolaou stain. Squamous cell carcinoma with classic 'tadpole' cell, a heavily keratinzed squamous cell (bright orange cytoplasm) with hyperchromatic, irregular nucleus

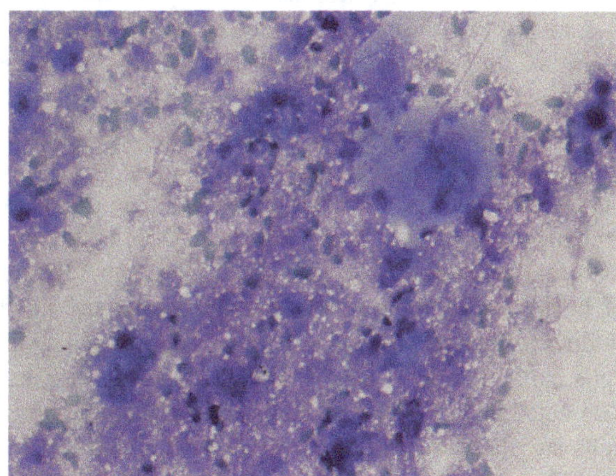

Fig. 4.10 Fine needle aspiration biopsy, lung nodule, 60X, Diff Quik®. Primary squamous cell carcinoma of the lung. Markedly atypical, squamous cells with characteristic dense cytoplasm; one with multiple nuclei. The background reveals abundant necrotic debris with dense, dark blue keratin blobs

4.8.3 Large Cell Carcinoma

Large cell carcinoma is a high grade undifferentiated neoplasm with an aggressive course. The cells lack morphologic features of squamous cell differentiation (intracellular bridges, keratin pearls and dense cytoplasm) or glandular differentiation (gland formation and mucin production); therefore, it is a diagnosis of exclusion. Electron microscopy has demonstrated large cell carcinomas express characteristic of both squamous and adenocarcinomas at an ultrastructural level. Currently, the WHO classification recognizes several microscopic variants of large cell carcinoma: basaloid, clear cell, lymphoepithelial-like, and large cell neuroendocrine carcinoma. The tumors tend to occur peripherally and many have cavitary changes. Cytologic specimens are usually cellular with small groups of loosely cohesive cells and numerous isolated cells. The cells typically have an increased nucleus to cytoplasmic ratio, ill-defined cytoplasm, irregular chromatin and multiple nucleoli, features that help to separate this tumor from the small cell carcinoma in cytologic preparations. As mentioned earlier the cells lack squamous or glandular differentiation.

4.8.4 Neuroendocrine Carcinoma

The neuroendocrine carcinomas comprise a spectrum of neoplasms with an array of morphology and biologic behavior, ranging from clinically insignificant carcinoid 'tumorlet' to undisputedly lethal small cell carcinoma. Even though a majority of neuroendocrine tumors occur centrally, the lesions are deep to the respiratory epithelium and therefore the neoplastic cells are not shed and hence not detectable by exfoliative methods. There has been considerable debate over the cell of origin in these lesions; in the past the resident neuroendocrine cell, the Kulchitsky cell, has been implicated as the cell of origin, however more recent literature suggests neuroendocrine differentiation is simply an expression of toti-potential cells.

Typical carcinoid (grade 1 NEC, well differentiated neuroendocrine carcinoma) is a rare neoplasm in the lung, accounting for about 3 % of primary ling neoplasms. Carcinoids were thought to be benign entities; however, it has been well recognized now that these neoplasms do have the ability to metastasize and therefore are regarded as low grade malignancies. Carcinoids may arise centrally or in the periphery in nearly equal amounts and nearly half will have radiologic findings of atelectasis. FNA smears of carcinoids reveal loosely cohesive sheets of cells, sometimes in vague rosette formations as well as numerous isolated cells. The cells are uniform and commonly plasmacytoid, although round to columnar cells are also seen. Ample amounts eosinophilic cytoplasm and uniform, granular nuclei are present. Importantly, carcinoids lack nuclear molding, mitotic activity or necrosis, all features consistent with a higher grade lesion [31]. Neuroendocrine differentiation is confirmed with immunohistochemical stains including chromogranin, synaptophysin and CD56. Differentiation of primary pulmonary carcinoid from non-pulmonary neuroendocrine tumor should be considered and can be accomplished with a panel of immunohistochemical stains including CK7, CK20, and TTF-1.

Atypical carcinoid (Grade 2 NEC) lies within the spectrum between grade 1 NEC and small cell carcinoma. Atypical carcinoids are less common than typical carcinoids, occur in both central and peripheral locations and show more aggressive behavior than typical carcinoids. The diagnosis in cytology is challenging and lies in finding necrosis, mitosis and variable degrees of nuclear molding [32, 33]. The nuclei are more hyperchromatic with coarser chromatin than the nuclei of typical carcinoids.

Large cell neuroendocrine carcinoma (Grade 3 NEC) is the most recently described variant of neuroendocrine carcinoma and is extremely aggressive. Most of the lesions occur peripherally and present with vague symptoms, similar to the other lung neoplasms. The lesions are difficult to diagnose on cytologic material and requires sufficient material to perform immunohistochemistry studies to demonstrate neuroendocrine differentiation. Large cell neuroendocrine carcinomas are typically immunopositive with cytokeratin 7 and approximately half are immunopositive with TTF-1. They are sometimes misdiagnosed as adenocarcinoma or squamous cell carcinoma by a less experienced cytopathologist.

Small cell (undifferentiated) carcinoma is regarded as a high grade neuroendocrine carcinoma and accounts for 20–25 % of all primary lung malignancies, and is reported to be decreasing in incidence. There is a strong association with cigarette smoking and a slight male predilection. Typically the lesions occur as centrally located bulky masses with evidence of metastatic disease at the time of diagnosis. Although response to chemotherapy and radiation therapy is favorable, relapse of disease is common and the overall prognosis is dismal with a 5–10 % survival rate at 5 years. Clinically the symptoms are reflective of the anatomic location; including coughing, shortness of breath, hemoptysis, pleural effusion, and superior vena cava syndrome. Paraneoplastic syndromes are not uncommon and include syndrome of inappropriate anti-diuretic hormone, Eaton-Lambert syndrome and Cushing's syndrome. FNA smears of small cell carcinomas are cellular with distinct morphologic features. The cells have high nuclear cytoplasmic ratios with very scant cytoplasm, dark nuclei, stippled nuclear chromatin, and inconspicuous nucleoli [32]. The malignant cells are extremely delicate; therefore nuclear molding and 'crush artifact' are typical findings (Fig. 4.11). Mitotic figures are found easily. Due to the invariable necrosis, a background of granular debris is to be expected. Lymphoproliferative malignancies and poorly differentiated adenocarcinoma should be considered in the differential diagnosis [3]. Majority of SCLCs show positivity for TTF-1 and neuroendocrine markers (synaptophysin, chromogranin and CD56). However, individual neuroendocrine markers may be negative in up to 30 % of SCLC and multiple markers may be negative in 10–15 % of cases.

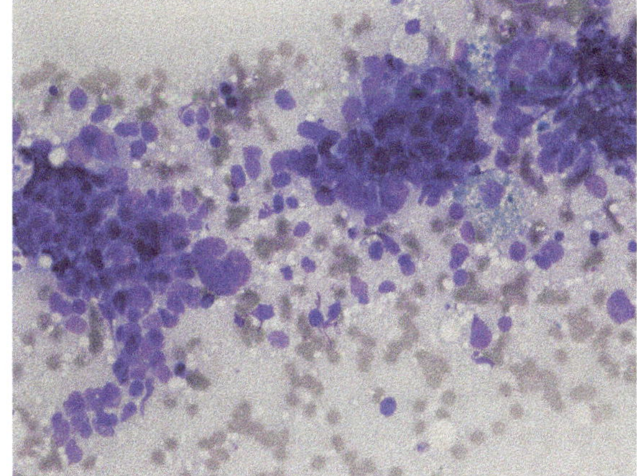

Fig. 4.11 Fine needle aspiration, lung nodule, 60X, Diff-Quik® stain. Small cell carcinoma. Atypical cells with prominent nuclear molding, scant cytoplasm and inconspicuous nucleoli with apoptotic cells in a background of necrosis

4.8.5 Metastatic Carcinomas to the Lung

Dual blood supply ensures the lung has ample opportunity to filter travelling tumor cells, indeed metastatic disease is always considered in mass lesions of the lung and suspicion for metastatic disease is a primary indication to perform transthoracic needle aspiration. It is reported that 14–26 % of transthoracic needle biopsies are metastatic lesions. Colon, breast, renal, bladder carcinomas, and melanoma are the most commonly encountered metastatic lesions in the lung, although there are differing reports as to the rank [4, 34].

The origin of metastatic lesions can be inferred by the architectural and cellular morphology. Certainly if there is history of a previously diagnosed neoplasm, it is helpful to compare the morphology of the original tumor to the material obtained at FNA. Immunohistochemistry can also be useful to support a diagnosis of metastasis (particularly if stains were performed on the original diagnostic specimen) or to distinguish a primary lung neoplasm from a metastatic lesion. Metastatic lesions with an unknown primary are worked up as such.

Additionally, in the current age, multiple primary malignancies in a single patient are becoming more frequent and thus the pathologist will usually confirm the morphologic impression by immunohistochemistry (IHC). Since material is limited in cytologic preparations, appropriate usage of IHC is warranted so that material remains for further molecular testing if required.

4.9 Malignant Mesenchymal Neoplasms

4.9.1 Epitheloid Haemangioendothelioma/Angiosarcoma

This unique vascular tumor can be seen in both lung and pleura. Pulmonary epitheloid haemangioendothelioma is a low to intermediate grade vascular tumor with a distinct predilection for younger females. The tumor cells forming the nodules are small, round to oval, and show intracytoplasmic vacuoles, which represent primitive vascular lumina. High grade epitheloid vascular tumors are called epitheloid angiosarcomas.

4.9.2 Synovial Sarcoma

Synovial sarcomas are uncommon malignant tumors of uncertain histogenesis arising commonly in the pleura, but also from lung. It is composed primarily of spindle cells with variable epithelial components. The tumor can be difficult to diagnose specifically on FNA or core biopsy specimens, especially if monophasic. Tissue can be sent to cytogenetics to confirm the SYT-SSX fusion gene, characteristic of this sarcoma.

4.10 Pleural Lesions

Tumors of the pleura are classified as diffuse and localized forms and secondarily localized tumors as benign or malignant. Diffuse tumors of the pleura include diffuse malignant mesothelioma, metastatic carcinomas, vascular sarcomas, and synovial sarcomas. Localized benign tumors or tumors of uncertain malignant potential include solitary fibrous tumor, lipoma, adenomatoid tumor and schwannoma. Localized malignant tumors include malignant mesothelioma, malignant solitary fibrous tumor, liposarcoma, and lymphoma.

Cytology specimens and small cores of tissue can be obtained by needle aspirations, but it is often difficult to make a diagnosis of mesothelioma due to sampling error and small sample size. The inability to assess for invasion is one of the potential drawbacks of exfoliative cytology in the diagnosis of diffuse malignant mesothelioma. However, on microscopic examination of the biopsy specimens, these neoplasms tend to be relatively monotonous and often deceptively bland, while the metastatic carcinomas to the pleura are often much more pleomorphic. A panel of IHC stains can be very useful in reaching a specific diagnosis.

4.11 Ancillary Testing

There are a variety of ancillary studies available for both diagnosis and prognostic purposes. The amount and type of material impacts which studies can be performed; therefore any clinical suspicions should be communicated to the pathology staff so that the appropriate amount and type of material can be collected and triaged at the time of procedure.

In addition to the standard Diff Quik® and Papaniculaou stains, there are a variety of special stains that can be utilized. Immunohistochemistry (IHC) utilizes the antibody-antigen binding relationship to identify cell differentiation (epithelial, mesenchymal, hematopoietic) and type. A full discussion of IHC is beyond the scope of this chapter (further details can be found in Chap. 2 of this book); suffice it to say that IHC is one of the most powerful and widely used tools used by pathologist. Core biopsy and cell block material are preferred for IHC as there are more cells and consistency of material. FNA smears can be used for IHC but are not optimal due to high background and non-specific staining. Additionally, duplicate slides of smears cannot be made as all the material at the time of biopsy is expelled onto the slide. Interpretation of immunohistochemical stains is not as simple as 'positive' or 'negative': the portion of the cell that stains (nucleus, cytoplasm, and cell membrane) and the intensity of staining need to be taken into consideration. Similarly, the choice of immunostains should be made carefully and ideally should support or refute a suspected diagnosis, which is based on morphologic features.

Flow cytometry is in extraordinarily sensitive modality employed in the identification of cells based on their cell surface receptors and proteins. It is used almost exclusively in the identification of hematopoietic cells in lymphoproliferative disorders. Most labs require cellular material to be submitted in a liquid-based medium (RPMI) therefore dedicated FNA passes or whole tissue should be placed in the appropriate medium at the time of collection if clinically indicated or as a result of on-site cytologic assessment.

Fluorescent in situ hybridization (FISH) employs fluorescently tagged probes to detect specific numeric and structural chromosomal abnormalities in specific malignancies and can be used as a diagnostic or prognostic biomarker. A variety of materials including cytologic material can be utilized for FISH.

PCR-based molecular studies are increasing in clinical use and are continually integrated into hospital laboratories. Many different types of specimens from fresh tissue to formalin-fixed paraffin embedded tissue can be utilized for molecular studies. Clear communication between clinicians and pathologists is essential as there are usually specific and stringent requirements for performance of these tests.

References

1. Linder J (2000) Lung cancer cytology. Something old, something new. Am J Clin Pathol 114(2):169–171
2. Mullan CP et al (2004) CT-guided fine-needle aspiration of lung nodules: effect on outcome of using coaxial technique and immediate cytological evaluation. Ulster Med J 73(1):32–36
3. Sidawy MK (2007) Fine needle aspiration cytology. In: Goldblum JR (ed) Foundations in diagnostic pathology. Churchill Livingstone, London, pp 159–199
4. DeMay R (1996) The art and science of cytopathology. American Society of Clinical Pathologists, Chicago, pp 948–981
5. Khajotia RR et al (1991) Induced sputum and cytological diagnosis of lung cancer. Lancet 338(8773):976–977
6. Larsen SS, Krasnik M, Vilmann P et al (2002) Endoscopic ultrasound guided biopsy of mediastinal lesions has a major impact on patient management. Thorax 57:98–103
7. Johnston WW (1984) Percutaneous fine needle aspiration biopsy of the lung. A study of 1,015 patients. Acta Cytol 28(3):218–224
8. Naryshkin S, Daniels J, Young NA (1992) Diagnostic correlation of fiberoptic bronchoscopic biopsy and bronchoscopic cytology performed simultaneously. Diagn Cytopathol 8(2):119–123
9. Zarbo RJ, Fenoglio-Preiser CM (1992) Interinstitutional database for comparison of performance in lung fine-needle aspiration cytology. A college of american pathologists Q-probe study of 5264 cases with histologic correlation. Arch Pathol Lab Med 116(5):463–470
10. Motherby H et al (1999) Diagnostic accuracy of effusion cytology. Diagn Cytopathol 20(6):350–357
11. Saad RS, Silverman JF (2009) Respiratory cytology: Differential diagnosis and pitfalls. Diagn Cytopathol 38:297–307
12. Roggli VL, Piantadosi CA, Bell DY (1986) Asbestos bodies in bronchoalveolar lavage fluid. A study of 20 asbestos-exposed individuals and comparison to patients with other chronic interstitial lung diseases. Acta Cytol 30(5):470–476

13. Edman JC et al (1988) Ribosomal RNA sequence shows Pneumocystis carinii to be a member of the fungi. Nature 334(6182):519–522
14. Maiese SC, Naryshkin S (1991) Diagnosis of Pneumocystis carinii by cytologic examination of Papanicolaou-stained sputum specimens. Diagn Cytopathol 7(1):111–112
15. Naryshkin S et al (1991) Cytology of treated and minimal Pneumocystis carinii pneumonia and a pitfall of the Grocott methenamine silver stain. Diagn Cytopathol 7(1):41–47
16. Ness MJ et al (1988) Detection of Candida antigen in bronchoalveolar lavage fluid. Acta Cytol 32(3):347–352
17. Weiss RL et al (1991) Diagnosis of cytomegalovirus pneumonitis on bronchoalveolar lavage fluid: comparison of cytology, immunofluorescence, and in situ hybridization with viral isolation. Diagn Cytopathol 7(3):243–247
18. Hughes JH et al (2005) Fine-needle aspiration of pulmonary hamartoma: a common source of false-positive diagnoses in the college of American pathologists interlaboratory comparison program in nongynecologic cytology. Arch Pathol Lab Med 129(1):19–22
19. Xiao S et al (1997) HMGI(Y) activation by chromosome 6p21 rearrangements in multilineage mesenchymal cells from pulmonary hamartoma. Am J Pathol 150(3):901–910
20. Siegel R, Naishadham D, Jemal A et al (2012) Cancer statistics. CA Cancer J Clin. 62(1):10–29
21. Travis WD, Brambilla E, Noguchi M, et al (2011) International association for the study of lung cancer/american thoracic society/european respiratory society international multidisciplinary classification of lung adenocarcinoma. J Thorac Oncol : official publication of the International Association for the Study of Lung Cancer. 6(2):244–285
22. Bell DW et al (2005) Epidermal growth factor receptor mutations and gene amplification in non-small-cell lung cancer: molecular analysis of the IDEAL/INTACT gefitinib trials. J Clin Oncol 23(31):8081–8092
23. Li AR et al (2008) EGFR mutations in lung adenocarcinomas: clinical testing experience and relationship to EGFR gene copy number and immunohistochemical expression. J Mol Diagn 10(3):242–248
24. Marty M et al (2005) Randomized phase II trial of the efficacy and safety of trastuzumab combined with docetaxel in patients with human epidermal growth factor receptor 2-positive metastatic breast cancer administered as first-line treatment: the M77001 study group. J Clin Oncol 23(19):4265–4274
25. Sequist LV et al (2007) Molecular predictors of response to epidermal growth factor receptor antagonists in non-small-cell lung cancer. J Clin Oncol 25(5):587–595
26. Atkins KA (2004) The diagnosis of bronchioloalveolar carcinoma by cytologic means. Am J Clin Pathol 122(1):14–16
27. Ohori NP, Santa Maria EL (2004) Cytopathologic diagnosis of bronchioloalveolar carcinoma: does it correlate with the 1999 World Health Organization definition? Am J Clin Pathol 122(1):44–50
28. Mukhopadhyay S, Katzenstein AL (2011) Subclassification of non-small cell lung carcinomas lacking morphologic differentiation on biopsy specimens: utility of an immunohistochemical panel containing TTF-1, napsin A, p63, and CK5/6. Am J Surg Pathol 35(1):15–25
29. Rekhtman N et al (2011) Suitability of thoracic cytology for new therapeutic paradigms in non-small cell lung carcinoma: high accuracy of tumor subtyping and feasibility of EGFR and KRAS molecular testing. J Thorac Oncol 6(3):451–458
30. Liu J, Farhood A (2004) Immunostaining for thyroid transcription factor-1 on fine-needle aspiration specimens of lung tumors: a comparison of direct smears and cell block preparations. Cancer 102(2):109–114
31. Soga J, Yakuwa Y (1999) Bronchopulmonary carcinoids: An analysis of 1,875 reported cases with special reference to a comparison between typical carcinoids and atypical varieties. Ann Thorac Cardiovasc Surg 5(4):211–219

32. Nicholson SA, Ryan MR (2000) A review of cytologic findings in neuroendocrine carcinomas including carcinoid tumors with histologic correlation. Cancer 90(3):148–161
33. Travis WD et al (1998) Survival analysis of 200 pulmonary neuroendocrine tumors with clarification of criteria for atypical carcinoid and its separation from typical carcinoid. Am J Surg Pathol 22(8):934–944
34. Johnston WW (1985) The malignant pleural effusion. A review of cytopathologic diagnoses of 584 specimens from 472 consecutive patients. Cancer 56(4):905–909

Chapter 5
Liver Cytology

Deborah J. Chute, Marc Sarti and Kristen A. Atkins

5.1 Introduction

Cytologic evaluation of the liver is largely restricted to focal, mass-forming lesions [1]. The diagnosis of diffuse parenchymal diseases of the liver relies in a large part upon the histologic architecture. For example, diagnosing and grading the activity of chronic hepatitis requires assessment of the pattern of lymphocytes infiltrating the portal tracts and/or lobules. A fine needle aspiration biopsy (FNAB) would contain hepatocytes and inflammatory cells but would lack the architecture necessary to assess the etiology and amount of hepatic damage. Conversely, a definitive diagnosis is often obtained in FNABs of discrete hepatic lesions.

As in other sites, FNAB has several advantages over traditional core biopsy. One of the greatest benefits is rapid on-site evaluation for adequacy of material. The cytologist can determine if lesional material is present and triage the material for additional studies such as flow cytometric analysis, microbiologic culture, or cytogenetics. FNAB also allows for increased sampling of large masses.

Liver FNAB is primarily used for diagnosis and staging. In general, diagnostic use occurs when FNAB is performed in a patient with a new liver mass and no history of prior disease. Staging FNAB typically occurs in a patient with a known malignancy, and confirmation of liver metastasis is needed for staging and treatment purposes (i.e., colon carcinoma metastasis to the liver). These cases less

D. J. Chute
Cleveland Clinic Department of Anatomic Pathology, 9500 Euclid Avenue L25,
Cleveland, OH 44195, USA

M. Sarti
Medical Director of Ultrasound and Cross-Sectional International Radiology Department
of Radiology, 1215 Lee Street, 800170, Charlottesville, VA 22908, USA

K. A. Atkins (✉)
Department of Pathology, University of Virginia Medical System,
1215 Lee St Office 3034, Charlottesville, VA 22908, USA
e-mail: kaa2p@virginia.edu

R. Nayar (ed.), *Cytopathology in Oncology,*
Cancer Treatment and Research 160, DOI: 10.1007/978-3-642-38850-7_5,
© Springer-Verlag Berlin Heidelberg 2014

Table 5.1 Clinical presentations to consider when evaluating hepatic lesions for tissue diagnosis

Clinical presentation	Suggested tissue procurement
Diffuse hepatic process	Proceed to core biopsy
Suspect primary liver process	
Background cirrhosis	Combined FNA and core biopsy for optimal sensitivity
Background normal	FNA with on-site assessment for triage, possible cell block or core biopsy based on these results
Suspect metastasis	
Known primary, need tissue diagnosis for staging	FNA with on-site assessment for adequacy, additional studies not likely needed
Known primary, need tissue for special studies	FNA with on-site assessment for adequacy with cell block or core biopsy
No known primary	FNA with on-site assessment for triage, likely will need cell block or core biopsy for special studies
Suspect hematolymphoid neoplasm	FNA with on-site assessment for triage, additional passes for flow cytometry and cytogenetics. If appears large cell, cell block or core biopsy needed for immunohistochemistry

FNA Fine needle aspiration

commonly require special studies, as comparison to the patient's prior material will frequently confirm the diagnosis. An exception to this is when special testing is desired (i.e., k-ras mutation in colon cancer, ER/PR/Her2Neu status in breast cancer). Discussion of the specific needs of the FNAB with the radiologist and/or pathologist, prior to the procedure, will help to ensure that adequate material is obtained for diagnosis and special studies.

The clinical assessment and radiologic findings can help assess the utility of FNAB. This can be summarized by a few questions:

- Is the process focal or diffuse?
- Does the patient have underlying cirrhosis?
- Is there a history of prior malignancy?

Table 5.1 shows general responses to these questions and their impact on the preferred type of tissue procurement.

5.2 Procuring a Cytologic Specimen

5.2.1 Patient Preparation for Biopsy

Adequate pre-procedure planning is necessary to minimize patient risk and limit the severity of biopsy-related complications. Platelet count, prothrombin time (PT), international normalized ratio (INR), partial thromboplastin time (PTT), and complete blood count (CBC) should be obtained within 4–6 weeks prior to biopsy.

A medical history review, with special attention paid to bleeding risk (i.e., medications, clotting disorders, liver or renal failure, etc.) should be performed at least 1 week in advance of the biopsy, as prolonged cessation of certain drugs may be necessary.

The only absolute contraindication to a percutaneous fine needle aspiration biopsy is lack of a safe access route. In practice, the majority of all liver lesions can be percutaneously sampled without transgression of a vital structure.

Several relative contraindications are recognized. An uncooperative patient will be at risk for a parenchymal tear during biopsy and conscious sedation or general anesthesia may be necessary. Biopsy in the setting of extrahepatic biliary obstruction is associated with an increased risk of biliary peritonitis, septicemia, and death; consequently, the benefit of cytologic diagnosis must significantly outweigh risk, and, if possible, a transjugular approach is preferable [2, 3]. Highly vascular tumors such as suspected hepatoma or hemangioma may be safely sampled, provided the biopsy needle traverses normal hepatic parenchyma, as this approach minimizes the risk of direct hemorrhage into the peritoneum. Anecdotal evidence of adverse outcomes in the setting of tense ascites, ranging from poor biopsy yield to increased bleeding, have not been substantiated in randomized, controlled trials; however, it is reasonable to perform a total paracentesis prior to biopsy in such cases.

The most commonly cited relative contraindication to liver biopsy is coagulopathy. Although opinions diverge regarding values at which abnormal coagulation indices become contraindications to biopsy, common practice is to ensure the INR is ≤ 1.5 and the platelet count is $>50,000$/ml [4, 5]. Correlation between INR and bleeding risk is poor in patients with cirrhosis; as such, biopsy may be performed in the setting of mild elevation of the INR (≤ 2.0), provided the platelet count is optimized ($>100,000$/ml) [6]. Aspirin or other nonsteroidal anti-inflammatory drugs must be avoided for 1 week prior to biopsy to ensure proper platelet function. Coumadin or heparin must be discontinued, with laboratory confirmation of normal coagulation parameters prior to biopsy. Although poor renal function is not a contraindication to biopsy, knowledge of renal impairment is critical, as patients on hemodialysis are at higher risk for hemorrhage, independent of bleeding time, due to abnormalities in platelet function.

5.2.2 Imaging Guidance: Ultrasound Versus Computed Tomography

Historically, ultrasound guidance was reserved for percutaneous biopsies of moderate to large peripheral hepatic lesions; computed tomography (CT) was used for lesions that were considered more difficult to access [7]. However, advances in ultrasound technology have led to tremendous improvements in the visualization of small and deep hepatic lesions, even in large patients. In a recent study of 64 consecutive patients with 74 hepatic lesions, all ≤1 cm, ultrasound-guided biopsy yielded a true-malignant diagnosis in 44 of 45 lesions (sensitivity of 98 %) [8].

Ultrasound has two distinct advantages over CT. First, ultrasound provides real-time visualization of the needle. This allows reorientation of the needle as it approaches the lesion, enables compensation for respiratory motion, and minimizes the risk of biopsy related injury. Furthermore, visualization of needle excursion during the biopsy itself facilitates sampling of distinct portions of a lesion. Real-time needle observation is possible with CT fluoroscopy, but this technique exposes both patient and operator to significant radiation and should be reserved for lesions which are very difficult to access, and only visible on CT. Second, ultrasound guided biopsy can be performed in any plane, including nonaxial planes, whereas CT guided biopsies are best performed in axial or near-axial planes. Consequently, ultrasound facilitates sampling of lesions in difficult locations, such as behind a rib or in the hepatic dome.

Computed tomography guidance is reserved for those lesions which are not visible sonographically. Most commonly, sonographically occult lesions are difficult to appreciate on noncontrast CT and only visible on contrast enhanced studies.

5.2.3 Biopsy Technique

Whether using ultrasound or CT, an image guided biopsy begins with finding the lesion. Pre-procedure scanning with ultrasound allows the operator to determine the safest access route and the optimal transducer; high frequency transducers (7–12 mHz) are preferred for shallow, peripheral lesions, and low frequency transducers (2–5 mHz) are preferred for deep lesions. When using CT, a non-contrast pre-procedure scan is performed through the liver. If the lesion is known to be occult on noncontrast CT, intravenous iodinated contrast is administered during the planning scan to facilitate visualization of the lesion and to provide guidance for the subsequent biopsy. Alternatively, if HCC is strongly suspected, intra-arterial administration of iodized oil such as lipiodol may be performed 6–13 days prior to the biopsy. If a lesion takes up lipiodol, it will have high density at CT, and intravenous administration of contrast will not be necessary; however, strong uptake of lipiodol is considered near diagnostic for HCC, sufficient to warrant treatment without biopsy.

Ultrasound guided biopsies are performed using the freehand technique or using a needle guide. When using the freehand technique, the transducer and needle are held in separate hands and positioned to allow simultaneous visualization of both needle and lesion. When using a needle guide, the needle is effectively attached to the transducer and directed along its imaging axis (Fig. 5.1). With either technique, both needle and lesion are visualized in real time as the needle is advanced to the lesion, allowing the operator to constantly correct the trajectory. The choice of technique depends on operator experience and comfort, and results are likely similar.

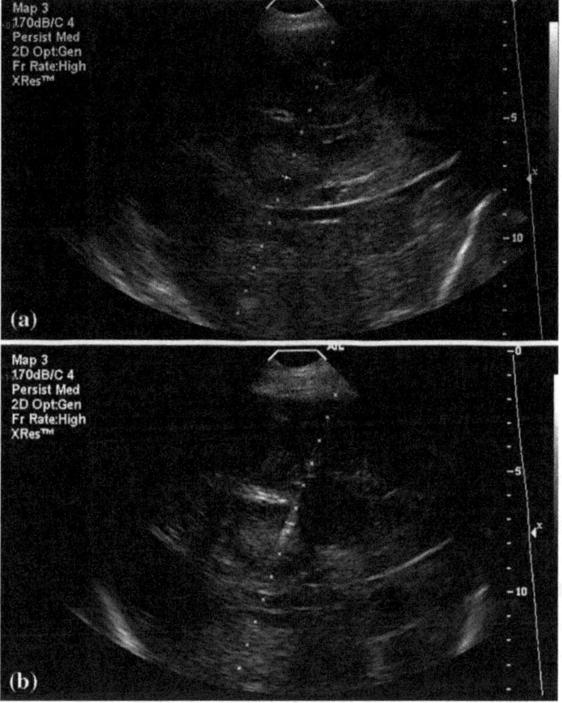

Fig. 5.1 Ultrasound image of a solid liver lesion (**a**) with needle attached to the transducer and visualized in the mass (**b**)

When using CT guidance, percutaneous access is determined by selecting the axial image from the planning scan which contains the lesion, and noting the level of the lesion along the cranio-caudad axis; this level is projected on the patient by a laser. Determining the percutaneous entry site in the left–right axis is performed by measuring distance from the midline on both the planning scan and the patient. As the planning scan is performed prior to the biopsy, it is essential that the patient should not move between the scan and the marking of the skin. The biopsy is then performed by advancing the needle stepwise, performing repeat scans through the needle to confirm advancement toward the lesion (Fig. 5.2). CT fluoroscopy allows visualization of the needle in real time as images are constantly acquired as the needle is advanced to the lesion, but results in a significant radiation to both the operator and patient.

FNAB or core biopsy may be performed using the coaxial technique, in which a single percutaneous pass is made by a large bore needle (17–20 gauge) and multiple biopsies are performed through this access needle, or the noncoaxial technique, in which multiple percutaneous passes are made with the biopsy needle (20–22 gauge). The theoretical disadvantage of the coaxial technique is an increased risk of bleeding, as the coaxial needle may be significantly larger than the biopsy needle. However, a retrospective study of 1,060 patients who underwent image-guided hepatic or renal biopsies showed no difference in complication rates between the noncoaxial or coaxial biopsy methods [9]. Another potential disadvantage of the

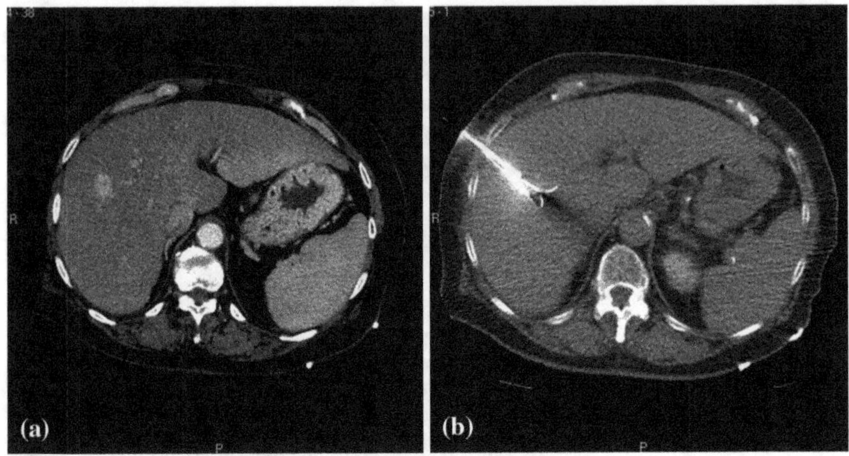

Fig. 5.2 CT scan of a hepatic mass (**a**) with needle seen transversing the lesion (**b**)

coaxial technique is that multiple biopsies are obtained along the same needle path, limiting the spatial distribution of the biopsies and possibly leading to sampling error. The theoretical advantage of the coaxial technique is decreased tumor seeding along the biopsy tract. Indeed, a recent retrospective study of 101 patients with coaxial percutaneous biopsy yielding HCC had a tumor seeding rate of 0 %, a significant result when compared to a meta-analysis showing a needle tract tumor seeding rate of 2.7 % following biopsy of HCC [10, 11].

The decision to perform FNA or core biopsy is in part determined by the presence or absence of a cytopathologist. It is recognized that an accurate cytologic diagnosis is more likely when a cytopathologist is present during the biopsy procedure [12]. Consequently, if FNAB yields a definitive diagnosis at the time of the biopsy, core biopsy is not necessary. However, if a cytopathologist is absent, both FNA and core biopsy should be performed, unless the patient is at increased risk of bleeding. The value of this approach is confirmed by evidence that FNA and core biopsy show increased diagnostic sensitivity in combination, when compared to either FNA or core biopsy alone (described in further detail below) [13].

5.2.4 Biopsy/Imaging Discordance and Management of HCC

It is necessary to confirm concordance of imaging and pathologic findings following the biopsy of any focal hepatic lesion. If discordance is present, i.e., a benign pathologic result when malignancy is strongly expected, a repeat biopsy is usually performed. Alternatively, if a focal hepatic lesion yields only hepatocytes or normal hepatic parenchyma, a repeat biopsy is performed, unless focal nodular hyperplasia or hepatic adenomas are strongly suspected.

If hepatocellular carcinoma is suspected at imaging, biopsy confirmation may not be necessary to initiate treatment. The European Association for the Study of the Liver has developed criteria for the diagnosis and clinical management of hepatocellular carcinoma; these criteria are currently in widespread use [14]. Characteristic imaging features of HCC in the cirrhotic liver include a focal hypo- or hyperechoic nodule at ultrasound, or focal arterial hypervascularity at CT, MRI, or angiography. As imaging is insufficiently accurate in the diagnosis of small HCCs (<2 cm) pathologic confirmation is recommended. Alternatively, very small lesions (<1 cm) may be closely followed at 3-month intervals, and sampled if growing. Lesions larger than 2 cm within a cirrhotic liver, imaging alone may confidently establish the diagnosis of HCC [15, 16]. Furthermore, a negative biopsy of a large nodule with imaging characteristics of HCC should not be used to rule out malignancy. Consequently, radiologic criteria were developed stating that in the setting of cirrhosis, detection of a focal lesion >2 cm having characteristic features of HCC on two separate imaging tests is sufficient to confirm the diagnosis. Alternatively, combined criteria were developed stating that in the setting of markedly elevated alpha-fetoprotein levels (>400 ng/ml) a single radiologic examination showing a focal lesion >2 cm with arterial hypervascularization is sufficient to confirm the diagnosis of HCC.

5.2.5 Diagnostic Accuracy of Liver FNA

The accuracy of liver FNAB of focal liver lesions ranges from 73 to 94 %, with sensitivities and specificities ranging from 80 to 95 % and 87 to 100 %, respectively. In comparison [17–27] , the diagnostic accuracy of liver core biopsy for focal liver lesions ranges from 67 to 95 %, with a sensitivity of 61–89 %, and specificity near 100 % [18, 19, 27, 28].

Some studies have focused specifically on the ability of FNAB to diagnose focal liver lesions suspicious for hepatocellular carcinoma in patients with underlying cirrhosis. The accuracy of liver FNAB in this setting ranges from 69 to 85 % sensitivity and 93 to 100 % specificity [17, 22, 29–31]. This is likely due in part to the difficulty of FNAB to distinguish well-differentiated hepatocellular carcinoma from a regenerative cirrhotic nodule. Comparisons to liver core biopsy in this setting show a similar sensitivity (66 %) and specificity (100 %). However, when FNAB and core biopsy are used in combination, the sensitivity and specificity increase to 90 % and 100 %, respectively [29–31].

The nondiagnostic rate for liver FNAB of focal masses is reported to range from 1 to 29 % [23, 24, 27]. The nearly 30 % nondiagnostic rate was observed in a community practice setting with radiologists and pathologists relatively new to the procedure [24]. A nondiagnostic sample is variably defined by authors as blood only, or can include normal-appearing hepatic parenchyma. When assessing the accuracy and sensitivity of liver FNAB, these nondiagnostic cases are not included, so the values reported above may be somewhat elevated; for example, the accuracy of liver

FNAB including all cases in one study was 78 %, but when nondiagnostic cases were excluded the accuracy was 93 % [27]. This indicates that when material is present, pathologists are good at making a diagnosis on liver aspirate material.

The primary causes of a nondiagnostic specimen are sampling errors and scant or noninterpretable specimens. This can be significantly improved with rapid on-site evaluation. The impact of on-site evaluation has been well established in other body sites, including breast, thyroid, head and neck, and lung and lymph nodes, but few studies have focused on this issue in liver diagnosis [26, 32–39]. One study that directly compared the unsatisfactory rate of focal liver lesion FNABs with and without immediate on-site assessment found the unsatisfactory rates were 17 % and 33 %, respectively [32]. When rapid on-site evaluation was implemented at our institution, the nondiagnostic rate dropped from 16 to 11 % (personal experience).

5.2.6 Complications of Liver FNA

Complications of percutaneous fine needle aspiration biopsy are rare, occurring in less than 0.5 % of patients (3 % if pain is included in complications), with death resulting in less than 0.03 % of patients [40, 41]. The majority of the fatal complications were secondary to hemorrhage [18, 41–44]. Other rare complications reported include bile peritonitis, bile-venous fistulas, anaphylaxis (after aspiration of a hydatid cyst), and carcinoid crisis [45–47]. Endoscopic trans-gastric FNA of the liver is similar, with a reported complication rate between 0.5 and 2 %, the most common of which is pain, followed by fever, hemorrhage, sepsis, and death (0.05 %) [48, 49].

One of the most worrisome potential complications in an oncology patient is tumor seeding along the needle tract, which has been reported to occur in approximately 2 % of patients [50–59]. More recent reports suggest this occurs even less frequently when needles of 21 gauge or smaller are used; earlier studies included patients who had procedures using 18-gauge needles [57].

The literature is mixed regarding whether patients with hepatocellular carcinoma have a higher risk of extrahepatic tumor spread after core needle biopsy and/or FNAB. Saborido et al. compared patients with and without preoperative FNAB who underwent orthotopic liver transplant for HCC. They found a significantly increased risk of extrahepatic HCC recurrence after transplant in patients who underwent FNAB (27 %) compared to those who did not have a preoperative biopsy (2 %) [60]. However, the patients who underwent FNABs had significantly larger intrahepatic tumors, higher tumor stage, and worse Childs classification. Overall survival was not significantly different between patients with and without preoperative FNAB. In addition, the primary site of extrahepatic involvement was lung metastasis, not needle tract seeding. Because of these risks, some authors have advocated diagnosis of HCC by radiologic and serologic studies, without definitive tissue diagnosis prior to surgery [61]. Ng et al. performed a similar study, but did not find a significant difference in patient outcome or tumor characteristics between patient groups. They found no statistical difference in extrahepatic recurrence after OLT in patients who underwent preoperative FNAB compared to those who did not undergo FNAB [62]. Due to the contradictory information available regarding FNAB in patient with hepatocellular carcinoma, it is unclear whether these patients are truly at increased risk of tumor seeding.

5.3 Cytologic Findings

5.3.1 Normal Liver

Normal liver is characterized by small irregular sheets of cells and single cells. Hepatocytes have a low nuclear to cytoplasmic ratio, a centrally placed round nucleus and often cytoplasmic bile pigment and lipofuscin (Fig. 5.3). Usually small clusters of bile epithelium are present. Bile duct epithelium is composed of sheets of cells with a high nuclear to cytoplasmic ratio. The cell borders are distinct, form a honeycomb pattern, and the nuclei are centrally placed. This uniformity to the bile duct cells is extremely important when evaluating for a bile duct lesion.

5.3.2 Benign Tumors

5.3.2.1 Focal Nodular Hyperplasia

Focal nodular hyperplasia is a benign liver lesion, which typically presents as a solitary liver mass in a young woman. The etiology of these lesions is unclear, but is thought to be a focal vascular lesion. The classic radiographic finding is a central scar, which when present allows for a presumptive diagnosis. Histologically, focal

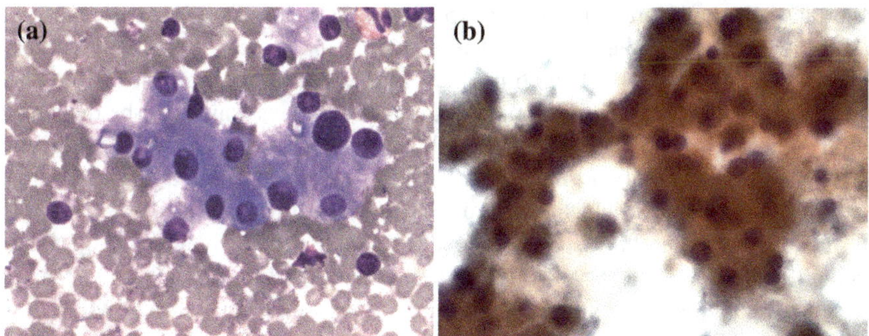

Fig. 5.3 Normal liver demonstrating large round nuclei, prominent nucleoli, and abundant granular cytoplasm (**a** Diff Quik, 400× and **b** Papanicolaou stain 400×)

nodular hyperplasia demonstrates nodules of normal hepatocytes separated by radiating fibrous septae from a central scar. The fibrous septae contain a bile duct proliferation and scattered vascular structures.

The cytologic appearance of focal nodular hyperplasia on fine needle aspiration is nonspecific. The aspirates will contain benign-appearing hepatocytes without significant atypia and scattered bile duct epithelium. This is identical to the cytologic appearance of normal liver, regenerating nodules in cirrhosis, and hepatic adenoma. Liver core biopsy suffers from similar difficulties, and the same differential diagnosis applies. Clinical and radiologic correlation is required for this diagnosis.

5.3.2.2 Hepatic Adenoma

Hepatic adenoma is a benign solitary liver neoplasm of young women, particularly those with a history of oral contraceptive use. The presenting complaint is most commonly abdominal pain. Occasionally, adenomas can rupture, resulting in severe intraperitoneal hemorrhage. Histologically, hepatic adenomas have a proliferation of benign-appearing hepatocytes with normal 2-cell-thick hepatic plate architecture, but lack portal tracts. Occasional veins and arteries are present, but there is a conspicuous lack of bile duct epithelium within the lesion.

The cytologic findings of hepatic adenoma on FNAB include a predominance of hepatocytes with minimal atypia, and an absence of bile duct epithelium. The differential diagnosis include normal liver, focal nodular hyperplasia, and well-differentiated hepatocellular carcinoma. While the absence of bile duct epithelium would appear to exclude normal liver and focal nodular hyperplasia, in practice bile duct epithelium may or may not be seen due to variable sampling in all these lesions. Clinical and radiologic correlation is required for this diagnosis.

5.3.2.3 Bile Duct Adenoma/Hamartoma (von Meyenburg Complex)

Bile duct adenomas are solitary, subcapsular nodules less than 1 cm. Because of the location and size, they are frequently found at the time of abdominal surgery for other conditions, at which time they mimic metastatic deposits. Bile duct hamartomas (von Meyenburg complex) are small nodules which can be dispersed throughout the liver. Histologically, both contain a proliferation of benign bile ducts which are typically arranged in a haphazard manner within a fibrous stroma.

Bile duct adenomas and hamartomas are infrequently aspirated for cytologic evaluation. Aspirates are usually hypocellular, and contain bland bile duct epithelium in cohesive sheets and forming glandular structures. Commonly, benign hepatocytes are also present due to sampling of the normal liver around the lesion. The differential diagnosis includes normal liver and a well-differentiated cholangiocarcinoma (which is usually larger and much more cellular).

5.3.3 Primary Malignant Hepatic Tumors

5.3.3.1 Hepatocellular Carcinoma

The majority of hepatocellular carcinomas (HCC) are seen in older patients in the setting of cirrhosis. HCCs can present as a solitary lesion or as multiple nodules. The prototypic histologic feature of HCC is loss of the normal liver architecture. Specifically, the hepatic cords are thickened (> 2 cells in thickness) with trabecular or acinar growth patterns and loss of portal tracts. The specific morphologic appearance of HCC on histology and cytology varies depending on the degree of differentiation of the tumor.

Well-differentiated hepatocellular carcinoma closely resembles normal liver (see Table 5.2). Histologically, the hepatic cords are thickened with prominent sinusoidal vessels. The hepatocytes typically show mild nuclear atypia. The cytologic correlate to this histology is highly cellular smears with cells that resemble normal hepatocytes, but which show an increased nuclear to cytoplasmic ratio (less cytoplasm) and large nuclei containing prominent nucleoli. The most specific finding on aspirate specimens is the presence of prominent spindled endothelial cells rimming groups of hepatocytes, highlighting the thickened hepatic cord architecture seen on histology [63–65] (Fig. 5.4). This imparts a smooth outline to the cellular groups, rather than the discohesive, frayed edge appearance seen in normal liver. However, this finding is not always present, which can cause significant difficulty in differentiating neoplastic liver from a benign process. The differential diagnosis of a well-differentiated hepatocellular carcinoma include hepatic adenoma, a regenerative nodule in cirrhosis, and focal nodular hyperplasia. A concurrent core biopsy and reticulin stain can be very useful in such cases.

Poorly differentiated hepatocellular carcinoma can have a variety of histologic appearances ranging from gland-like structures to spindled cells. The cytologic diagnosis of poorly differentiated hepatocellular carcinoma encounters similar difficulties as the histologic diagnosis; the aspirates are clearly malignant, but determining hepatocellular differentiation can be difficult. The aspirate smears are typically highly cellular, and the neoplastic cells form sheets, gland-like structures, or may be single cells with moderate to severe atypia and numerous mitotic figures (see Table 5.3). Tumor giant cells are commonly seen. The most helpful cytologic features to suggest poorly differentiated hepatocellular carcinoma are polygonal cells with centrally placed nuclei, and intracytoplasmic bile. Spindled endothelial cells separating neoplastic groups, similar to that seen in well-differentiated hepatocellular carcinoma is often lost in more poorly differentiated tumors.

The differential diagnosis of poorly differentiated hepatocellular carcinoma includes, but is not limited to cholangiocarcinoma, metastatic carcinoma, and malignant melanoma. In this setting, cell block material or core biopsy for immunohistochemical stains can be particularly useful in distinguishing hepatocellular carcinoma from other tumors (see Table 5.2). Hepatocyte paraffin 1 (HepPar1) antibody is highly sensitive and specific for normal liver and hepatic

Table 5.2 Comparison of the cytologic features of hepatocytic lesions

	Architecture	Cells	Other features
Normal liver	Large tissue fragments with frayed edges Thin ribbons Single cells	Polygonal cells Low N/C ratio Abundant granular cytoplasm Central round nuclei Prominent nucleoli	Occasional pigment (bile, lipofuscin, iron)
Cirrhosis	Similar to normal liver	Similar to normal liver Focal atypia with marked variation in nuclear size, prominent nucleoli	Pigment frequently prominent (bile, lipofuscin, iron)
HCC—Well-differentiated	Cords, nests and sheets Thickened trabeculae (>3 cells) rimmed by spindle-shaped endothelial cells Smooth tissue fragment contours	Polygonal cells Central nuclei Increased N/C ratio Monomorphous appearance Macronucleoli Mitotic figures	Background containing large naked nuclei Intracytoplasmic bile
HCC—Poorly differentiated	Cords, nests, sheets, glands, and single cells Rarely show endothelial cell rimming	Polygonal cells High N/C ratio Moderate to marked pleomorphism May have vacuolated or clear cytoplasm	Presence of intracytoplasmic bile
Cholangiocarcinoma	Sheets, 3-dimensional clusters and single cells Acinar arrangements with lumen formation	Cuboidal/columnar cells Increased N/C ratio Large eccentric nuclei with variable pleomorphism Scant cytoplasm	No bile Mucin may be present Benign hepatocytes in background

HCC hepatocellular carcinoma *N/C* nuclear to cytoplasmic

neoplasms [66, 67]. In situ hybridization for albumin RNA is similarly highly sensitive and specific for hepatic processes [68, 69]. Hepatocellular carcinoma is negative for keratin antibodies (i.e., AE1/3, MOC31), which will stain metastatic carcinomas and cholangiocarcinoma, and is not immunoreactive for antibodies typically used to highlight melanoma (S100, HMB45, MelanA) [70–74].

Fibrolamellar hepatocellular carcinoma is an uncommon variant of HCC that occurs in younger patients (20–30 s) without underlying parenchymal liver disease. This subtype of HCC should be distinguished from well-differentiated HCC, as the prognosis is better [75]. The histologic appearance of fibrolamellar hepatocellular carcinoma is distinctive; dense bands of fibrosis surround extremely large, polygonal cells with abundant eosinophilic cytoplasm. On cytology specimens, fibrolamellar HCC shows large single cells with abundant cytoplasm and large nuclei with prominent nucleoli. Intra-nuclear inclusions and binucleated cells are frequent. These cells are much larger than normal hepatocytes and well-differentiated

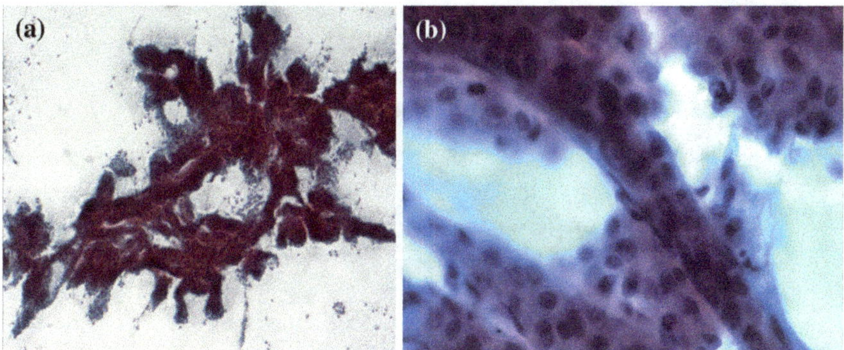

Fig. 5.4 Hepatocellular carcinoma demonstrating the smooth contours to the cellular aggregates (**a** Papanicolaou stain 100×) and the flattened endothelial cells wrapping around the aggregates of hepatocytes (**b** Papanicolaou stain 400×)

Table 5.3 Immunohistochemical and histochemical stains useful in the differential diagnosis of liver tumors

	Hepatocellular carcinoma	Cholangiocarcinoma	Metastatic colon carcinoma	Metastatic lung adenocarcinoma
Bile	+	−	−	−
Mucin	−	+	+	±
CAM5.2	+	+	+	+
CK 7	−	+	−	+
CK 20	−	−	+	−
CEA	p+[a]	m+[a]	m+[a]	m+[a]
TTF-1	−[b]	−	−	+
HepPar1	+	−	−	−
AFP	+	−	−	−
ISH albumin	+	−	−	−

[a] Polyclonal CEA (p) will show a canalicular pattern in hepatocellular carcinoma; monoclonal CEA (m) will be negative in hepatocellular carcinoma and will be positive in cholangiocarcinoma and other metastatic adenocarcinomas
[b] TTF-1 frequently shows a high cytoplasmic background in hepatocytes, but will not show nuclear staining as seen with pulmonary and thyroid carcinomas

hepatocellular carcinoma. The nuclear to cytoplasmic ratio is reduced, which is the opposite of well-differentiated usual type HCC. The cytoplasm of fibrolamellar carcinoma may contain intracytoplasmic globules, and occasionally the aspirate may obtain fibrous tissue.

5.3.3.2 Cholangiocarcinoma

Cholangiocarcinoma arises in the extrahepatic or intrahepatic bile ducts. When in the liver, cholangiocarcinoma can present as a solitary mass or as multiple lesions.

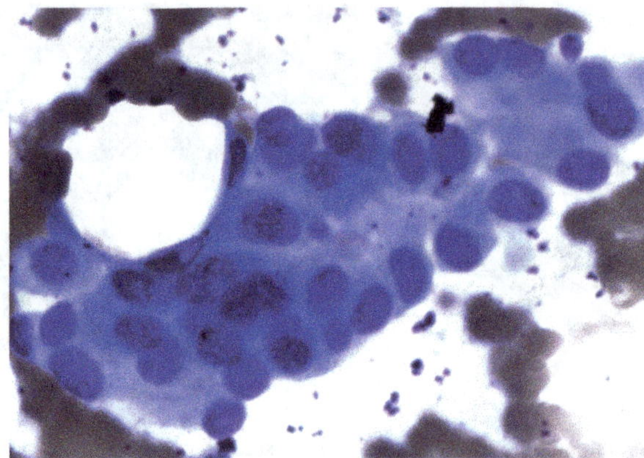

Fig. 5.5 Gland formation characteristic of adenocarcinoma/cholangiocarcinoma (Diff Quik, power?)

Histologically, the tumor cells form irregular glands infiltrating a fibrous, desmoplastic stroma. Cytologically, the neoplastic cells are generally columnar or cuboidal, forming sheets, three dimensional clusters, or glandular structures (Fig. 5.5). Well-differentiated cholangiocarcinomas often show minimal atypia, and are difficult to distinguish by morphology from benign ductal epithelium. However, even in benign bile duct proliferations, the cellularity of the aspirate is low, while cholangiocarcinomas generally have much more material and the groups are larger. Bile is not a component of cholangiocarcinomas, as typically the tumor cells do not have a connection with the normal biliary system. Intracytoplasmic bile supports hepatocellular carcinoma. Benign hepatocytes are often present in the background, but represent a minority of the cells (Fig. 5.6).

Moderately and poorly differentiated cholangiocarcinomas are cytologically indistinguishable from metastatic adenocarcinomas. A panel of immunohistochemical stains can help in differentiating cholangiocarcinoma from some other

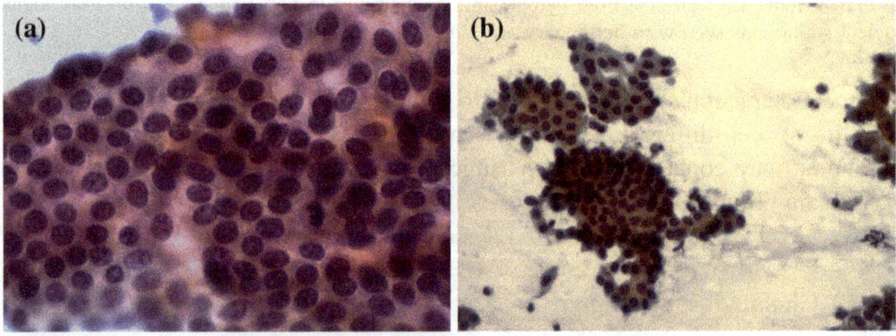

Fig. 5.6 Well-differentiated cholangiocarcinoma is characterized by sheets of cells with only mild atypia (**a** Papanicolaou stain 400×). The sheer volume of bile duct epithelium aids in making the diagnosis (**b** Papanicolaou stain 100×)

primary sites (see Table 5.2), but certain tumors (i.e., pancreatic ductal adeno-carcinoma) are indistinguishable even with ancillary studies. Poorly differentiated hepatocellular carcinoma is also in the differential diagnosis of cholangiocarci-noma, but positive immunohistochemistry with antibodies against alpha fetal protein and HepPar1 are highly sensitive and specific for HCC [66, 67].

Rarely a combined hepatocellular carcinoma/cholangiocarcinoma can be seen.

5.3.3.3 Hepatic Vascular Tumors

Vascular tumors are the most common nonepithelial tumor of the liver; the majority of these are cavernous hemangiomas which are often diagnosed by radiology alone. Histologically, cavernous hemangiomas have large, blood-filled spaces lined by bland endothelial cells. FNAB of hemangiomas typically yields only blood and very infrequently benign spindled endothelial cells. Bleeding complications and rarely death have been reported after fine needle aspiration or core biopsy of vascular lesions, so careful consideration should be given to whether tissue diagnosis is needed in these cases [44].

Angiosarcoma is an uncommon malignant vascular tumor that is associated with cirrhosis and exposure to high levels of vinyl chloride monomers or thorium dioxide. Angiosarcoma is characterized histologically by malignant spindle cells, which can range in architecture from well-formed vascular channels to solid, epithelioid sheets. When aspirated, the cytology shows abundant blood with similar variability in the cellular component. Well-differentiated angiosarcomas often have elongated spindle cells forming groups and syncytia, while poorly differentiated angiosarcomas can have spindled or epithelioid cells with large pleomorphic nuclei and tumor giant cells (Fig. 5.7). The presence of intracyto-plasmic lumens (which appear as well-demarcated cytoplasmic bubbles) can be helpful in suggesting this diagnosis. Cell block preparations and core biopsies

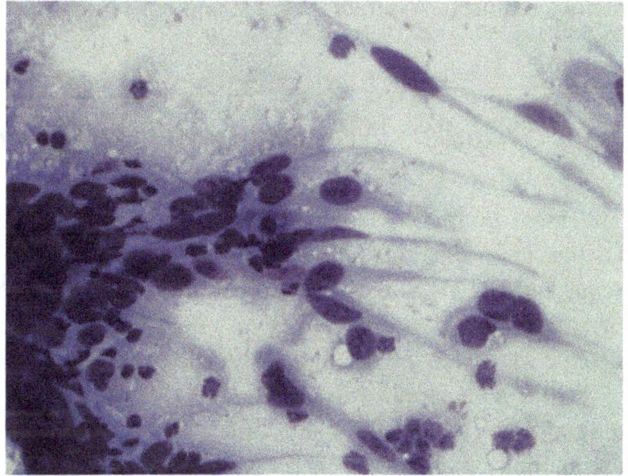

Fig. 5.7 Vascular tumors can be challenging to aspirate given their inherent blood volume. Solid areas in high grade lesions, however, often yield diagnostic atypical spindled cells (Diff Quick stain 200×)

assist in recognizing an anastomosing vascular architecture and allow immuno-histochemical staining for vascular markers.

Epithelioid hemangioendothelioma is a rare tumor that can occur in the liver and is found in women more frequently than men. It has an intermediate prognosis between cavernous hemangiomas (benign) and angiosarcoma (malignant). These tumors are typically solid and multifocal, often inciting a sclerotic tissue response. Histologically the cells appear epithelioid (round rather than spindled) and vascular spaces are difficult to appreciate. Because of the sclerotic background, cytology aspirates are commonly hypocellular. When present, the neoplastic cells are large, epithelioid, and often bizarre, mimicking a poorly differentiated hepatocellular carcinoma. Immunohistochemical stains on cell block preparations or core biopsy are often essential to make this diagnosis.

5.3.3.4 Hepatoblastoma

Hepatoblastoma, albeit rare, is the most common primary hepatic malignancy in children. It most commonly affects children less than 2 years of age. Unlike HCC in the pediatric population, hepatoblastoma is not associated with cirrhosis, viruses, or storage diseases. Hepatoblastomas sometimes secrete HCG and children may present with precocious puberty. Survival depends on the completeness of excision, and is over 70 % when tumors are stage 1 or stage 2 [76, 77].

Histologically hepatoblastoma presents as three subtypes which are often mixed. These include fetal, embryonal, and small cell undifferentiated subtypes. The cytologic features will depend on the type of pattern sampled. Additionally, hepatoblastoma often contains heterologous elements (bone and smooth muscle) and extramedullary hematopoiesis; if these components are sampled they can lead to misdiagnosis. When small cell undifferentiated forms are seen, the cytologic differential diagnosis includes many other pediatric small blue cell tumors (metastatic Wilms tumor, neuroblastoma, rhabdomyosarcoma, Ewing's sarcoma, hematolymphoid malignancies). For pediatric tumors, tissue for ancillary studies is almost always required. Aspirate material and core biopsy are ideal in tissue procurement.

5.3.4 Secondary Neoplasms (Metastatic Tumors)

The most common diagnosis on liver FNAB is metastatic disease [78]. Liver lesions are frequently identified during staging of malignancies by PET or CT scan, and FNAB is a quick and minimally invasive method to obtain tissue confirmation of metastasis. However, not infrequently, fine needle aspiration of a hepatic mass may be the first diagnosis of advanced disease from another location.

While any neoplasm can involve the liver, the most common tumors to be diagnosed by FNAB are metastatic colon cancer, pancreatic adenocarcinoma, lung carcinoma, melanoma, and lymphoma. Mesenchymal tumor metastasis is

Fig. 5.8 Metastatic colon adenocarcinoma demonstrating the characteristic glands with tall columnar cells. Note the extensive granular debris ("dirty necrosis") in the background (Papanicolaou stain, 200×)

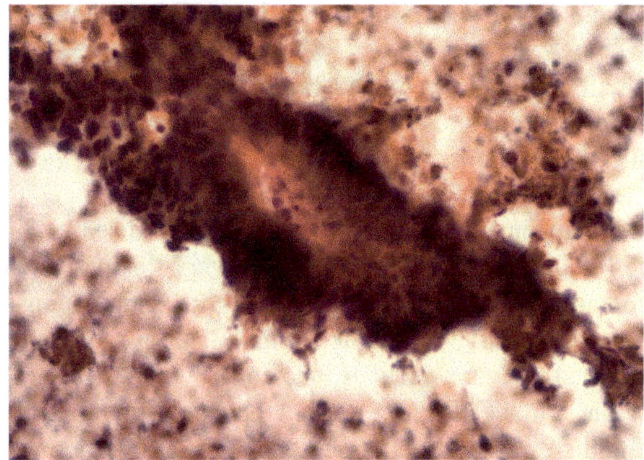

extremely uncommon, but when present are most commonly gastrointestinal stromal tumors (GISTs) or leiomyosarcomas. The cytologic appearance of metastatic tumors is very similar to that seen at other sites. The following section will briefly describe the cytologic findings in the most frequent metastatic tumors to the liver; the reader is directed to the appropriate chapter for any given neoplasm for a more in-depth discussion of the clinical and cytologic features.

5.3.4.1 Metastatic Colon Carcinoma

Colon carcinoma is the most common liver metastasis. The cytologic features are distinctive: tall columnar epithelium with hyperchromatic, elongated, and oval nuclei which are basally located forming a so-called "picket fence" arrangement, in a background of extensive necrosis (Fig. 5.8). Colon carcinomas frequently produce extracellular and intracytoplasmic mucin. When poorly differentiated, the morphology can be nonspecific; in this instance immunohistochemistry can be helpful in distinguishing colorectal carcinoma from other adenocarcinomas.

5.3.4.2 Pancreatic Ductal Carcinoma

Pancreatic ductal carcinoma frequently metastasizes to lymph nodes and liver. The cytologic features of pancreatic ductal carcinoma include three dimensional groups of cuboidal or low columnar cells with mild to severe nuclear atypia. As discussed previously, the cytologic and immunohistochemical features of well-differentiated pancreatic ductal carcinoma can be indistinguishable from cholangiocarcinoma. In this situation, comparison of prior pathology to the liver lesion or correlation with imaging findings is most helpful in determining the primary site.

5.3.4.3 Small Cell Undifferentiated Carcinoma

Small cell undifferentiated carcinoma most commonly arises in the lung, but can occur in other sites such as pancreas, colon, and cervix. Regardless of the primary site, these tumors are aggressive and frequently present at high stage with nodal metastasis and/or liver metastasis. Therefore, liver FNAB is often employed for simultaneous initial diagnosis and stage of disease. The cytologic features of small cell undifferentiated carcinoma are very distinctive. A typical aspirate smear will contain small oval to spindled cells with scant, inconspicuous cytoplasm which are loosely cohesive or isolated. The nuclei are hyperchromatic with finely granular chromatin, inconspicuous nucleoli, and classically show nuclear molding and crush artifact (Fig. 5.9). The major differential diagnosis is with lymphoma, although poorly differentiated non-small cell carcinomas (i.e., basaloid squamous cell carcinoma) need to be excluded if the cells are larger and have a more cohesive appearance.

5.3.4.4 Melanoma

Melanoma has variable cytomorphology and can mimic other neoplasms. It can appear as a small round cell tumor, a large pleomorphic multinucleated neoplasm, or a spindle cell neoplasm. The liver is one of the most common sites of metastasis after lymph node spread (even from distant sites such as ocular melanoma). The classic appearance of malignant melanoma on fine needle aspiration is large, discohesive epithelioid cells with abundant cytoplasm, and large nuclei with prominent nucleoli. Binucleation is common, and often the nuclei are eccentrically placed imparting a plasmacytoid appearance (Fig. 5.10). Occasionally, the nuclei appear to protrude from the cells. When present, melanin pigment is particularly helpful in confirming the diagnosis, although it can be confused with bile pigment.

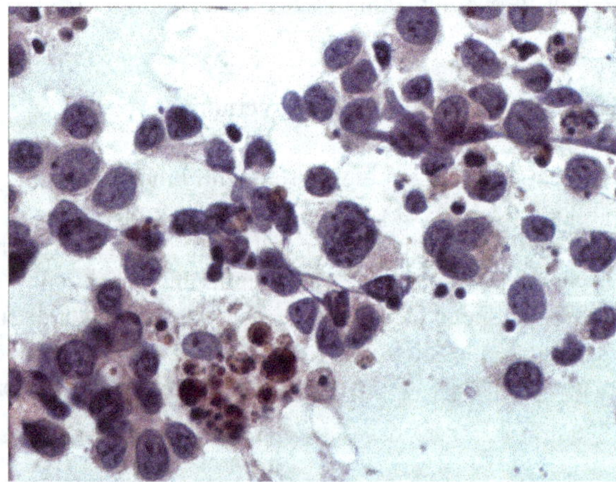

Fig. 5.9 Small cell carcinoma is a small blue cell tumor due to its very high nuclear to cytoplasmic ratio. Often, small cell carcinoma has abundant nuclear streaking artifact, nuclear molding, and single cell apoptosis (Papanicolaou stain 400×)

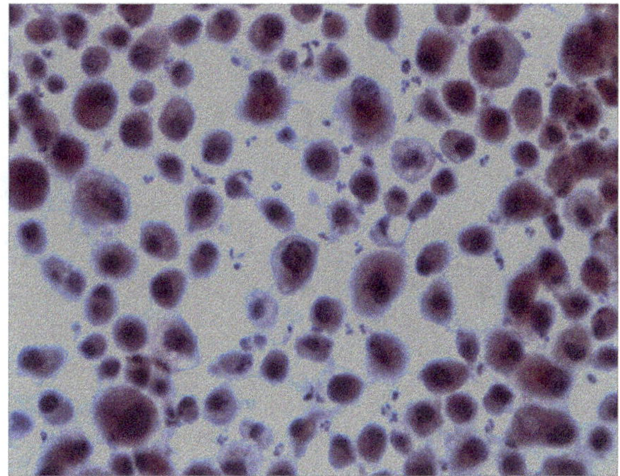

Fig. 5.10 Melanoma can look like hepatocytes but often has a markedly discohesive pattern (Papanicolaou stain 400×)

5.3.4.5 Lymphoma

Lymphomas rarely arise primarily in the liver, but most often secondarily involve the liver as part of a disseminated process. This can occur with both non-Hodgkin and Hodgkin lymphomas, and may present as a mass lesion or a diffuse infiltrate. Involvement of the liver can be patchy, and may be missed by both FNA and core needle biopsies. The cytomorphology of various lymphomas ranges widely; almost all subtypes have discohesive cells with scant cytoplasm, but they can range in size from small uniform cleaved cells to large atypical pleomorphic cells with prominent nucleoli. Primary hepatic lymphomas are very uncommon, and are most commonly of B cell type. If lymphoma is suspected on rapid on-site assessment or from clinical parameters, additional passes should be obtained for flow cytometric analysis.

5.3.4.6 Mesenchymal Neoplasms

Primary sarcomas of the liver are very uncommon, and most are vascular tumors. The most commonly diagnosed sarcoma of the liver is metastatic gastrointestinal stromal tumor (GIST), although any sarcoma can involve the liver. The cytologic appearance of GIST ranges from spindle cells with mild to marked pleomorphism and mitotic activity, to epithelioid round cells with clear cytoplasm (Fig. 5.11). Leiomyosarcoma is the second most common sarcoma of the liver, most frequently of gynecologic origin. The appearance of leiomyosarcoma on FNAB of the liver often shows spindle cells with marked pleomorphism, an appearance which is nonspecific. Knowledge of a prior sarcoma is particularly helpful. If comparison material is not available, immunohistochemistry on cell block material will be required for definitive diagnosis.

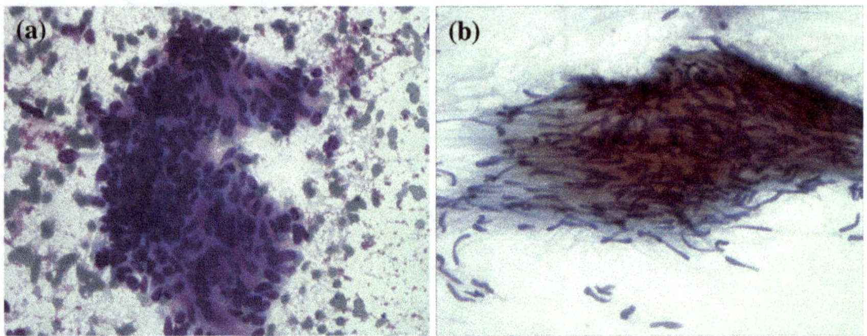

Fig. 5.11 Classic spindle cell morphology of a gastrointestinal stromal tumor. Cytologically, GIST resembles leiomyosarcoma and distinction requires ancillary testing. (**a** Diff Quick 200×, **b** Papanicolaou stain 200×)

5.3.5 Cysts

True hepatic cysts are those with an epithelial lining. Simple hepatic cysts form de novo and in the setting of polycystic kidney disease. Most of these aspirates are acellular or small clusters of bland bile ducts epithelial cells are found. Biliary cystadenomas usually have internal septations and may be suggested on imaging.

Abscesses can cause cystic spaces, are characterized by abundant neutrophils and reactive hepatocytes, and occasionally giant cells, histiocytes, and granulomas. When abscess material is found or is suspected clinically, a separate aspirate should be sent to microbiology. This material needs to be sent in a sterile tube, to decrease any chance of contamination. The most common reasons for liver abscesses in the United States are bacterial, usually secondary to biliary disease (*Escherichia coli* and *Klebsiella pneumoniae*) [79]. Bacterial and fungal abscesses will have similar cytologic findings but occasionally fungal organisms can be seen, even at the time of on-site evaluation. Aspirate material can be sent for microbiological assessment so appropriate treatment can be given.

Although rare in the United States, liver is a common location for parasitic cysts. *Echinococcus granulosus* causes hydatid disease characterized by a single cyst. It is often asymptomatic unless it gets over 10 cm. The cysts have a lamellated wall and often calcify in the periphery. FNAB of *Echinococcus* involving the liver has the greatest notoriety due to early reports of anaphylaxis. In reports where needle size is recorded, the needles were often 18 G [80]. Other case series have shown no allergic response after accidental aspiration of hydatid cysts [81, 82]. Because long-standing infections of *Echinococcus* form a laminated fibrous cyst wall, they can present as cystic masses and inadvertently be sampled by FNAB. If just the wall is aspirated, the aspirate may be dry or demonstrate only fibroblasts. If the cyst contents are aspirated, daughter cysts, protoscolices, and hooklets might be seen. Inflammation is distinctly absent and can aid in the

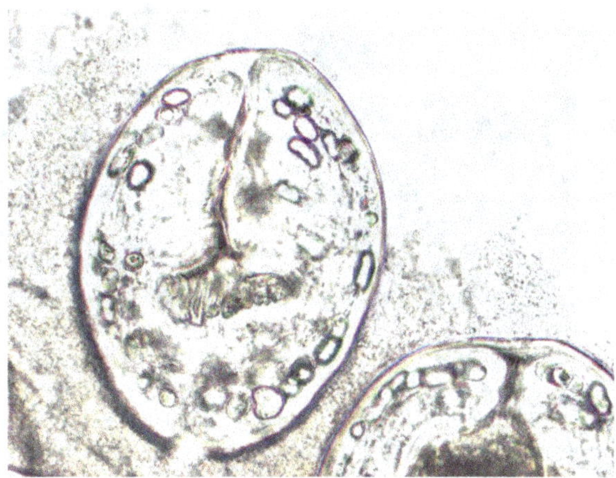

Fig. 5.12 Characteristic scolices of *Echinococcus* (wet mount preparation 600×)

differential between an amebic cysts or other infectious abscesses (which would have neutrophils). Unstained slides are often easier on which to visualize the organisms (Fig. 5.12).

Entamoeba histolytica can also cause hepatic cysts and are often symptomatic resulting in abdominal pain, fever, and hepatomegaly. The classic aspirate material will be thick and orange-brown. Amoebae are most numerous on the edge of the cyst but can sometimes be found within the necrotic cyst contents. The organisms are approximately 10–60 µm, have a small round nucleus, and often have phagocytosed red blood cells in their cytoplasm [83]. They can easily be mistaken for histiocytes. Even if no organisms are identified, the presence of marked necrotic debris should raise the possibility of *Entamoeba*, particularly in someone who had antecedent gastrointestinal symptoms or the appropriate travel history, so material can be sent for DNA analysis if clinically indicated [83, 84].

5.3.6 Bile Duct Cytology

With the advent of esophageal ultrasound-guided FNA and esophageal retrograde cholangiopancreatography procedure (ERCP), bile duct strictures and masses can be sampled. Distinguishing benign from malignant strictures is challenging clinically and radiographically and bile duct brushings allow for minimally invasive means for sampling the area of concern. While most benign and malignant processes can be accurately distinguished cytologically, there is a large gray zone of dysplastic and reactive changes that are problematic even for experienced cytologists.

Benign bile duct cells on a brushing are characterized by a sheets of cells with a low nuclear to cytoplasmic ratio, centrally placed round nuclei and a small but conspicuous nucleolus (Fig. 5.13a). The chromatin is fine and evenly dispersed

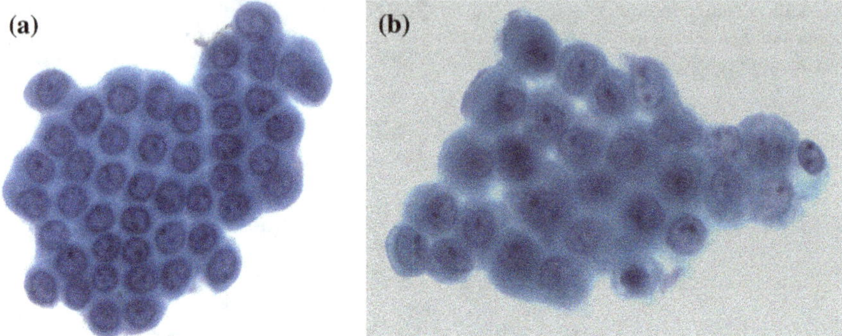

Fig. 5.13 Bile duct brushings showing: normal bile duct epithelium showing a sheet of bland homogeneous cells (**a** Papanicolaou stain 400×) and reactive epithelium with some nuclear variability and overlap and small nucleoli (**b** Papanicolaou stain 400×)

throughout the nucleus. In the setting of inflammation, the cells demonstrate enlarged nuclei with some nuclear overlap, small and sometimes multiple nucleoli, and granular chromatin (Fig. 5.13b) [85]. All of these changes become more pronounced in the setting of a stent or chronic inflammation. In contrast, cholangiocarcinoma is characterized as disordered clusters and single cells with a high nuclear to cytoplasmic ration, irregular nuclear contours, coarse chromatin, and prominent nucleoli (Fig. 5.14). In one study, the most useful features in differentiating benign from malignant cells were nuclear molding, high nuclear to cytoplasmic ratio, and chromatin clumping [86]. However, the previously mentioned criteria are frequently found and are used as well in the diagnosis of adenocarcinoma. Bile duct epithelium responds dramatically to chronic irritation

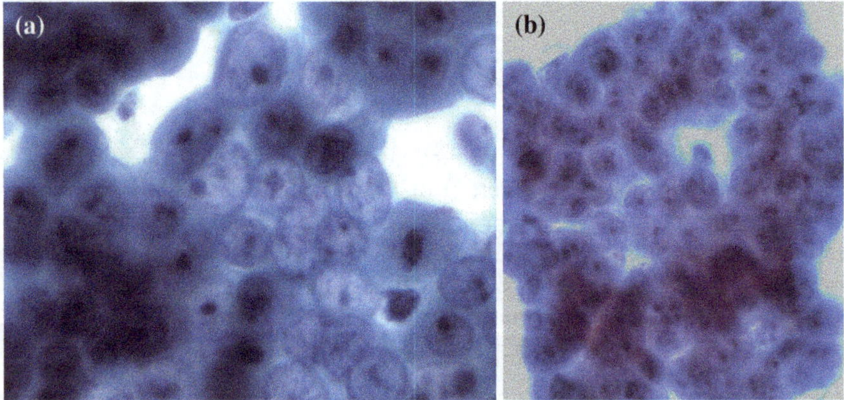

Fig. 5.14 Bile duct brushings from a cholangiocarcinoma. Note the markedly high nuclear to cytoplasmic ratio, prominent nucleoli, and nuclear size variability and overlap (**a, b** Papanicolaou stain, 600×)

such as a stent or chronic inflammation such as in primary sclerosing cholangitis. In these settings, the duct epithelium frequently demonstrates some markedly atypical cells. Often there is a spectrum of cytologic changes that suggests a reactive process. However, not infrequently reactive atypia cannot be discriminated from carcinoma.

Most studies report a low to intermediate sensitivity and a high specificity for carcinoma. The low sensitivity is usually secondary to sampling error, benign epithelium overlying the malignancy, interpretive errors, poor cell preservation, or limited cellularity [87]. As stated in a review article by Selvaggi, "a diagnosis of malignancy should be made in conjunction with the patient's complete medical history and the appropriate radiographic procedures. Communication between the cytologist and the referring doctor/gastroenterologist is essential..." [88]

References

1. Perry MD, Johnston WW (1985) Needle biopsy of the liver for the diagnosis of non neoplastic liver diseases. Acta Cytol 29(3):385–390
2. LoIudice T, Buhac I, Balint J (1977) Septicaemia as a complication of percutaneous liver biopsy. Gastroenterology 72:949–951
3. Morris JS, Gallo GA, Scheuer PJ et al (1975) Percutaneous liver biopsy in patients with large bile duct obstruction. Gastroenterology 68:750–754
4. Grant A, Neuberger J (1999) Guidelines on the use of liver biopsy in clinical practice. Gut 45:iv1–iv11
5. Sue M, Caldwell SH, Dickson RC et al (1996) Variation between centres in technique and guidelines for liver biopsy. Liver 16:267–270
6. Tripodi A, Caldwell SH et al (2007) Review article: the prothrombin time test as a measure of bleeding risk and prognosis in liver disease. Aliment Pharmacol Ther 26:141–148
7. Gazelle GS, Haaga JR (1989) Guided percutaneous biopsy of intra abdominal lesions. AJR Am J Roentgenol 153:929–935
8. Yu SC, Liew CT et al (2001) US-guided percutaneous biopsy of small ($\leq$ 1-cm) hepatic lesions. Radiology 218:195–199
9. Hatfield MK, Beres RA, Sane SS et al (2008) Percutaneous imaging-guided solid organ core needle biopsy: coaxial versus non coaxial method. Am J Roentgenol 190:413–417
10. Maturen KE, Nghiem HV, Marrero JA et al (2006) Lack of tumor seeding of hepatocellular carcinoma after percutaneous needle biopsy using coaxial cutting needle technique. Am J Roentgenol 187:1184–1187
11. Silva MA, Hegab B, Hyde C et al (2008) Needle tract seeding following biopsy of liver lesions in the diagnosis of hepatocellular cancer: a systematic review and meta-analysis. Gut 57:1592–1596
12. Austin JHM, Cohen MB (1993) Value of having a cytopathologist present during percutaneous fine-needle aspiration biopsy of lung: report of 55 cancer patients and meta analysis of the literature. Am J Roentgenol 160:175–177
13. Stewart CJR, Coldewey J, Stewart IS (2002) Comparison of fine needle aspiration cytology and needle core biopsy in the diagnosis of radiologically detected abdominal lesions. J Clin Pathol 55(2):93–97
14. Bruix J, Sherman M, Llovet JM et al (2001) Clinical management of hepatocellular carcinoma. Conclusions of the Barcelona-2000 EASL conference. J Hepatol 35:421–430

15. Torzilli G, Minagawa M, Takayama T et al (1999) Accurate preoperative evaluation of liver mass lesions without fine-needle biopsy. Hepatology 30:889–893
16. Lim JH, Kim CK, Lee WJ et al (2000) Detection of hepatocellular carcinomas and dysplastic nodules in cirrhotic livers: accuracy of helical CT in transplant patients. Am J Roentgenol 175:693–698
17. Bru C, Maroto A, Bruix J, Faus R, Bianchi L, Calvet X et al (1989) Diagnostic accuracy of fine-needle aspiration biopsy in patients with hepatocellular carcinoma. Dig Dis Sci 34(11):1765–1769
18. Buscarini L, Fornari F, Bolondi L, Colombo P, Livraghi T, Magnolfi F et al (1990) Ultrasound-guided fine-needle biopsy of focal liver lesions: Techniques, diagnostic accuracy and complications. A retrospective study on 2091 biopsies. J Hepatol 11(3):344–348
19. Bell DA, Carr CP, Szyfelbein WM (1986) Fine needle aspiration cytology of focal liver lesions. Results obtained with examination of both cytologic and histologic preparations. Acta Cytol 30(4):397–402
20. Cochand-Priollet B, Chagnon S, Ferrand J, Blery M, Hoang C, Galian A (1987) Comparison of cytologic examination of smears and histologic examination of tissue cores obtained by fine needle aspiration biopsy of the liver. Acta Cytol 31(4):476–480
21. Droese M, Altmannsberger M, Kehl A, Lankisch PG, Weiss R, Weber K et al (1984) Ultrasound-guided percutaneous fine needle aspiration biopsy of abdominal and retroperitoneal masses. Accuracy of cytology in the diagnosis of malignancy, cytologic tumor typing and use of antibodies to intermediate filaments in selected cases. Acta Cytol 28(4):368–384
22. Fornari F, Filice C, Rapaccini GL, Caturelli E, Cavanna L, Civardi G et al (1994) Small (< or = 3 cm) hepatic lesions. results of sonographically guided fine-needle biopsy in 385 patients. Dig Dis Sci 39(10):2267–2275
23. Bognel C, Rougier P, Leclere J, Duvillard P, Charpentier P, Prade M (1988) Fine needle aspiration of the liver and pancreas with ultrasound guidance. Acta Cytol 32(1):22–26
24. Leiman G, Leibowitz CB, Dunbar F (1989) Fine-needle aspiration of the liver: out of the ivory tower and into the community. Diagn Cytopathol 5(1):35–39
25. Samaratunga H, Wright G (1992) Value of fine needle aspiration biopsy cytology in the diagnosis of discrete hepatic lesions suspicious for malignancy. Aust N Z J Surg 62(7):540–544
26. Guo Z, Kurtycz DF, Salem R, De Las Casas LE, Caya JG, Hoerl HD (2002) Radiologically guided percutaneous fine-needle aspiration biopsy of the liver: retrospective study of 119 cases evaluating diagnostic effectiveness and clinical complications. Diagn Cytopathol 26(5):283–289
27. Franca AV, Valerio HM, Trevisan M, Escanhoela C, Seva-Pereira T, Zucoloto S et al (2003) Fine needle aspiration biopsy for improving the diagnostic accuracy of cut needle biopsy of focal liver lesions. Acta Cytol 47(3):332–336
28. Stewart CJ, Coldewey J, Stewart IS (2002) Comparison of fine needle aspiration cytology and needle core biopsy in the diagnosis of radiologically detected abdominal lesions. J Clin Pathol 55(2):93–97
29. Caturelli E, Bisceglia M, Fusilli S, Squillante MM, Castelvetere M, Siena DA (1996) Cytological vs microhistological diagnosis of hepatocellular carcinoma: comparative accuracies in the same fine-needle biopsy specimen. Dig Dis Sci 41(12):2326–2331
30. Longchampt E, Patriarche C, Fabre M (2000) Accuracy of cytology vs. microbiopsy for the diagnosis of well-differentiated hepatocellular carcinoma and macroregenerative nodule. Definition of standardized criteria from a study of 100 cases. Acta Cytol 44(4):515–523
31. Rapaccini GL, Pompili M, Caturelli E, Fusilli S, Trombino C, Gomes V et al (1994) Ultrasound-guided fine-needle biopsy of hepatocellular carcinoma: comparison between smear cytology and microhistology. Am J Gastroenterol 89(6):898–902
32. Klapman JB, Logrono R, Dye CE, Waxman I (2003) Clinical impact of on-site cytopathology interpretation on endoscopic ultrasound-guided fine needle aspiration. Am J Gastroenterol 98(6):1289–1294

33. Baloch ZW, Tam D, Langer J, Mandel S, LiVolsi VA, Gupta PK (2000) Ultrasound-guided fine-needle aspiration biopsy of the thyroid: role of on-site assessment and multiple cytologic preparations. Diagn Cytopathol 23(6):425–429

34. Dixon JM, Clarke PJ, Crucioli V, Dehn TC, Lee EC, Greenall MJ (1987) Reduction of the surgical excision rate in benign breast disease using fine needle aspiration cytology with immediate reporting. Br J Surg 74(11):1014–1016

35. Eisele DW, Sherman ME, Koch WM, Richtsmeier WJ, Wu AY, Erozan YS (1992) Utility of immediate on-site cytopathological procurement and evaluation in fine needle aspiration biopsy of head and neck masses. Laryngoscope 102(12 Pt 1):1328–1330

36. Austin JH, Cohen MB (1993) Value of having a cytopathologist present during percutaneous fine-needle aspiration biopsy of lung: report of 55 cancer patients and metaanalysis of the literature. AJR Am J Roentgenol 160(1):175–177

37. Stewart CJ, Stewart IS (1996) Immediate assessment of fine needle aspiration cytology of lung. J Clin Pathol 49(10):839–843

38. Nasuti JF, Gupta PK, Baloch ZW (2002) Diagnostic value and cost-effectiveness of on-site evaluation of fine-needle aspiration specimens: review of 5,688 cases. Diagn Cytopathol 27(1):1–4

39. Miller DA, Carrasco CH, Katz RL, Cramer FM, Wallace S, Charnsangavej C (1986) Fine needle aspiration biopsy: the role of immediate cytologic assessment. AJR Am J Roentgenol 147(1):155–158

40. Montali G, Solbiati L, Croce F, Ierace T, Ravetto C (1982) Fine-needle aspiration biopsy of liver focal lesions ultrasonically guided with a real-time probe. Report on 126 cases. Br J Radiol 55(658):717–723

41. Smith EH (1991) Complications of percutaneous abdominal fine-needle biopsy. Review. Radiology 178(1):253–258

42. Martinez-Noguera A, Donoso L, Coscojuela P (1991) Fatal bleeding after fine-needle aspiration biopsy of a small hepatocarcinoma. AJR Am J Roentgenol 156(5):1114–1115

43. Mingoli A, Marzano M, Sgarzini G, Nardacchione F, Corzani F, Modini C (1995) Fatal bleeding after fine-needle aspiration biopsy of the liver. Ital J Gastroenterol 27(5):250–251

44. Hertzanu Y, Peiser J, Zirkin H (1990) Massive bleeding after fine needle aspiration of liver angiosarcoma. Gastrointest Radiol 15(1):43–46

45. Patel RI, Shapiro MJ (1995) Biliary venous fistula: an unusual complication of fine-needle aspiration biopsy of the liver. J Vasc Interv Radiol 6(6):953–956

46. Nasseri Moghaddam S, Abrishami A, Malekzadeh R (2006) Percutaneous needle aspiration, injection, and reaspiration with or without benzimidazole coverage for uncomplicated hepatic hydatid cysts. Cochrane Database Syst Rev (2):003623

47. Bissonnette RT, Gibney RG, Berry BR, Buckley AR (1990) Fatal carcinoid crisis after percutaneous fine-needle biopsy of hepatic metastasis: case report and literature review. Radiology 174(3 Pt 1):751–752

48. tenBerge J, Hoffman BJ, Hawes RH, Van Enckevort C, Giovannini M, Erickson RA et al (2002) EUS-guided fine needle aspiration of the liver: indications, yield, and safety based on an international survey of 167 cases. Gastrointest Endosc 55(7):859–862

49. Wiersema MJ, Vilmann P, Giovannini M, Chang KJ, Wiersema LM (1997) Endosonography-guided fine-needle aspiration biopsy: diagnostic accuracy and complication assessment. Gastroenterology 112(4):1087–1095

50. van Leeuwen DJ, Wilson L, Crowe DR (1995) Liver biopsy in the mid-1990s: questions and answers. Semin Liver Dis 15(4):340–359

51. Kosugi C, Furuse J, Ishii H, Maru Y, Yoshino M, Kinoshita T et al (2004) Needle tract implantation of hepatocellular carcinoma and pancreatic carcinoma after ultrasound-guided percutaneous puncture: clinical and pathologic characteristics and the treatment of needle tract implantation. World J Surg 28(1):29–32

52. Durand F, Regimbeau JM, Belghiti J, Sauvanet A, Vilgrain V, Terris B et al (2001) Assessment of the benefits and risks of percutaneous biopsy before surgical resection of hepatocellular carcinoma. J Hepatol 35(2):254–258

53. de Sio I, Castellano L, Calandra M, Del Vecchio-Blanco C (2002) Subcutaneous needle-tract seeding after fine needle aspiration biopsy of pancreatic liver metastasis. Eur J Ultrasound 15(1–2):65–68

54. Isobe H, Imari Y, Sakai H, Sakamoto S, Nawata H (1993) Subcutaneous seeding of hepatocellular carcinoma following fine-needle aspiration biopsy. J Clin Gastroenterol 17(4):350–352

55. McGrath FP, Gibney RG, Rowley VA, Scudamore CH (1991) Cutaneous seeding following fine needle biopsy of colonic liver metastases. Clin Radiol 43(2):130–131

56. Nakamuta M, Tanabe Y, Ohashi M, Yoshida K, Hiroshige K, Nawata H (1993) Transabdominal seeding of hepatocellular carcinoma after fine-needle aspiration biopsy. J Clin Ultrasound 21(8):551–556

57. Navarro F, Taourel P, Michel J, Perney P, Fabre JM, Blanc F et al (1998) Diaphragmatic and subcutaneous seeding of hepatocellular carcinoma following fine-needle aspiration biopsy. Liver 18(4):251–254

58. Park YM, Lee CD, Yoon KH, Han NI, Cho HM, Yook KS et al (1989) A case of subcutaneous seeding of hepatocellular carcinoma after fine needle aspiration biopsy. Korean J Intern Med 4(1):96–100

59. Yamada N, Shinzawa H, Ukai K, Wakabayashi H, Togashi H, Takahashi T et al (1993) Subcutaneous seeding of small hepatocellular carcinoma after fine needle aspiration biopsy. J Gastroenterol Hepatol 8(2):195–198

60. Saborido BP, Diaz JC, de Los Galanes SJ, Segurola CL, de Usera MA, Garrido MD et al (2005) Does preoperative fine needle aspiration-biopsy produce tumor recurrence in patients following liver transplantation for hepatocellular carcinoma? Transpl Proc 37(9):3874–3877

61. Torzilli G, Minagawa M, Takayama T, Inoue K, Hui AM, Kubota K et al (1999) Accurate preoperative evaluation of liver mass lesions without fine-needle biopsy. Hepatology 30(4):889–893

62. Ng KK, Poon RT, Lo CM, Liu CL, Lam CM, Ng IO et al (2004) Impact of preoperative fine-needle aspiration cytologic examination on clinical outcome in patients with hepatocellular carcinoma in a tertiary referral center. Arch Surg 139(2):193–200

63. Pitman MB, Szyfelbein WM (1995) Significance of endothelium in the fine-needle aspiration biopsy diagnosis of hepatocellular carcinoma. Diagn Cytopathol 12(3):208–214

64. Sole M, Calvet X, Cuberes T, Maderuelo F, Bruix J, Bru C et al (1993) Value and limitations of cytologic criteria for the diagnosis of hepatocellular carcinoma by fine needle aspiration biopsy. Acta Cytol 37(3):309–316

65. Soyuer I, Ekinci C, Kaya M, Genc Y, Bahar K (2003) Diagnosis of hepatocellular carcinoma by fine needle aspiration cytology. Cellular features. Acta Cytol 47(4):581–589

66. Zimmerman RL, Burke MA, Young NA, Solomides CC, Bibbo M (2001) Diagnostic value of hepatocyte paraffin 1 antibody to discriminate hepatocellular carcinoma from metastatic carcinoma in fine-needle aspiration biopsies of the liver. Cancer 93(4):288–291

67. Siddiqui MT, Saboorian MH, Gokaslan ST, Ashfaq R (2002) Diagnostic utility of the HepPar1 antibody to differentiate hepatocellular carcinoma from metastatic carcinoma in fine-needle aspiration samples. Cancer 96(1):49–52

68. Kakar S, Muir T, Murphy LM, Lloyd RV, Burgart LJ (2003) Immunoreactivity of hep par 1 in hepatic and extrahepatic tumors and its correlation with albumin in situ hybridization in hepatocellular carcinoma. Am J Clin Pathol 119(3):361–366

69. Krishna M, Lloyd RV, Batts KP (1997) Detection of albumin messenger RNA in hepatic and extrahepatic neoplasms. A marker of hepatocellular differentiation. Am J Surg Pathol 21(2):147–152

70. Maeda T, Kajiyama K, Adachi E, Takenaka K, Sugimachi K, Tsuneyoshi M (1996) The expression of cytokeratins 7, 19, and 20 in primary and metastatic carcinomas of the liver. Mod Pathol 9(9):901–909

71. Wieczorek TJ, Pinkus JL, Glickman JN, Pinkus GS (2002) Comparison of thyroid transcription factor-1 and hepatocyte antigen immunohistochemical analysis in the

differential diagnosis of hepatocellular carcinoma, metastatic adenocarcinoma, renal cell carcinoma, and adrenal cortical carcinoma. Am J Clin Pathol 118(6):911–921

72. Onofre AS, Pomjanski N, Buckstegge B, Bocking A (2007) Immunocytochemical diagnosis of hepatocellular carcinoma and identification of carcinomas of unknown primary metastatic to the liver on fine-needle aspiration cytologies. Cancer 111(4):259–268

73. Kakar S, Gown AM, Goodman ZD, Ferrell LD (2007) Best practices in diagnostic immunohistochemistry: Hepatocellular carcinoma versus metastatic neoplasms. Arch Pathol Lab Med 131(11):1648–1654

74. Terada T, Sugiura M (2008) Metastatic hepatocellular carcinoma of skin diagnosed with hepatocyte paraffin 1 and a-fetoprotein immunostainings. Int J Surg Pathol 18:433–436

75. Torbenson M (2007) Review of the clinicopathologic features of fibrolamellar carcinoma. Adv Anat Pathol 14(3):217–223

76. Andres AM, Hernandez F, Lopez-Santamaría M et al (2007) Surgery of liver tumors in children in the last 15 years. Eur J Ped Surg 17(6):387–392

77. D'Antiga L, Vallortigara F, Cillo U (2007) et al Features predicting unresectability in hepatoblastoma. Cancer 110(5):1050–1058

78. Hertz G, Reddy VB, Green L, Spitz D, Massarani-Wafai R, Selvaggi SM et al (2000) Fine-needle aspiration biopsy of the liver: a multicenter study of 602 radiologically guided FNA. Diagn Cytopathol 23(5):326–328

79. Fang C, Lai S, Yi W et al (2007) Klebsiella pneumoniaegenotype K1: an emerging pathogen that causes septic ocular or central nervous system complications from pyogenic liver abscess. Clin Infect Dis 45:284–293

80. Agarwal PK, Husain N, Singh BN (1989) Cytologic findings in aspirated hydatid fluid. Acta Cytol 33(5):652–654

81. Singh A, Singh Y, Sharma VK, Agarwal AK, Bist D (1999) Diagnosis of hydatid disease of abdomen and thorax by ultrasound guided fine needle aspiration cytology. Indian J Pathol Microbiol 42(2):155–156

82. Das DK, Bhambhani S, Pant CS (1995) Ultrasound guided fine-needle aspiration cytology: diagnosis of hydatid disease of the abdomen and thorax. Diagn Cytopathol 12(2):173–176

83. Washington K, Harris E (2009) Liver. In: Mills E (ed) Sternberg's diagnostic surgical pathology 5th edn. Lippincott Williams and Wilkins, Philadelphia, pp 1535–1544

84. Salles JM, Salles MJ, Moraes LA, Silva MC (2007) Invasive amebiasis: an update on diagnosis and management. Expert Rev Anti Infect Ther 5(5):893–901

85. Wright C, Zaitoun A, Boulton-Jones J, Dunkley C, Beckingham I, Ryder S (2004) Improving diagnostic yield of biliary brushings cytology for pancreatic cancer and cholangiocarcinoma. Cytopathology 15:87–92

86. Cohen M, Wittchow R, Bottles K, Raab S (1995) Brush cytology of the intrahepatic biliary tract: comparison of cytologic features of adenocarcinoma and benign biliary strictures. Mod Pathol 8:498–502

87. Kocjan G, Smith A (1997) Bile duct brushing cytology: potential pitfalls in diagnosis. Diagn Cytopathol 16:358–363

88. Selvaggi S (2004) Biliary brushing cytology, review article. Cytopathology 15:74–79

Chapter 6
Esophagus, Stomach, and Pancreas

Xiaoqi Lin and Srinadh Komanduri

Cytologic examination using fine needle aspiration (FNA), exfoliative brushings, and needle core biopsy are essential tests in the diagnosis of esophageal, gastric and pancreatic lesions, staging of malignancy, and follow-up of patients. The sensitivity and specificity of cytology is increased by the concurrent use of radiologic imaging (endoscopic ultrasound (EUS), ultrasound, computed tomography (CT) and magnetic resonance imaging (MRI), immuno-cytochemistry, and molecular studies.

6.1 Utility of Cytology in Esophageal, Gastric and Pancreatic Lesions

6.1.1 Diagnostic Methodology

The following techniques can be used to obtain samples from the esophagus, stomach and pancreas, and their surrounding tissues or lymph nodes for cytologic examination of neoplastic, infectious, or inflammatory lesions.

X. Lin (✉)
Department of Pathology, Northwestern University/Northwestern Memorial Hospital,
675 N St. Claire St, Galter Pavillion 7-132F, Chicago, IL 60611, USA
e-mail: xlin@northwestern.edu

S. Komanduri
Department of Gastroenterology, Northwestern University, 676 N. St. Claire St, 14th floor,
Chicago, IL 60611, USA
e-mail: koman1973@gmail.com

R. Nayar (ed.), *Cytopathology in Oncology*,
Cancer Treatment and Research 160, DOI: 10.1007/978-3-642-38850-7_6,
© Springer-Verlag Berlin Heidelberg 2014

6.1.1.1 Esophageal, Common Bile Duct and Pancreatic Duct Brushing Cytology

Brush cytology is used for superficial mucosal lesions or lesions involving the mucosa [1–4]. Brushing cytology is more routinely used in the setting of pancreaticobiliary malignancy. In this setting, common bile duct and pancreatic duct brushings can be obtained during ERCP [3].

6.1.1.2 Ultrasound, CT or MRI-Guided Percutaneous FNA or Needle Core Biopsy

These techniques are used for gastric and pancreatic lesions, lesions surrounding the stomach and pancreas for diagnosis, and mediastinal, peri-gastric, and peri-pancreatic lymph nodes for staging.

6.1.1.3 EUS-Guided Fine Needle Aspiration

In conjunction with FNA, EUS has become a very effective tool for tissue acquisition for many malignant and benign processes both within and outside the gastrointestinal tract (e.g., lymph nodes) [5]. While ultrasound and CT-guided FNA biopsies are also alternative techniques for tissue acquisition, EUS-FNA has become the gold standard and offers greater efficacy with less complications.

6.1.1.4 Abrasive Balloons for Gastroesophageal Lesions

Although this less costly cancer surveillance method for gastroesophageal diseases is not used in USA, it is used in other countries [6, 7]. The sensitivity for detecting high-grade dysplasia or carcinoma in high incidence areas is 80 %, while the sensitivity for detecting low-grade dysplasia is much lower, at 25 % [6].

6.1.2 Diagnostic Application

Optimal tissue acquisition techniques as described above are essential to procure good cytologic samples for establishing a diagnosis of malignancy, infectious and inflammatory processes, as well as in the assessment for dysplasia in non-neo-plastic entities (e.g., Barrett's esophagus, primary sclerosing cholangitis).

6.1.3 Staging Application

Utilization of cytologic samples is an important aspect of cancer staging. In many clinical scenarios, EUS-FNA and CT/ultrasound-FNA are utilized to improve cancer staging in the esophagus, stomach, and pancreaticobiliary trees. EUS-FNA allows for sampling of local and metastatic lymph nodes and ascitic fluid to stage gastrointestinal malignancies. CT/ultrasound-FNA allows sampling of many sites further away from the gastrointestinal tract to assess for metastatic disease. Both of these diagnostic modalities have become a mainstay in locoregional and distant cancer staging.

6.2 Esophagus

6.2.1 Non-Neoplastic Conditions: Esophagitis

The most common non-neoplastic disease of the esophagus is esophagitis. Esophagitis can be caused by gastroesophageal reflux disease (GERD), infections (e.g., bacteria, cytomegalovirus (CMV) [8], Herpes simplex virus (HSV) [8, 9], Candida spp. [9], and human papilloma virus (HPV) [10], irritants (e.g., alcohol, smoking, and hot drinks), trauma, radiation/chemotherapy, and autoimmune diseases (e.g., Crohn's disease, sarcoidosis, and eosinophilic esophagitis). Infectious esophagitis is commonly encountered in immunocompromised patients.

6.2.1.1 Diagnostic Challenges and Techniques

There are many challenges in diagnosis of esophagitis. The most difficult area for diagnosis occurs with infectious etiologies. While in some circumstances, there be numerous organisms present (Candida spp.), in other situations we may struggle to find more than a single organism or virus-infected cell. While endoscopic biopsy has largely replaced cytology in esophagitis, a combination of modalities may in fact provide the greatest yield [9]. Special and immunohistochemical (IHC) stains can be performed on smears, cytospin slides, cell blocks, or biopsies. Gram stain is for bacteria, GMS and PAS stains for fungi, and acid fast or FITE stains for mycobacteria. IHC stains for CMV, HSV and *Helicobacter pylori* are available for confirmation. Cultures are also useful for identification of infectious agents and are used to detect sensitivity/resistance to medications.

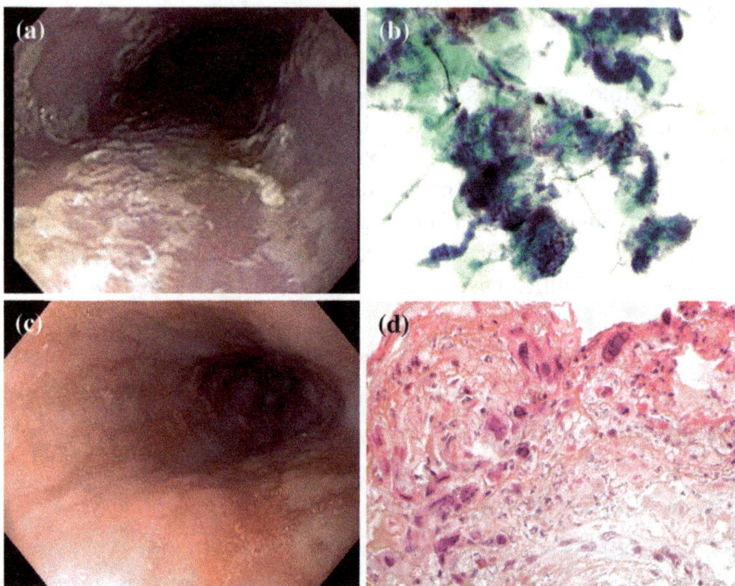

Fig. 6.1 **a** Endoscopy image of esophageal candidiasis. **b** Brushing cytology of esophageal candidiasis, ThinPrep, Pap stain, 600×. **c** Endoscopy image of esophageal HSV infection. **d** Biopsy of esophageal HSV infection, H and E stain, 600×

6.2.1.2 Application of Endoscopy and Cytology in Esophagitis

Esophageal candidiasis is the most common cause of infectious esophagitis and is often seen in immunosuppressed or antibiotic-treated patients. Endoscopy reveals a white plaque on an erythematous mucosa, and possibly erosion or ulceration (Fig. 6.1a). Brushing cytology is more sensitive than biopsy for diagnosing Candida esophagitis (sensitivity of 100 and 67 %, respectively), and shows typical budding yeasts and pseudohyphae (Fig. 6.1b) [9]. The clinician needs to distinguish disease from oral contamination. Inflammatory cells (predominantly neutrophils), necrotic debris, and reactive/reparative cells can be seen. GMS stain on smeared slides or cellblock and culture can be ordered for any suspicious cases, but is usually not necessary.

Herpes virus infection is more often seen with immunosuppression. Endoscopy may reveal vesicles and ulcers (Fig. 6.1c). Biopsy is similar or more sensitive than brushing cytology for Herpes esophagitis [8, 9]. Virus-infected cells are found at the edge of ulcers versus the base. Infected cells show intranuclear inclusions with multinucleation, nuclear molding, chromatin margination, and ground glass appearance (Fig. 6.1d). Reactive and reparative changes, inflammatory cells, necrotic debris, and granulation tissue may be seen. IHC staining should be ordered for suspicious cases, but culture is not helpful for diagnosis [8].

CMV esophagitis is generally associated with immunodeficiency. Endoscopic biopsy is the best method for diagnosis, while brushing cytology and culture add little to diagnose CMV (sensitivity, 0 and 27 %, respectively) [8]. Endoscopy generally reveals ulcers; contrary to Herpes infection, CMV-infected cells are found in the base of the ulcer. It is therefore imperative that the center and edges of all ulcers are sampled endoscopically to ensure adequate diagnosis. CMV infects glandular cells and endothelial cells. The infected cells are enlarged with large intranuclear or cytoplasmic inclusions with halos (Fig. 6.1). IHC stain for CMV can be used if there is suspicion for CMV infection.

HPV infection causes esophagitis [10], squamous papillomas [11], flat condylomas [12], and squamous cell carcinoma [13]. However, some studies showed no association between HPV infection and esophageal squamous cell carcinoma [14]. Cytologic features of HPV infection are koilocytes similar to those seen in cervical Pap tests. IHC p16 stain is helpful for confirming HPV infection and grading dysplasia.

6.2.2 Barrett's Esophagus

Barrett's esophagus is defined as "a change in the esophageal epithelium of any length that can be recognized at endoscopy and is confirmed to have intestinal metaplasia by biopsy" [11]. GERD is the most common type of esophagitis in the USA and may result in Barrett's esophagus, dysplasia, and adenocarcinoma with an odds ratio of 7 in chronic reflux and 43.5 in longstanding and severe reflux [15–17]. Long-term surveillance of patients with Barrett's esophagus is recommended to detect the occurrence of dysplasia and adenocarcinoma.

6.2.2.1 Diagnostic Challenges and Techniques

Tissue acquisition in Barrett's esophagus has numerous limitations. The endoscopist should utilize methods of sampling that allow for maximal surface area coverage. Despite the fact that endoscopic biopsy has largely replaced brushing cytology in dysplasia surveillance, it still remains suboptimal. Endoscopic sampling error accounts for much difficulties in dysplasia assessment in Barrett's esophagus (Fig. 6.2a). The majority of dysplasia in Barrett's esophagus may be unrecognizable from the surrounding intestinal metaplasia endoscopically. While enhanced endoscopic imaging modalities (e.g., narrow band imaging and confocal endomicroscopy) have been promising, their role is still unclear [18]. It is therefore essential to follow a methodical technique in tissue sampling (e.g., Seattle protocol) to minimize sampling error [19].

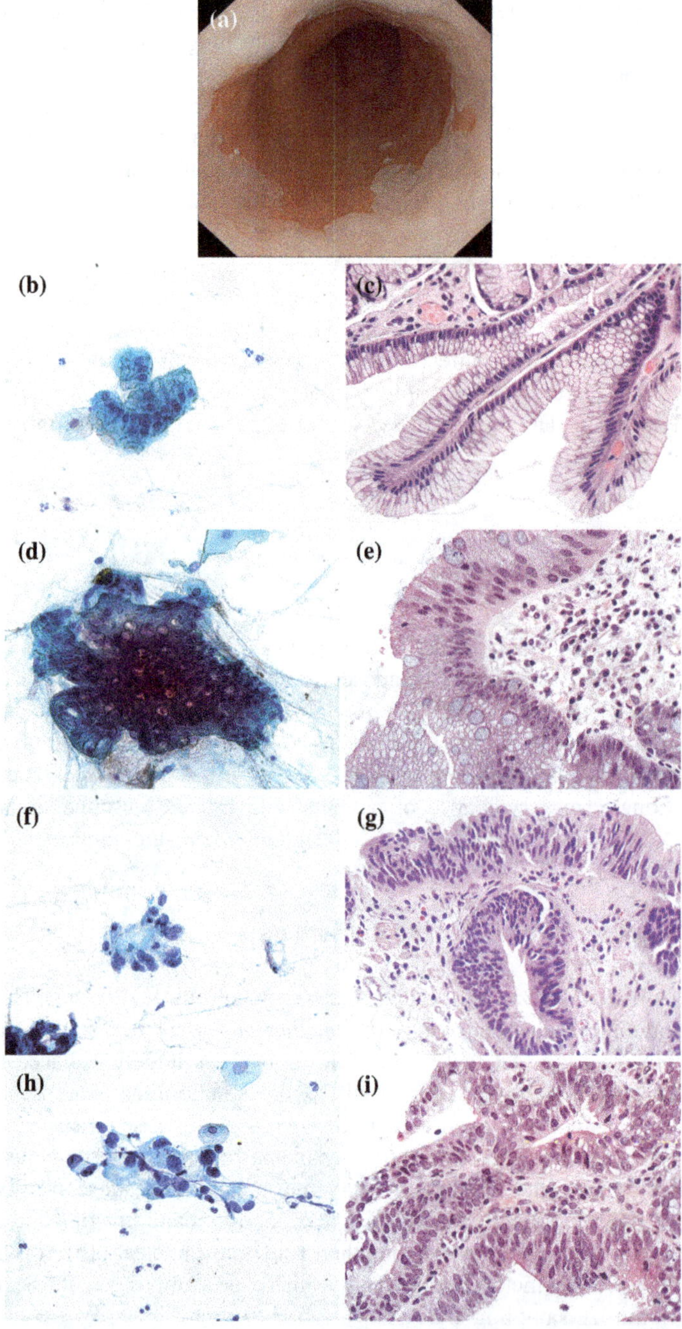

Fig. 6.2 **a** Endoscopic image of Barrett's esophagus. **b** Brushing cytology of normal mucosa, Pap stain, 600×. **c** Biopsy of normal mucosa, H and E stain, 400×. **d** Brushing cytology of Barrett's esophagus, Pap stain, 600×. **e** Biopsy of Barrett's esophagus, H and E stain, 400×. **f** Brushing cytology of low-grade dysplasia, Pap stain, 600×. **g** Biopsy of low-grade dysplasia, H and E stain, 400×. **h** Brushing cytology of high-grade dysplasia, Pap stain, 600×. **i** Biopsy of high-grade dysplasia, H and E stain, 400x

6.2.2.2 Application of Cytology in Barrett's Esophagus

Nowadays, most institutes in the USA utilize endoscopic biopsies to diagnose Barrett's esophagus and follow up the patients, as it is more sensitive and specific than brushing cytology to diagnose Barrett's esophagus (sensitivity, 92 vs. 60 %) [9]. Esophageal brushing cytology combined with detection of a broad panel of loss of heterozygosity (LOH) targeting tumor suppressor genes is more sensitive and accurate to diagnose Barrett's esophagus, low-, high-grade dysplasia and adenocarcinoma than biopsy histomorphology, brushing cytology, and combination of biopsy histomorphology with detection of the same panel of LOH [1]. As compared with brushing cytology, FISH targeting oncogenes and tumor suppressor genes increases sensitivity to detect low-grade dysplasia (from 5 to 50 %), high-grade dysplasia (from 32 to 82 %) and carcinoma (from 45 to 100 %) [20, 21]. The sensitivity of DNA ploidy analysis for these lesions is similar to that of cytology [20].

Barrett's Esophagus

The features of Barrett's esophagus detected by endoscopic biopsy are the presence of intestinal metaplasia including goblet cells (Fig. 6.2e). Proliferation of basal and parabasal cells, extension of papillae of connective tissue close to the mucosal surface (GERD), and an acute and/or chronic inflammation in the mucosa (reflux esophagitis) may be also seen. The features of Barrett's esophagus in brushing cytology (smears, cytospin, or ThinPrep) are the presence of goblet cells (large cytoplasmic vacuoles compressing the nuclei to one side) embedded in cuboidal or columnar intestinal metaplastic cells arranged in small nests or acini (Fig. 6.2d) [9, 22, 23]. Reactive/reparative epithelial cells, inflammatory cells (neutrophils, lymphocytes, and possibly eosinophils), and gastric epithelial cells may be seen. Alcian blue stain may be helpful to confirm the presence of goblet cells in intestinal metaplasia.

Low-Grade Dysplasia

Endoscopic biopsy histomorphology is much more sensitive for diagnosing low-grade dysplasia than brushing cytology (sensitivity, 97 vs. 20 %) [9]. The features of LGD on biopsy are the presence of columnar cells with crowded, enlarged, elongated, pseudostratified (confined to the lower half of the glandular epithelium), and hyperchromatic nuclei with mild pleomorphism, increased nuclear to cytoplasmic ratio, decreased cytoplasmic mucin, and minimal architectural changes (Fig. 6.2g) [17, 22]. The features of LGD on brushing cytology are the presence of small clusters or acini of columnar cells with crowded, enlarged, elongated and hyperchromatic nuclei, and increased nuclear to cytoplasm ratio (Fig. 6.2f) [22,

23] Differential diagnosis includes benign gastroesophageal junctional mucosa, Barrett's esophagus, and high-grade dysplasia.

High-Grade Dysplasia

Endoscopic biopsy histomorphology shows marked architectural aberrations including cribriform glands, marked pleomorphism, nuclear stratification extending to the upper part of the cells and glands, and decrease in or loss of mucin secretion, and frequent mitosis (Fig. 6.2i) [17, 22]. On brushing cytology, HGD shows two- to three-dimensional small clusters or acini of cuboidal to columnar cells with crowded, pleomorphic, enlarged and hyperchromatic nuclei with irregular nuclear membranes and prominent nucleoli, and increased nuclear to cytoplasm ratio (Fig. 6.2h) [22, 23]. Few single atypical glandular cells and rare mitoses may be seen. Tumor diathesis is absent. The differential diagnosis of HGD on cytology includes reactive and reparative atypia, LGD, and invasive adenocarcinoma.

6.2.2.3 Therapeutic Impact

Adequate tissue sampling in Barrett's esophagus has been a limitation. Utilization of jumbo biopsy forceps, addition of cytology to biopsy, enhanced imaging techniques (e.g., narrow band imaging), and emphasis to all endoscopists to follow some sampling protocol may ultimately improve our diagnostic yield. In an era of improved endoscopic therapies for Barrett's esophagus with dysplasia (e.g., radiofrequency ablation), it is more essential to improve our diagnostic technique. Improving our abilities to identify dysplasia early will allow for endoscopic therapies to be more effective in reducing the rise of esophageal adenocarcinoma.

6.2.3 Neoplastic Conditions

6.2.3.1 Esophageal Adenocarcinoma

The incidence of esophageal adenocarcinoma is estimated to be between 1 and 4 per 100,000 per year in the USA and approaches or exceeds that of squamous cell esophageal cancer [17]. There is a distinct predominance in white males (male: female ratio 7:1). Barrett's esophagus is the single most important precursor lesion and risk factor for distal esophageal adenocarcinoma [17]. Other etiologies include tobacco, obesity, alcohol, and *H. pylori* [17].

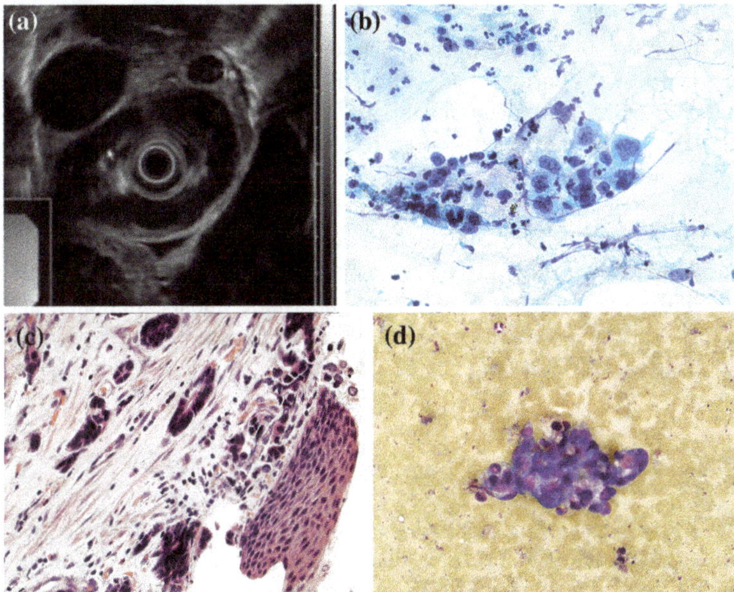

Fig. 6.3 Gastroesophageal junctional adenocarcinoma. **a** Endoscopy image. **b** Brushing cytology, Pap stain, 600×. **c** Biopsy, H and E stain, 400×. **d** EUS-FNA smear of metastatic gastroesophageal junctional adenocarcinoma in an enlarged 1.1-cm peri-esophageal lymph node, Diff Quik stain, 400×

Role of EUS-FNA in Staging Esophagus Adenocarcinoma

EUS has become an integral component of initial esophageal cancer staging (Fig. 6.3a). The accuracy of EUS for T-staging is 89 % [24]. The sensitivity and specificity for regional lymph node metastasis is 80 and 70 %, respectively and for celiac lymph node metastasis it is 85/96 % [25]. While EUS-FNA provides the most accurate locoregional staging, CT and PET are essential to assess for metastatic disease. Additional studies have demonstrated EUS-FNA to be cost-effective for preoperative staging of esophageal cancer [26]. Of note, EUS-FNA is not very effective in staging after neoadjuvant therapy.

Application of Cytology in Diagnosis of Esophageal Adenocarcinoma

Brushing cytology has similar sensitivity as biopsy for diagnosis of adenocarcinoma (96 vs. 91 %) [9]. The diagnostic accuracy of touch smear in esophageal malignancy was significantly higher (94.12 %) than brushing and crush smears (89.71 % each), and endoscopic biopsy had diagnostic accuracy of 88.24 % [27]. The diagnostic accuracy of combined brushing and biopsy was 100 %; it was 97.06 % for touch smears combined with biopsy [27].

Brushing and FNA cytology of adenocarcinoma is characterized by the presence of pleomorphic cuboidal, columnar or polygonal cells present singly or arranged in loosely cohesive and crowded three-dimensional clusters, acini or papillae (Fig. 6.3b) [23]. The nuclei are enlarged and hyperchromatic, with abnormal chromatin and one or more prominent nucleoli [23]. The cytoplasm is delicate, granular or vacuolar, and may contain mucin. More single pleomorphic cells and tumor diathesis are seen. Signet ring cell adenocarcinoma is characterized by the presence of single or loosely cohesive tumor cells with cytoplasmic mucin pushing hyperchromatic dysplastic nuclei to one side. Differential diagnosis includes HGD, reactive/reparative atypia, metastatic adenocarcinoma, and non-keratinizing squamous cell carcinoma. The tumor cells are positive for CK7 and possibly positive for CK20 and CDX2.

Therapeutic Impact

Accurate T and N staging is essential for optimizing therapy in esophageal cancer. In patients with potentially operable disease, the median survival strongly correlates with disease stage (AJCC). EUS-FNA allows for stratification based on locoregional staging. Patients with locally advance disease (T3 or greater) and/or evidence of lymph node involvement generally will be treated with neoadjuvant chemotherapy and radiation (Fig. 6.3d). Those patients with locally limited disease as determined by EUS-FNA (T2 or less without LN) potentially would be offered curative resection.

6.2.3.2 Squamous Cell Carcinoma

The annual incidence of squamous cell carcinoma does not exceed 5 per 100,000 in males and 1 per 100,000 in females [28]. It is 2–3 times more frequent in blacks [28]. The median age is 65. Contrary to the rise of esophageal adenocarcinoma, squamous cell carcinoma has decreased in incidence significantly [29]. Etiologies include tobacco, alcohol, nutrition, hot beverages, and HPV.

Diagnostic Challenges and Techniques

Similar diagnostic dilemmas exist in accurately diagnosing this disease [29]. While intestinal metaplasia can be clearly visualized in the esophagus, squamous dysplasia may be very subtle and require adjuvant imaging techniques. Endoscopy may reveal polypoid, flat, or ulcerative masses (Fig. 6.4a). Using iodine staining with the pink sign as a diagnostic index for endoscopy to diagnose high-grade intra-epithelial squamous neoplasia and squamous cell carcinoma, sensitivity is 91.9 % and specificity is 94.0 % [30]. Most cases can be diagnosed by cytology [31]. Biopsy and cytologic screening (brushing or esophageal balloon)

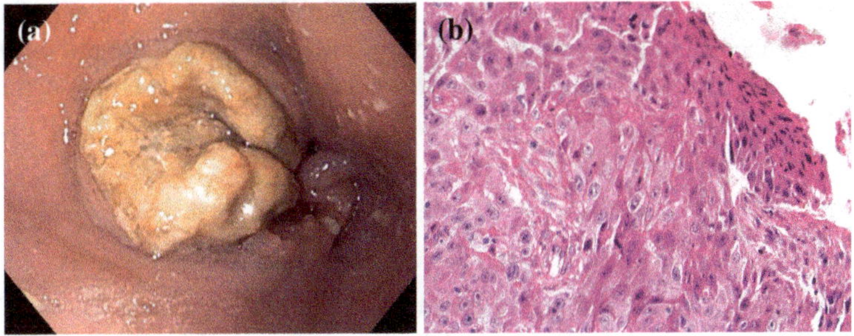

Fig. 6.4 Esophageal squamous cell carcinoma. **a** Endoscopy image. **b** Biopsy, H and E stain, 400×

of high-risk populations could decrease the mortality by facilitating early detection of the disease (Fig. 6.4b) [32].

Application of Cytology in Diagnosis of Esophageal Squamous Cell Carcinoma

Squamous cell carcinoma can be keratinizing or non-keratinizing. Keratinizing SCC is characterized by the presence of single- or three-dimensional clusters of marked pleomorphic (polygonal, bizarre, and spindle in shape) keratinizing squamous cells (Fig.6.4b). Non-keratinizing squamous cell carcinoma is characterized by the presence of single- or three-dimensional clusters of polygonal or spindle cells arranged like streams of fish or swirls and with high nuclear to cytoplasm ratios. Basaloid squamous cell carcinoma is characterized by the presence of cohesive three-dimensional clusters of cells with basaloid appearance (small, round to oval, hyperchromatic nuclei, and scant cytoplasm). Spindle squamous cell carcinoma is characterized by the presence of spindle-shaped non-keratinizing squamous cell carcinoma cells.

Differential diagnosis includes poorly differentiated adenocarcinoma, reactive/reparative squamous cells, radiation and chemotherapy effects, and squamous cell dysplasia. Basaloid squamous cell carcinoma should be distinguished from small cell carcinoma. Spindle squamous cell carcinoma should be distinguished from sarcoma or GIST. Immunohistochemical markers, p63, CK5/6, and K903 can be used to confirm squamous cell carcinoma.

Squamous cell dysplasia and carcinoma in situ are the precursors of invasive squamous cell carcinoma. Endoscopy may reveal normal mucosa, white plaques, or red areas. Using iodine staining, endoscopy can diagnose high-grade squamous dysplasia with high sensitivity [30]. Biopsy can accurately evaluate the degree of dysplasia. Brushing cytology may show atypical squamous cells with no tumor diathesis. Differential diagnosis includes reactive/reparative squamous cells, chemotherapy or radiation effect, and squamous cell carcinoma.

Combination of brushing cytology and molecular analysis targeting tumor suppressor genes and oncogenes as well as microRNA will increase the sensitivity and specificity to early diagnose precursor lesions (dysplasia and carcinoma in situ).

Therapeutic Impact

The role of EUS in squamous cell carcinoma of the esophagus is similar to adenocarcinoma as described above. Adequate locoregional staging has similar impact on management and ultimate outcome.

6.2.3.3 Other Esophageal Neoplasms

Benign or malignant mesenchymal tumors (e.g., leiomyoma, leiomyosarcoma, gastrointestinal stromal tumor (GIST), etc.), low- and high-grade endocrine neoplasms (carcinoid, endocrine carcinoma, and small cell carcinoma), low- and high-grade lymphomas, melanoma, and metastases (e.g., carcinoma, sarcoma, thymic carcinoma, etc.) can be seen in esophagus or paraesophageal lymph nodes or tissue, which should be included in the differential diagnosis based on the cytomorphology. IHC stains should be ordered based on the cytomorphology and clinical information (history, imaging studies, etc.).

Diagnostic Challenges and Techniques

The other neoplasms seen in the esophagus can be divided into mucosal and submucosal lesions. The mucosal lesions are generally endoscopically visible and diagnosis made with mucosal biopsy and/or brushing cytology. Submucosal lesions provide a diagnostic dilemma as they are generally not amenable to simple mucosal biopsy or brushing cytology. EUS-FNA is essential in obtaining tissue for diagnosis and IHC [33]. Submucosal lesions are easily identified by EUS and amenable to FNA. The most common clinical scenario is distinction between leiomyoma and GIST. This requires demonstration of not only a spindle cell neoplasm but also adequate IHC for desmin versus CD117 and CD34. The sensitivity of EUS-FNA for diagnosis of GIST is 78 % [33]. The addition of core biopsy does not appear to significantly improve diagnostic yield [33]. The introduction of tunneled jumbo biopsies in ulcerated lesions can be very effective [34].

Therapeutic Impact

EUS-FNA diagnosis and immunohistochemical studies are essential in management of submucosal lesions of the esophagus. EUS-FNA and biopsy may facilitate preoperative diagnosis of these tumors. Application of cytology (cytomorphology and ancillary tests) and therapeutic impact will be discussed in the following section.

6.3 Stomach

6.3.1 Non-Neoplastic Conditions

6.3.1.1 Gastritis

Diagnostic Challenges and Techniques

Gastritis is generally discovered on upper endoscopy. The majority of causes of gastritis can be diagnosed with standard mucosal biopsy or brushing. Most gastroenterologists utilize mucosal biopsy to make the diagnosis of *H. Pylori* gastritis or other causes. Occasionally, there may be an infiltrative cause of gastritis (e.g., eosinophilic gastroenteritis or amyloidosis). In these circumstances, jumbo biopsy forceps may improve diagnostic yield.

Cytology Application in Gastritis

Brushings and exfoliate cytology are not commonly used in gastric lesions. EUS-FNA and endoscopic biopsy are the techniques for tissue acquisition.

H. pylori infection is an important factor of acute and chronic gastritis, peptic ulcer, gastric adenocarcinoma, and gastric MALT lymphoma [35]. Gastric brushing cytology provides a sensitive, inexpensive, accurate, and easy technique for rapid detection of *H. pylori* infection, although it is not often used in diagnosis of gastritis [36]. Sensitivity of brushing cytology to identify *H. pylori* (95 %) was higher than that of biopsy histology (80.5 %) and rapid urease test (RUT) (72 %) [36]. *H. pylori* is 1–3-μm-curved or "seagull"-shaped bacteria. Markedly increase in neutrophils and/or lymphocytes, and a reactive/reparative glandular epithelium can be seen in brushing cytology, and superficial acute and chronic inflammation, erosion or an ulcer can be seen in gastric biopsy. The differential diagnosis includes Gastrospirillum hominis, which is longer and more tightly coiled. IHC stain for *H. pylori* or special Giemsa stain should be ordered for suspicious cases.

If abundant neutrophils are seen on smears from brushing and FNA specimens without the presence of atypical epithelial, mesenchymal or lymphoid cells, acute gastritis of varied causes is favored. If abundant lymphoid cells are seen, differential diagnosis includes chronic gastritis and lymphoma. If atypical lymphoid cells are identified, an aliquot of sample should be sent for flow cytometry analysis for lymphoma and a biopsy specimen should be obtained for histology examination and possible IHC studies. The sensitivity of gastric brushing cytology in diagnosis of gastric lymphoma was approximately 48 % in one study, all of which were large B cell lymphoma [37]. If abundant foamy macrophages are seen, differential diagnosis should include atypical mycobacteria infection (MAI) and xanthelasma, and an aliquot of the specimen should be sent for culture or special studies for mycobacteria. If inflammatory cells as well as atypical epithelial or mesenchymal cells are seen, a biopsy or FNA specimen for cellblock should be obtained for histologic examination and possible IHC studies to distinguish neoplasia from reactive/reparative atypia due to inflammatory processes. IHC studies can also be performed on smear slides.

Therapeutic Impact

While endoscopy with biopsy generally can provide a diagnosis of gastritis and its etiology, only 63 % of patients biopsied for gastritis truly had histologic evidence of gastritis [38]. Therapy is dependent on histologic or cytologic assessment. Early eradication of *H. Pylori* is essential to decrease risk for gastric cancer and MALT lymphoma [38].

6.3.1.2 Polyps

Gastric polyps are divided into non-neoplastic and neoplastic [39] and the majority are benign in nature. Most of them measure less than 1 cm [40]. Hyperplastic polyps were the most frequent (71.3 %), whereas fundic gland polyps accounted for 16.3 % and adenomatous polyps for 12.4 % [40]. Hyperplastic and adenomatous polyps were primarily single, whereas fundic gland polyps tended to be multiple [40]. Adenocarcinoma was detected in 0.9 % of hyperplastic polyps and in 10.5 % adenomatous polyps [40]. High-grade dysplastic foci were found in 21 % adenomatous polyps [40]. Histopathological identification is not possible by endoscopic impression thus diagnosis and treatment will depend on biopsy results [40].

Diagnostic Challenges and Techniques

As polyps are mucosal in nature, they are amenable to mucosal biopsy or endoscopic polypectomy. Cytology is seldom used in evaluation of gastric polyps. In general, there is limited challenge with gastric polyps. If the polyp is large or has any suspicion for adenoma, it can be removed in its entirety with snare polypectomy or endoscopic mucosal resection [41].

6.3.2 Neoplastic Conditions

6.3.2.1 Gastric Adenocarcinoma

Gastric cancer was the second commonest cancer in the world, but its incidence and mortality rate declined steadily worldwide [42]. The incidence increases with age in both males and females [42]. The etiology includes diet, bile reflux, *H. pylori* infection, excessive cell proliferation, oxidative stress, interference with antioxidant functions, and DNA damage [42].

Role of EUS-FNA in Diagnosis and Staging of Gastric Adenocarcinoma

EUS is an essential component of T and N staging in gastric adenocarcinoma. This has become increasingly important with the advent of endoscopic submucosal resection in the eastern world. The accuracy of T and N staging is near 90 % in gastric adencocarcinoma [43]. Similar to esophageal cancer staging, EUS-FNA is excellent for locoregional staging and LN sampling (Fig. 6.5c). It is essential to combine EUS-FNA with CT imaging to assess for metastatic disease. Endoscopy may show polypoid, fungating, or ulcerated lesions (Fig. 6.5a). It tends to occur on the greater curvature of the stomach.

Cytology Application in Gastric Adenocarcinoma

Cytology is seldom used in the diagnosis of gastric adenocarcinoma. Endoscopic biopsy and EUS-FNA are the techniques to acquire specimens for diagnosis (Fig. 6.5b). The diagnostic accuracy in gastric malignancy was 75 % for brushing alone, which was significantly lower than touch smear (87.5 %) and endoscopic biopsy (87.5 %) [27]. The diagnostic yield for crush smear was 81.25 %. A combination of touch smears and biopsy had a diagnostic yield of 100 %; it was 93.75 % for combined brushings and biopsy [27].

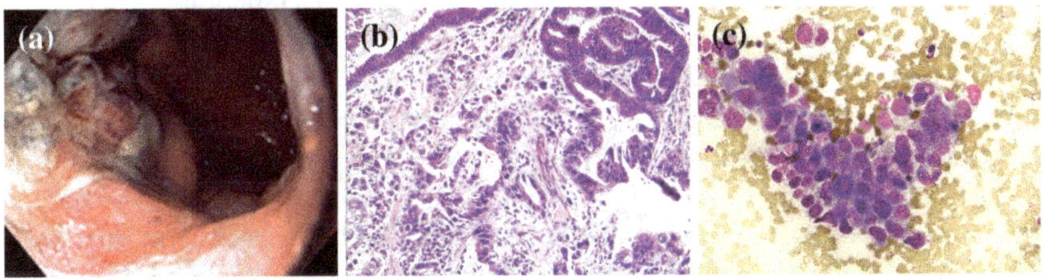

Fig. 6.5 **a** Endoscopy image of fungating gastric adenocarcinoma. **b** Biopsy of severe dysplasia and invasive gastric adenocarcinoma, H and E stain, 200×. **c** EUS-FNA smear of an enlarged 1.5-cm peri-gastric lymph node of metastatic gastric adenocarcinoma, Diff Quik stain, 400×

Brushing and FNA cytomorphology of gastric adenocarcinoma is similar to that seen in esophageal adenocarcinoma. Tumor cells are positive for CK7, possibly for CK20 and CDX-2.

Differential diagnosis includes reactive atypia, dysplasia, endocrine neoplasm, and metastatic adenocarcinoma. Presence of single, viable dysplastic epithelial cells, and tumor diathesis is helpful to establish a diagnosis of adenocarcinoma.

Therapeutic Impact

Tissue acquisition and accurate staging are important in the management of gastric cancer. This includes endoscopic and surgical resection for early lesions and chemotherapy and radiation for more advanced lesions. Perhaps the biggest diagnostic dilemma in gastric cancer lies in patients with premalignant conditions. There is a constant struggle in patients with gastric intestinal metaplasia and/or atrophic gastritis with surveillance [44]. It remains unclear what the optimal biopsy strategy and surveillance interval should be in these patients [45].

6.3.2.2 Lymphoma

The gastrointestinal tract, particularly the stomach, is the most common extranodal site of non-Hodgkin lymphoma, particularly B cell types [46]. Stomach lymphomas are considered primary if the main bulk of disease is present in the stomach. Gastrointestinal tract lymphomas account for 4–18 % of all non-Hodgkin lymphoma in Western countries, 25 % of cases in the Middle East, and 10 % of all gastric malignancies [46]. The majority of gastric lymphomas are high-grade B-cell lymphomas, some of which have developed through progression from low-grade lymphomas of mucosa associated lymphoid tissue (MALT) [46]. MALT lymphoma is most common in patients over 50 years at presentation. Predisposing factors include *H. pylori*, immunocompromised states, celiac disease, and chronic inflammatory bowel disease [46].

Role of EUS-FNA in Diagnosis and Staging of Gastric Lymphoma

The diagnosis of gastric lymphoma is generally made by mucosal biopsy. However, CT and upper endoscopy do not allow for accurate locoregional staging. EUS has been shown high accuracy in assessing gastric wall thickness and involvement by gastric lymphoma and for assessment of treatment response (Fig. 6.6a). In addition, utilization of FNA for cytologic analysis improves accuracy in nodal staging in advance disease (Fig. 6.6c) [47].

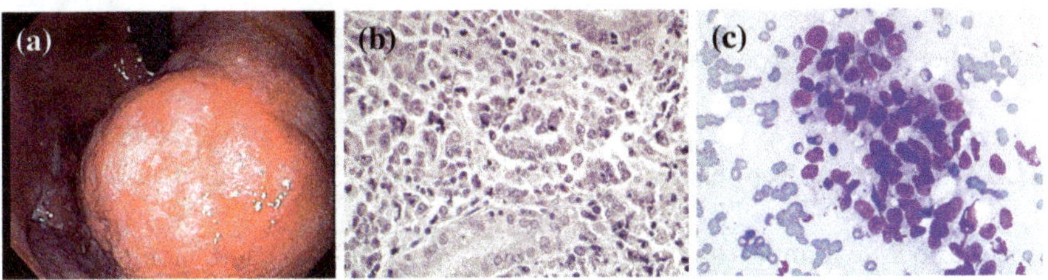

Fig. 6.6 Gastric large B cell lymphoma. **a** Endoscopy image. **b** Biopsy, H and E stain, 600×. **C** EUS-FNA cytology of metastatic gastric large B cell lymphoma in an enlarged peri-gastric lymph node, Diff Quik stain, 600×

Cytology Application in Gastric Lymphoma

Biopsy is a more commonly used technique than FNA and brushing cytology to obtain tissue for diagnosis (Fig. 6.6b). EUS-FNA can also obtain tissue for diagnosis of gastric lymphoma [48, 49]. FNA cytology of MALT lymphoma is characterized by the presence of monotonous to polymorphic, small to medium-sized lymphoid cells with minimal nuclear membrane irregularity, scant to abundant cytoplasm, plasmacytoid or monocytoid features [48, 49]. Large cell transformation is characterized by the presence of large atypical lymphoid cells with irregular nuclear membranes, vesicular chromatin and one or multiple prominent nucleoli, and moderate cytoplasm (Fig. 6.6b). Necrosis, mitotic, DNA strings, and apoptotic figures may be seen.

Differential diagnosis includes chronic gastritis, endocrine neoplasms, and poorly differentiated adenocarcinoma. FNA specimens can be used to make cell-block for histologic examination, immunohistochemistry or molecular studies, or submitted for flow cytometry analysis. MALT lymphoma cells are positive for CD20, CD19, CD79a, PAX-5, and CD43, while negative for CD5, CD10, and CD23. Molecular studies demonstrate 11:18(q21:q21) translocation, which can be detected by FISH on smears or cytospin slides. Large cell lymphoma cells are positive for CD19 and CD20, and possibly positive for CD10 and BCL-6. Immunohistochemistry and in situ hybridization for Kappa and Lambda light chain may show light chain restriction. Flow cytometry may not show a clonal proliferation of abnormal lymphoid cells in large B cell lymphoma, and thus may be not useful in the diagnosis of large B cell lymphoma.

Therapeutic Impact

Mucosal biopsies are generally obtained for diagnosis of MALT lymphoma. However, similar to other lymphomas for optimal staging, additional sampling (cytology with brushing or EUS-FNA) may improve overall yield. Detecting the presence of *H. Pylori* is essential for both diagnostic and therapeutic purposes. Adequate tissue sampling along with proper staging (EUS and endoscopy) allows for patients to be treated appropriately from simple *H. Pylori* eradication to systemic chemotherapy for advanced disesase [50].

6.3.2.3 Endocrine Neoplasms

Most endocrine tumors of the stomach are well differentiated, nonfunctioning enterochromaffin-like cell carcinoids arising from oxyntic mucosa in the corpus or fundus [51]. Carcinoid of stomach is composed of three types: (1) type I, associated with autoimmune chronic atrophic gastritis; (2) type II, associated with multiple endocrine neoplasia type-1 (MEN-1) and Zollinger–'Ellison syndrome; and (3) type III, sporadic, i.e., not associated with hyper gastrinaemia or autoimmune chronic atrophic gastritis. Carcinoid is the second most common epithelial tumor of the stomach and accounts for 11–41 % of all gastrointestinal carcinoids [51]. Gastric carcinoids are often multiple. Early diagnosis of carcinoid tumors in the gastrointestinal tract allows for possible endoscopic mucosal resection. EUS examination can determine the depth of this subepithelial lesion and determine if it is amenable for endoscopic mucosal resection or surgery. Endoscopic biopsy is much more commonly used technique than EUS-FNA for gastric endocrine tumor. The FNA cytology characteristics of endocrine tumors are discussed in the pancreas section.

6.3.2.4 Subepithelial Mesenchymal Neoplasms

Stomach is the most common site for gastrointestinal mesenchymal neoplasms [52]. The most common gastrointestinal mesenchymal neoplasms are GIST or smooth muscle neoplasms [52].

Diagnostic Challenges and Techniques

Submucosal lesions provide a diagnostic dilemma as they are generally not amenable to simple mucosal biopsy or brushing cytology. Submucosal lesions are easily identified by EUS and amenable to FNA. EUS-FNA is essential in obtaining tissue for diagnosis and immunohistochemistry [33, 48]. The sensitivity of EUS-FNA for diagnosis of GIST is 78 % [33]. The addition of core biopsy does not appear to significantly improve diagnostic yield [33]. The introduction of tunneled jumbo biopsies in ulcerated lesions can be very effective [34].

Cytology Application in Subepithelial Mesenchymal Neoplasms

GIST

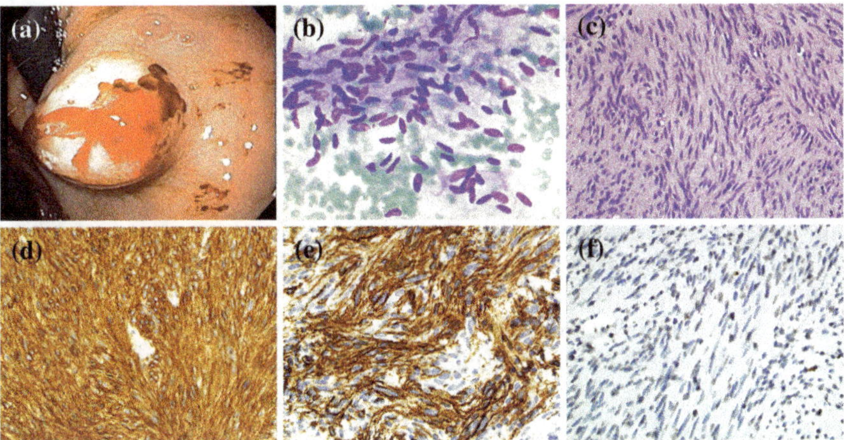

Fig. 6.7 Gastrointestinal stromal tumor of stomach. **a** Endoscopy image. **b** Touch preparation of a percutaneous needle core biopsy of 4 cm mass attached to gastric wall of a 58-year-old male patient, Diff Quik stain, 600×. **c** Needle core biopsy, H and E stain, 400×. **d** IHC stain for CD117, 400×. **e** IHC stain for CD34, 400×. **f** IHC stain for desmin, 400×

GIST accounts for 2.2 % of malignant gastric tumors with no gender preference. Patients are generally older than 60 years of age. The sensitivity of EUS-FNA cytology to diagnose gastric GIST was 84.4–100 % and is influenced by size, location, shape, and layer of origin [33, 48, 53]. Diagnostic FNA cytology samples were characterized by spindle cells (about 86 %), spindle and epithelioid mixture (7–12 %) and epithelioid cells (7 %) that present in either loosely cohesive or tight aggregates with irregular borders [33, 53]. Tumor cells are mostly well organized in one direction and focally palisading with ill-defined cytoplasmic borders (Fig. 6.7) [53]. The nuclei are either spindle or ovoid, and contain fine and evenly distributed chromatin and inconspicuous nucleoli, with or without atypia. Tumor cells are positive for CD117(c-kit), CD34, and vimentin. They are occasionally positive for S100 and smooth muscle actin. Grading of GIST depends on the tumor size and mitoses/50 high power fields [52]. The differential diagnosis includes normal smooth muscle, smooth muscle neoplasms, and fibromatosis.

Smooth Muscle Neoplasms

Well-documented true gastric leiomyomas and leiomyosarcomas are infrequent [52]. They are usually asymptomatic. The cytologic features of EUS-FNA smears and touch preparations of core biopsy are the presence of spindle cells that are well organized in one direction, have "cigar-shaped" nuclei containing fine evenly distributed chromatin, and scant to moderate cytoplasm without clear cytoplasmic borders. Hypercellularity, atypical mitoses, necrosis, and markedly pleomorphism can be seen in leiomyosarcoma. Smooth muscle neoplasms are positive for desmin and smooth muscle actin, and negative for CD117 and CD34. Differential diagnosis includes normal smooth muscle, fibromatosis, and GIST.

Other Mesenchymal Neoplasms
Glomus tumor, Schwannomas, lipoma, granular cell tumor, and Kaposi sarcoma can occur in the stomach.

Therapeutic Impact

Differentiation between leiomyoma and GIST is essential for targeted therapy of subepithelial neoplasms of the stomach. Adequate tissue for IHC is essential to make this distinction. In general, GIST is offered surgical resection or therapy with tyrosine kinase inhibitor, Gleevac. In addition to tissue sampling, EUS staging allows for assessment of size and intralesional features that may predict malignancy [54].

6.4 Pancreaticobiliary System

6.4.1 Non-Neoplastic Diseases: Benign Biliary and Pancreatic Strictures

Benign biliary and pancreatic strictures can be caused by primary sclerosing cholangitis (PSC), pancreatitis, cholangitis, and other inflammatory processes. Benign strictures may mimic ductal adenocarcinoma clinically.

6.4.1.1 Role of ERCP and Brushings in Benign Strictures

Brushings of the common bile duct and pancreatic duct are important in distinguishing benign from malignant disease. Brushing cytology has had low sensitivity (42–88 %) and high specificity (97–100 %) [55]. This can be problematic in inflammatory conditions such as PSC. Atypical brushings may result from regenerative atypia. As a result, other factors are incorporated into this diagnosis such as serum tumor markers (CA19-9). The recent improvement in techniques of peroral cholangioscopy has allowed for direct and improved sampling. However, longitudinal studies are still underway to delineate the role of cholangioscopic directed tissue sampling in benign biliary and pancreatic strictures. In the setting of pancreatitis, endoscopic tissue sampling has a limited role. CT-guided FNA can be important in identifying infection in patients with necrotizing pancreatitis. In chronic pancreatitis, brushing cytology is again utilized to assess for malignant progression, however, is fraught with limitations similar to that seen with PSC. Further investigations are underway to assess the role of both cholangioscopy and pancreatoscopy in improving diagnostic yield in benign disease.

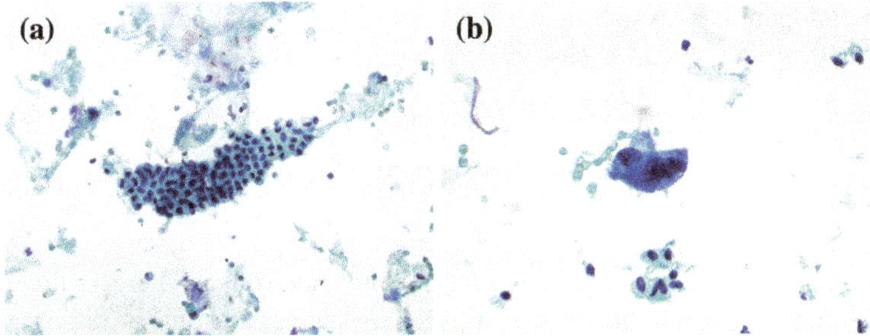

Fig. 6.8 a Brushing cytology image of benign stricture of common bile duct, ThinPrep, Pap stain, 400×. **b** Brushing cytology of cholangiocarcinoma of common bile duct, adenocarcinoma cells and benign bile duct epithelial cells, ThinPrep, Pap stain, 600×

6.4.1.2 Cytology Application in Benign Biliary and Pancreatic Strictures

Brushing cytology, biopsy, and FNA are commonly used in evaluation of common bile duct or pancreatic duct stricture. The cytologic features of benign stricture in brushing and FNA cytology are the presence of glandular epithelial cells with reactive atypia that are present in cohesive flat "honeycomb" sheets with maintenance of polarity (Fig. 6.8a). The nuclei may be hyperchromatic, vesicular, degenerative, enlarged, and varied in size, contain prominent single or multiple nucleoli and evenly distributed chromatin, and show smooth nuclear membranes. Normal mitotic figures and inflammatory cells can be seen. The differential diagnosis of reactive atypia includes dysplasia and adenocarcinoma.

6.4.1.3 Therapeutic Impact

In inflammatory conditions such as PSC and chronic pancreatitis, there is a small but true increase in the incidence of malignancy. Identification of cholangiocarcinoma in PSC would potentially allow a patient to be considered for liver transplant. Identification of early malignancy in chronic pancreatitis would potentially allow a patient to be considered for curative pancreaticoduodenectomy.

6.4.2 Cystic Lesions of the Pancreas

Pancreatic cystic lesions are often found incidentally and divided into non-neoplastic (pseudocyst, lymphoepithelial cyst, retention cysts, mucinous non-neoplastic cyst, etc.) and neoplastic lesions (mucinous cystic neoplasms (MCNs), intraductal papillary mucinous neoplasms (IPMNs), serous microcystic adenoma, solid pseudopapillary cystic neoplasm, teratoma, etc.). Endocrine neoplasms and acinar cell carcinoma can occasionally present as a cystic mass.

6.4.2.1 Role of EUS-FNA in Diagnosis of Cystic Lesions of the Pancreas

A combination of clinical and radiologic features, analysis of the cyst fluid, FNA biopsy, immunohistochemistry, and molecular studies is useful in differentiating the various types of pancreatic cysts [56]. The mainstay of assessment of pancreatic cysts is CT and MRI [57]. Accurate differentiation of cystic neoplasms of the pancreas is essential when considering surgical management. Preoperative distinction between mucinous and non-mucinous, and benign and malignant neoplasms is essential for planning an appropriate treatment strategy [56]. Endosonography allows for detailed characterization of cystic neoplasms and with the addition of FNA provides fluid for biochemical analysis and cytology. EUS examination allows for accurate assessment of size, presence of septation, presence of mural nodularity, and calcification. Increasing size and presence of any of these EUS features are more predictive of malignancy. ERCP is useful to determine the relationship between cystic lesions and the pancreatic duct.

Fluid analysis is generally sent for CEA, amylase, and cytology. A CEA level exceeding 192 has a specificity of 84 % for mucinous neoplasm [58]. Cytologic evaluation in general has had low sensitivity but high specificity for mucinous neoplasms. Recently, cytology has been coupled with molecular analysis. The addition of molecular analysis (e.g., KRAS and LOH) increases sensitivity and specificity of cyst fluid analysis significantly [56]. All patients with pancreatic cystic lesions must be thoroughly investigated to ascertain the underlying nature of the cyst. Small asymptomatic cysts (<3 cm) with no suspicious features on imaging or FNA may be safely followed up [57]. Follow-up should continue for at least 4 years, with a repeat FNA if needed [57].

6.4.2.2 Role Of Cytology in Cystic Lesions of the Pancreas

Pseudocyst

Pseudocyst results from pancreatitis, and is the most common cystic lesion in the pancreas (up to 75 %) [57]. Pseudocysts mostly occur in the tail, are usually unilocular, and lack lining epithelial cells (Fig. 6.9). Clinical presentation and image studies may mimic pancreatic cancer. The FNA-aspirated cyst content is low viscosity, hemorrhagic, dark and opaque [56], and has high amylase and low CEA [56]. The features of FNA cytology are the presence of rare benign appearing or reactive ductal epithelial cells or no epithelial cells, macrophages, hemosiderin/ bile pigment, necrotic amorphous debris, inflammatory cells, calcification, fatty necrosis, cholesterol crystals, granulation tissue, and fibrous tissue (Fig. 6.9). Islet

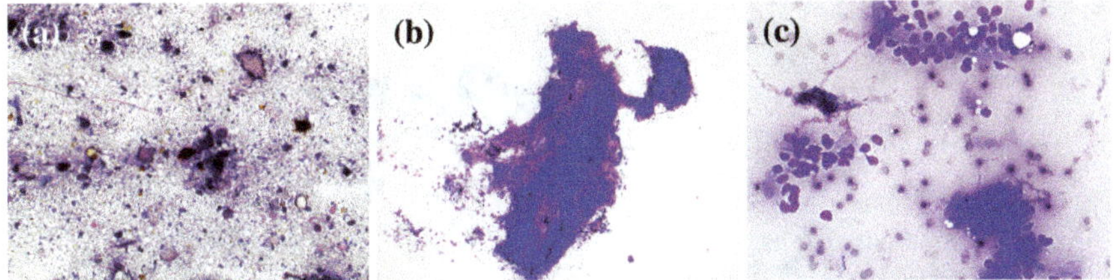

Fig. 6.9 Pancreatic pseudocyst, EUS-FNA. **a** Cyst aspiration, Diff Quik stain, 400×. **b** Fibrous tissue fragment containing chronic inflammation, islet cells and benign bile duct cells, Diff Quik, 100×. **c** Two clusters of islet cells and one cluster of benign bile duct cells, Diff Quik stain, 400×

cells may be present due to hyperplasia, which should not be misinterpreted as endocrine neoplasm. Atypical reactive and reparative ductal cells aspirated from chronic pancreatitis should be distinguished from dysplasia or ductal adenocarcinoma. Atypical reactive and reparative mesenchymal cells and histiocytes should not be mistaken for sarcoma.

Lymphoepithelial Cyst

Lymphoepithelial cyst of the pancreas is a rare non-neoplastic cystic lesion that occurs predominantly in male adults (usually in the 5th and 6th decade) with or without symptoms [59, 60]. The features of FNA cytology are presence of benign squamous cells, keratinous debris, predominantly small and mature lymphocytes, histiocytes, germinal center fragments, multinucleated giant cells, and cholesterol crystals [60, 61] (Fig. 6.10). Differential diagnosis includes benign cystic teratomas including dermoid cyst and epidermal cyst, squamous cell carcinoma [59], and adenosquamous carcinoma.

Mucinous Non-Neoplastic Cyst

Mucinous non-neoplastic cyst is a recently described pancreatic cystic lesion that presents as an isolated unilocular or multilocular mucinous cyst. The cyst is lined by single layer of cuboidal to columnar mucinous epithelium supported by hypocellular stroma and does not communicate with pancreatic ducts [62]. The features of FNA are presence of flat nests or sheets of cuboidal to columnar mucinous cells and abundant background mucus (Fig. 6.11). The mucinous cells have basally located small round to oval nuclei containing fine granular chromatin, and possible small nucleoli. Slightly nuclear membrane irregularity, nuclear grooves, and intranuclear inclusions may be seen. The epithelial cells are positive for MUC-1 and MUC5AC, and negative for MUC-2. Cyst fluid CEA levels are >500 ng/ml.

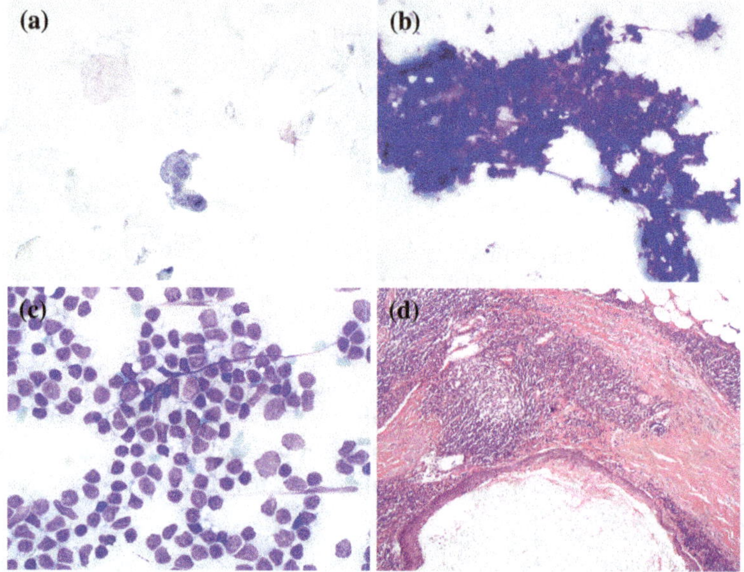

Fig. 6.10 Pancreatic lymphoepithelial cyst, EUS-FNA and excision of cystic mass. **a** Nucleated and anucleated squamous cells, Pap stain, 600×. **b** Necrosis, Diff Quik stain, 600×. **c** Polymorphous lymphocytes, predominantly small mature lymphocytes, Diff Quik, 600×. **d** Excision of cystic mass, H and E stain, 100×

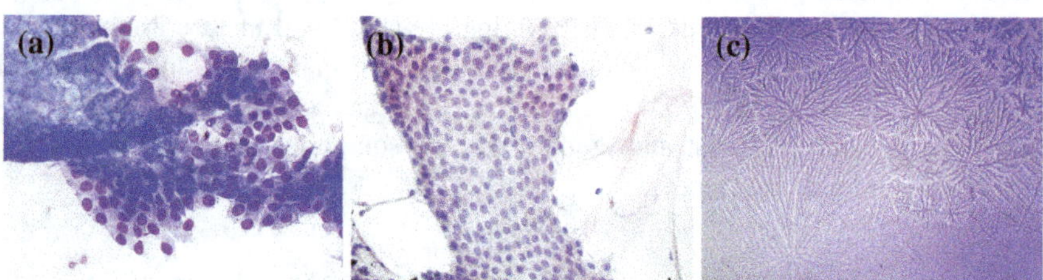

Fig. 6.11 Pancreatic mucinous non-neoplastic cyst, EUS-FNA. **a** Diff Quik stain, 400×. **b** Pap stain, 400×. **c** Extracellular mucin, Diff Quik stain, 100x

Serous Cystic Neoplasms

Serous cystic neoplasms (serous microcystic adenoma, serous oligocystic adenoma, and serous cystadenocarcinoma) are cystic epithelial neoplasms composed of glycogen-rich, ductular-type epithelial cells that produce a watery fluid similar to serum [63]. Most are benign with or without clinical symptoms, and may occur as part of the von Hippel-Lindau syndrome. FNA gives clear fluid. Serous epithelial cells were identified in <20–100 % of FNA specimens with a sensitivity ranging from 3.6 to 100 % [64–66]. The features of FNA cytology are the presence of loose flat nests or "honeycombed" sheets of bland cuboidal epithelial cells with small and round nuclei containing fine chromatin and possibly containing nucleoli [64, 67]. The cytoplasm is moderate in amount and clear to finely granular or vacuolar with indistinct cell borders. Mitotic figures and necrosis are absent. CEA levels are <5 ng/ml, CA-19.9 levels are low, and amylase levels range from 11 to 90 U/L [64, 67].

Mucinous Cystic Neoplasms

MCNs are composed of columnar, mucin-producing epithelium supported by the ovarian-type stroma with no communication with the pancreatic ductal system. MCNs are rare and usually found in the pancreatic body or tail of middle-aged women [57]. The aspirated cystic contents are usually thick, but may be hemorrhagic or necrotic [57]. The features of FNA cytology are the presence of nests, sheets, or papillae of cohesive mucinous columnar cells with or without atypia and loss of polarity, and abundant extracellular mucin (Fig. 6.12). Stroma seen in cellblock or core is typically ovarian-type stroma, which may be immunohistochemically positive for ER, PR, and inhibin and is useful to separate mucinous neoplasm from mucinous non-neoplastic cysts and IPMN. The epithelial cells are positive for CDX-2 (67 %), PDX-1 (100 %), CK7 (83 %), and CK20 (100 %), which is similar to ovarian mucinous cystic neoplasm of intestinal type [68].

Intraductal Papillary Mucinous Neoplasm

IPMNs commonly occur in old men, and most commonly involve the main pancreatic duct but may also affect the branches or a combination of the two [57]. There are three subtypes such as intestinal, pancreaticobiliary, and gastric foveolar subtype. Invasive adenocarcinoma arising from intestinal subtype has better prognosis than that arising from pancreaticobiliary subtype. Gastric foveolar subtype is seen in branch-type IPMN, which rarely progresses toward frank malignancy [69]. Communication with the pancreatic duct may be visualized on

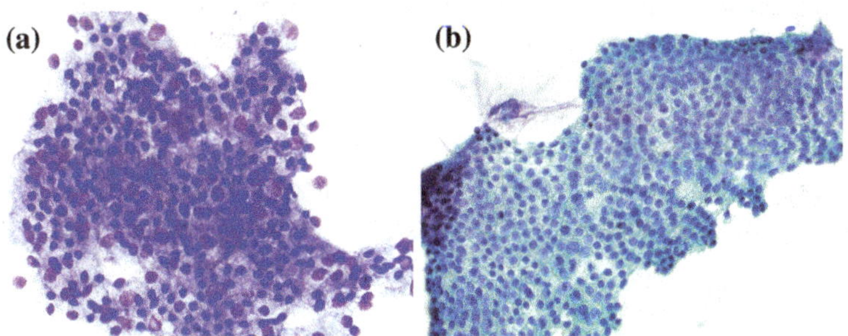

Fig. 6.12 Pancreatic mucinous cystic neoplasm, EUS-FNA. **a** Diff Quik stain, 400×. **b** Pap stain, 400×

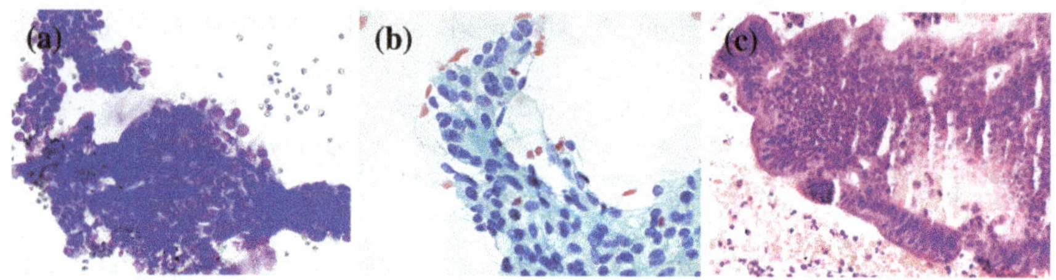

Fig. 6.13 Pancreatic intraductal papillary mucinous neoplasm, EUS-FNA. **a** and **b** EUS photos. **a** Diff Quik stain, 400×. **b** Pap stain, 400×. **c** Cellblock, H and E stain, 400×

endoscopic retrograde cholangiopancreatography (ERCP), magnetic resonance cholangiopancreatography (MRCP), or EUS [70]. The EUS-FNA technique in diagnosing IPMNs has been recognized to be of great importance in recent years. The features on FNA cytology are presence of papillae or sheets of cuboidal to columnar cells with round to ovoid, basally or eccentrically located nuclei containing fine evenly distributed granular to irregularly distributed coarse chromatin and small to prominent nucleoli (Fig. 6.13) [71]. Irregular clustering, complex papillae, and discohesiveness with single atypical cells were features of borderline and highly suspicious malignant lesions. Micropapillary clusters and single markedly atypical cells were seen in malignant cases [71]. The abundant background mucus obtained from IPMNs is thicker and more gelatinous than the watery mucin associated with a normal duodenal epithelium. Three main patterns of IHC stains with CDX-2, MUC-1, and MUC-2 are noted depending on the subtypes of IPMNs [71, 72]. Increased cytoplasmic expression of caspase-3 is seen in IPMNs with invasive adenocarcinoma [73].

6.4.2.3 Therapeutic Impact

Despite increased utilization of EUS-FNA for classifying pancreatic cystic lesions, a majority are managed conservatively. Serous cystadenomas are managed conservatively unless they become symptomatic or have demonstrated propensity to grow between serial imaging studies. In general, mucinous cystadenomas should be resected due to malignant potential. A distal pancreatectomy is performed for lesions in the body and tail and pancreaticoduodenectomy for lesions in the head and uncinate process. IPMN lesions which are main duct in nature should undergo surgical resection. This may require localized resection or even total pancreatectomy in severe cases. IPMN lesions limited to side branches of the pancreatic duct can be monitored. However, significant growth between imaging studies should prompt resection [74].

6.4.3 Solid Pancreatic Neoplasms

Pancreatic ductal adenocarcinoma, endocrine neoplasm, acinar cell carcinoma, solid pseudopapillary neoplasm, pancreatoblastoma, mesenchymal tumors, lymphoma, and metastatic malignancies are commonly present as a solid mass, but some of them may be present as a cystic mass or with cystic degeneration.

6.4.3.1 Ductal Adenocarcinoma

Ductal adenocarcinoma is the most common type of pancreatic cancer, representing 85–90 % of all pancreatic neoplasms, mostly affects older patients (60–80 years), and is mostly found in the head of the pancreas (60–70 %) [75].

Role of FNA and Brushing Cytology in Diagnosis and Staging of Pancreatic Ductal Adenocarcinoma

FNA biopsy is a more sensitive and reliable diagnostic technique than endoscopic brushing cytology and biopsy. The needle can be guided with a variety of diagnostic imaging techniques, including endoscopic retrograde cholangiopancreatography (ERCP), percutaneous transhepatic cholangiography (PTC), ultrasound, computed tomography, and MRI. EUS-FNA has provided significant improvements in locoregional staging for pancreatic adenocarcinoma. In direct comparison to Helical CT, EUS-detected significantly more tumors (97 vs. 73 %), more accurately determines respectability (91 vs. 83 %), and is more sensitive for assessment of vascular invasion (91 vs. 64 %) [76]. Addition of FNA increases the accuracy of acquiring tissue for diagnosis. In contrast to CT-FNA or other imaging-guided tissue sampling, a significant risk of tumor seeding is not seen. A majority of seeding occurs in the skin which is not traversed with EUS-FNA. The advent of EUS-FNA has significantly improvement staging and diagnosis of pancreatic adenocarcinoma. Brushing cytology is an alternative technique to obtain sample for superficial mucosal lesions or lesions involving mucosa [2–4]. The sensitivity, specificity, positive predictive values, negative predictive value, and diagnostic accuracy are 53–96.6 100, 100, 25–96.2, and 56–97.6 %, respectively, which are similar to those of biopsy and can be improved by simultaneous biopsy [2, 4, 77, 78].

Cytology in Diagnosis of Pancreatic Ductal Adenocarcinoma

FNA cytology characteristically presence of single, "drunken honeycomb" sheets or loosely cohesive two- or three-dimentional glandular clusters of pleomorphic polygonal, cuboidal or columnar cells with loss of polarity (Fig. 6.14). The nuclei are enlarged and pleomorphic, show irregular and thicken nuclear membranes, and

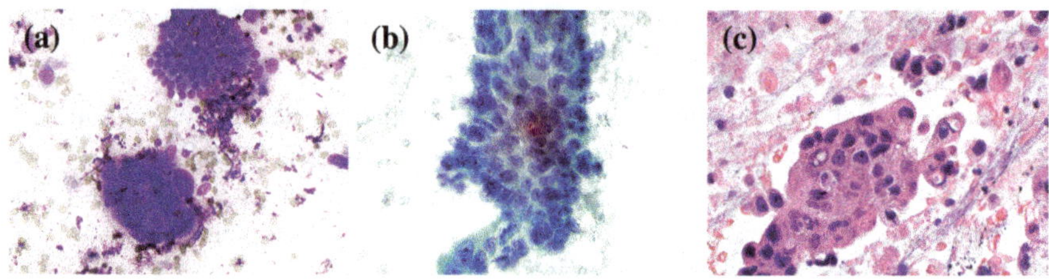

Fig. 6.14 Pancreatic ductal adenocarcinoma, EUS-FNA. **a** EUS image. **b** Diff Quik stain, 400×. **c** Pap stain, 600×. **d** Cellblock, H and E stain, 400×

contain hyperchromatic, coarse, or vesicular, unevenly distributed chromatin and prominent nucleoli. The cytoplasm is delicate, vacuolated or squamoid, is variable in amount, and may contain mucin. Bizarre cells, signet ring cells, binucleated or multinucleated cells, osteoclast-like giant cells, mitoses, necrosis, and mucin can be seen.

FNA cytology of mucinous (colloid) adenocarcinoma shows single or small clusters of malignant ductal cells floating in extensive extracellular mucin. Clear cell variants of ductal carcinoma is not uncommon, and FNA cytology shows clear cytoplasm, which should be separated from mucin production. FNA cytology of adenosquamous carcinoma shows glandular and squamous differentiation. Giant cell carcinoma is characteristically by presence of significant proportion of bizarre, pleomorphic, multinucleated tumor giant cells. Presence of abundant osteoclast-like giant cells raises the diagnosis of undifferentiated carcinoma with osteoclast-like giant cells.

Differential diagnosis includes degenerative changes, reactive atypia, mucinous cystadenocarcinoma, endocrine neoplasm, and metastatic adenocarcinoma. The tumor cells are positive for CK7, CK20, CK19, and rarely CDX-2.

Therapeutic Impact

The introduction of EUS-FNA in staging pancreatic malignancies has significantly altered management. Resectable lesions in the tail are amenable to distal pancreatectomy while lesions in the head to pancreatico-duodenectomy. Increasing accuracy for vascular invasion and lymph node metastasis has allowed for significant improvements in detection of respectability. In one study, EUS and EUS-FNA precluded surgery in 27 % patients with a cost-reduction of $3300 per patient [79]. Preoperative staging combining CT and EUS-FNA provides the most effective method to assess patients for surgical resection or chemotherapy and radiation.

6.4.3.2 Pancreatic Endocrine Neoplasms

Pancreatic endocrine neoplasms predominantly occur in older adults. They may present as part of MEN, and may be associated with a variety of clinical syndromes, depending hormones secreted.

Role of EUS-FNA in Diagnosis and Staging of Endocrine Neoplasms

EUS is also essential in localization of pancreatic endocrine tumors. EUS has been demonstrated have 82 % sensitivity, 95 % specificity, and 90 % accuracy for localization of these tumors [80, 81]. In addition, FNA can be done in lesions as small as 5 mm to obtain tissue diagnosis of pancreatic endocrine tumors when desired.

Cytology in Diagnosis of Pancreatic Endocrine Neoplasms

The FNA cytology of endocrine neoplasms is characterized by the presence of single, loosely cohesive sheets or clusters, and rosettes of monotonous cells that contain round or oval and eccentrically located nuclei (plasmacytoid) with characteristic "salt and pepper" chromatin, smooth nuclear membrane, and no or small nucleoli (Fig. 6.15). The cytoplasm is small-to-moderate in amount, finely granular, or delicate. Abundant naked nuclei with granular background are often seen and occasionally, significant pleomorphic cells (endocrine atypia) can be seen. Number of mitotic figures, tumor size measured by CT, and degree of nuclear atypia are related to the grade of the endocrine neoplasm. Small cell carcinoma is rare in pancreas.

Tumor cells are positive for pan-cytokeratin, CD56, chromagranin, synaptophysin, NSE, and hormones. Electron microscopy can demonstrate dense core neurosecretory granules.

The differential diagnosis includes islet cell hyperplasia, solid pseudopapillary neoplasm, acinar carcinoma, ductal carcinoma, metastatic small cell carcinoma, and malignant lymphoma including plasmacytoma.

6.4.3.3 Solid Pseudopapillary Neoplasm

Solid pseudopapillary neoplasm is a rare, usually benign neoplasm with predominant manifestation in the pancreatic body or tail of young women [82]. The diagnostic accuracy of EUS-FNA is 75 % [83]. The characteristics of FNA cytology are the presence of single or dyscohesive clusters of plasmacytoid cells surrounding branching vasculature (pseudopapillae) and myxoid stroma (metachromatic matrix) (Fig. 6.16) [83–85]. The relatively uniform cells have scant to moderate, delicate or granular cytoplasm with occasional many small or large clear

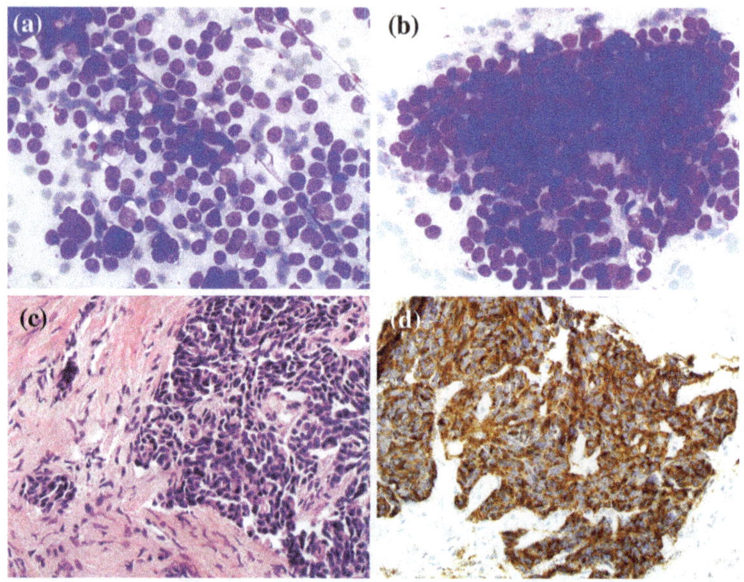

Fig. 6.15 Pancreatic endocrine neoplasm, percutaneous needle core biopsy. **a** and **b** Touch preparation, Diff Quik stain, 600×. **c** Core, H and E stain, 400×. **d** IHC for chromogranin, 400×

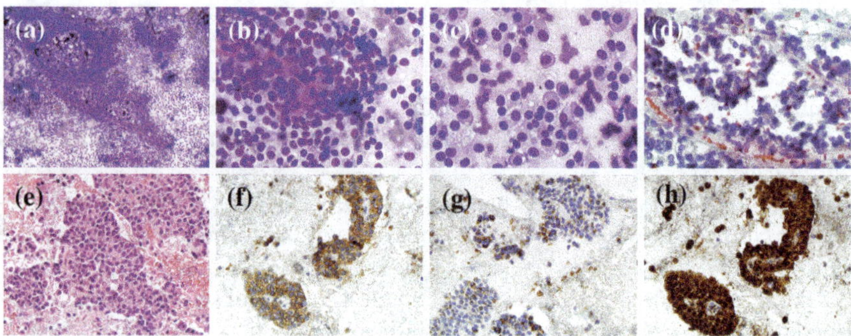

Fig. 6.16 Pancreatic solid pseudopapillary neoplasm, EUS-FNA. **a** Diff Quik stain, 100×. **b** and **c** Diff Quik stain, 600×. **d** Pap stain, 600×. **e** Cellblock, H and E stain, 400×. **f** IHC for CD10, 400×. **g** IHC for chromogranin, 400×. **i** IHC for β-catenin, 400×

cytoplasmic vacuoles and ill-defined cytoplasmic borders, and round or oval nuclei containing fine, evenly distributed chromatin and small nucleoli, showing smooth, regular nuclear membrane, and rarely showing nuclear grooves [84, 85]. Macrophages and necrosis may be seen [85]. Differential diagnosis includes endocrine neoplasms [83]. Large, clear cytoplasmic vacuolation, and IHC stains can be used to separate solitary pseudopapillary neoplasm from endocrine neoplasms [83, 84]. Tumor cells are positive for CD10, vimentin, beta-catenin, NSE, α-1 antitrypsin, CD56, and progesterone receptors, and focally positive for cytokeratin, chromogranin, and synaptophysin.

6.4.3.4 Acinar Cell Carcinoma

Acinar cell carcinoma is composed of relatively uniform neoplastic cells that are arranged in solid and acinar patterns and produce pancreatic enzymes [86]. Acinar cell carcinomas represent 1–2 % of all exocrine pancreatic neoplasms in adults with a mean age of 62 and may arise in any portion of the pancreas [86]. The FNA cytology is characterized by presence of abundant single or loosely cohesive clusters of malignant epithelial cells with vaguely acinar and trabecular formations (Fig. 6.17) [87, 88]. The pleomorphic nuclei show fine granular chromatin and small or prominent nucleoli. There are scant to moderate amounts of granular cytoplasm. Scattered, strikingly large tumor cells with giant nuclei, prominent mitoses, associated necrosis, and granular background released from cytoplasm due to preparation artifact may be seen. The differential diagnosis includes endocrine neoplasm, solid pseudopapillary neoplasm, and benign acinar cells from needle track. Tumor cells are positive for trypsin, chymotrypsin, lipase, and elastase. Tumor cells may also be focally positive for chromgranin, synaptophysin, CEA, B72.3, and AFP.

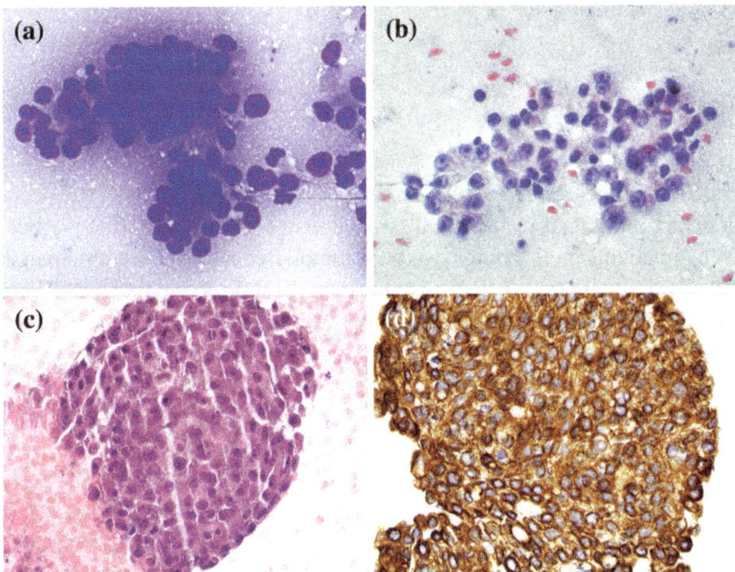

Fig. 6.17 Pancreatic acinar cell carcinoma, EUS-FNA. **a** Diff Quik stain, 600×. **b** Pap stain, 600×. **c** Cellblock, H and E stain, 400×. **d** IHC for CK7, 400×

6.5 Extrahepatic Biliary Tract: Cholangiocarcinoma

6.5.1 Role of ERCP Brushings and EUS-FNA in Diagnosis of Cholangiocarcinoma

Tissue acquisition in cholangiocarcinoma has been a longstanding dilemma. Brushing cytology has low accuracy of 65 % in malignant strictures [89]. In combination with tumor markers (CA19-9), sensitivity and specificity increase to 88 % [90]. The advent of EUS-FNA has allowed for improvements in patients with locally advanced disease and lymph nodes or overt mass lesions. Peroral cholangioscopy appears to significantly improve tissue diagnosis in cholangiocarcinoma in preliminary investigations. This allows for direct visualization of the stricture or mass lesion and targeted biopsies. Ultimately, the utilization of cholangioscopy and enhanced ductal imaging techniques will significantly improve diagnosis in cholangiocarcinoma.

6.5.2 Cytology in Diagnosis of Cholangiocarcinoma

FNA cytology and brushing cytology of the extrahepatic biliary tract, common bile duct and pancreatic duct, can be used in the diagnosis of cholangiocarcinoma. The characteristics of FNA and brushing cytology of cholangiocarcinoma are similar to those of pancreatic ductal adenocarcinoma (Fig. 6.8).

6.5.3 Therapeutic Impact

In general cholangiocarcinoma has a poor 5-year survival of 5–10 %. Respectability rates for distal, intrahepatic, and perihilar lesions are 91, 60, and 56 %, respectively [91]. Even in patients undergoing resection, tumor-free margins are obtained in only 20–40 % of proximal and 50 % of distal tumors [92]. Preoperative ERCP not only allows for tissue diagnosis but provides opportunity for biliary decompression and ultimately may be the only treatment option. In unresectable cholangiocarcinoma, chemotherapy and radiation is an option, but has very limited efficacy.

6.6 Other Pancreaticobiliary Malignancies

6.6.1 Role of ERCP Brushings and EUS-FNA in Diagnosis of Other Pancreaticobiliary Malignancies

ERCP and EUS can be effective in patients with other pancreaticobiliary malignancies. ERCP with brushings and or cholangioscopy with targeted biopsies are very effective in patients with metastatic malignancy and biliary strictures. EUS-FNA allows for tissue sampling with FNA and core biopsy sampling. In cases of suspected, lymphoma, core biopsy provides large samples for flow cytometry and proper lymphoma staging. In general, EUS-FNA is very effective in obtaining tissue diagnosis is non-adenocarcinoma pancreatic mass lesions and for metastatic malignancies with lymphadenopathy adjacent to the gastrointestinal tract.

6.6.2 Cytology in Diagnosis of Other Pancreaticobiliary Malignancies

Malignancies of the lung, kidney, breast, liver, gastrointestinal cancers, melanoma, and sarcoma may metastasize to pancreas. Pancreatic involvement by malignant lymphoma is almost always secondary rather than primary. Rare entities and metastases should be considered once cytomorphology and IHC stains do not support the diagnosis of common primary pancreatic neoplasms. Communication with clinicians and imaging study results are important to make a definitive diagnosis.

6.6.3 Therapeutic Impact

Adequate tissue diagnosis allows for appropriate therapeutic strategies. This is especially important in lymphoma. The diagnosis of lymphoma by EUS-FNA would preclude unnecessary surgery and allow for proper chemotherapy. EUS-FNA diagnosis of metastatic adenocarcinoma can provide the primary diagnosis and allow again for selection of the appropriate chemotherapeutic agents.

References

1. Lin X, Finkelstein SD, Zhu B, Ujevich BJ, Silverman JF (2009) Loss of heterozygosities in Barrett esophagus, dysplasia, and adenocarcinoma detected by esophageal brushing cytology and gastroesophageal biopsy. Cancer Cytopathol 117:57–66
2. Elek G, Gyokeres T, Schafer E, Burai M, Pinter F, Pap A (2005) Early diagnosis of pancreatobiliary duct malignancies by brush cytology and biopsy. Pathol Oncol Res 11:145–155

3. Urbano M, Rosa A, Gomes D, Camacho E, Calhau CA, Leitao M (2008) Team approach to ERCP-directed single-brush cytology for the diagnosis of malignancy. Rev Esp Enferm Dig 100:462–465
4. Uchida N, Kamada H, Tsutsui K, Ono M, Aritomo Y, Masaki T, Kushida Y, Haba R, Nakatsu T, Kuriyama S (2007) Utility of pancreatic duct brushing for diagnosis of pancreatic carcinoma. J Gastroenterol 42:657–662
5. Yamao K, Bhatia V, Mizuno N, Sawaki A, Shimizu Y, Irisawa A (2009) Interventional endoscopic ultrasonography. J Gastroenterol Hepatol 24:509–519
6. Falk GW, Chittajallu R, Goldblum JR, Biscotti CV, Geisinger KR, Petras RE, Birgisson S, Rice TW, Richter JE (1997) Surveillance of patients with Barrett's esophagus for dysplasia and cancer with balloon cytology. Gastroenterology 112:1787–1797
7. Adams L, Roth MJ, Abnet CC, Dawsey SP, Qiao YL, Wang GQ, Wei WQ, Lu N, Dawsey SM, Woodson K (2008) Promoter methylation in cytology specimens as an early detection marker for esophageal squamous dysplasia and early esophageal squamous cell carcinoma. Cancer Prev Res (Phila Pa) 1:357–361
8. Wilcox CM, Rodgers W, Lazenby A (2004) Prospective comparison of brush cytology, viral culture, and histology for the diagnosis of ulcerative esophagitis in AIDS. Clin Gastroenterol Hepatol 2:564–567
9. Saad RS, Mahood LK, Clary KM, Liu Y, Silverman JF, Raab SS (2003) Role of cytology in the diagnosis of Barrett's esophagus and associated neoplasia. Diagn Cytopathol 29:130–135
10. Quarto G, Sivero L, Somma P, De Rosa G, Mosella F, Nunziata G, Solimeno G, Benassai G (2008) A case of infectious esophagitis caused by human papilloma virus. Minerva Gastroenterol Dietol 54:317–321
11. Sampliner RE (2002) Updated guidelines for the diagnosis, surveillance, and therapy of Barrett's esophagus. Am J Gastroenterol 97:1888–1895
12. Syrjanen KJ (1982) Histological changes identical to those of condylomatous lesions found in esophageal squamous cell carcinomas. Arch Geschwulstforsch 52:283–292
13. Yao PF, Li GC, Li J, Xia HS, Yang XL, Huang HY, Fu YG, Wang RQ, Wang XY, Sha JW (2006) Evidence of human papilloma virus infection and its epidemiology in esophageal squamous cell carcinoma. World J Gastroenterol 12:1352–1355
14. Gao GF, Roth MJ, Wei WQ, Abnet CC, Chen F, Lu N, Zhao FH, Li XQ, Wang GQ, Taylor PR, Pan QJ, Chen W, Dawsey SM, Qiao YL (2006) No association between HPV infection and the neoplastic progression of esophageal squamous cell carcinoma: result from a cross-sectional study in a high-risk region of China. Int J Cancer 119:1354–1359
15. Pera M, Cameron AJ, Trastek VF, Carpenter HA, Zinsmeister AR (1993) Increasing incidence of adenocarcinoma of the esophagus and esophagogastric junction. Gastroenterology 104:510–513
16. Haggitt RC (1994) Barrett's esophagus, dysplasia, and adenocarcinoma. Hum Pathol 25:982–993
17. Werner M, Flejou JF, Hainaut P, Hofler H, Lambert R, Keller G, Stein HJ (2000) World health organization classification of tumors: Pathology and Genetics: Tumors of the digestive system. In: Hamilton SR, Aaltonen LA (eds) Adenocarcinoma of the esophagus, IARC Press, Lyon, pp 20–26
18. Goda K, Tajiri H, Ikegami M, Urashima M, Nakayoshi T, Kaise M (2007) Usefulness of magnifying endoscopy with narrow band imaging for the detection of specialized intestinal metaplasia in columnar-lined esophagus and Barrett's adenocarcinoma. Gastrointest Endosc 65:36–46
19. Wolfsen HC, Crook JE, Krishna M, Achem SR, Devault KR, Bouras EP, Loeb DS, Stark ME, Woodward TA, Hemminger LL, Cayer FK, Wallace MB (2008) Prospective, controlled tandem endoscopy study of narrow band imaging for dysplasia detection in Barrett's Esophagus. Gastroenterology 135:24–31
20. Fritcher EG, Brankley SM, Kipp BR, Voss JS, Campion MB, Morrison LE, Legator MS, Lutzke LS, Wang KK, Sebo TJ, Halling KC (2008) A comparison of conventional cytology

DNA ploidy analysis, and fluorescence in situ hybridization for the detection of dysplasia and adenocarcinoma in patients with Barrett's esophagus. Hum Pathol 39:1128–1135

21. Brankley SM, Wang KK, Harwood AR, Miller DV, Legator MS, Lutzke LS, Kipp BR, Morrison LE, Halling KC (2006) The development of a fluorescence in situ hybridization assay for the detection of dysplasia and adenocarcinoma in Barrett's esophagus. J Mol Diagn 8:260–267

22. Antonioli DA, Wang HH (1997) Morphology of Barrett's esophagus and Barrett's-associated dysplasia and adenocarcinoma. Gastroenterol Clin North Am 26:495–506

23. Wang HH, Doria MI Jr, Purohit-Buch S, Schnell T, Sontag S, Chejfec G (1992) Barrett's esophagus. The cytology of dysplasia in comparison to benign and malignant lesions. Acta Cytol 36:60–64

24. Rosch T (1995) Endosonographic staging of esophageal cancer: a review of literature results. Gastrointest Endosc Clin N Am 5:537–547

25. van Vliet EP, Heijenbrok-Kal MH, Hunink MG, Kuipers EJ, Siersema PD (2008) Staging investigations for oesophageal cancer: a meta-analysis. Br J Cancer 98:547–557

26. Harewood GC, Wiersema MJ (2002) A cost analysis of endoscopic ultrasound in the evaluation of esophageal cancer. Am J Gastroenterol 97:452–458

27. Batra M, Handa U, Mohan H, Sachdev A (2008) Comparison of cytohistologic techniques in diagnosis of gastroesophageal malignancy. Acta Cytol 52:77–82

28. Gabbert HE, Shimoda R, Hainaut P, Nakamura Y, Field JK, Inoue H (2000) World health organization classification of tumors: Pathology and Genetics: Tumors of the digestive system. In: Hamilton SR, Aaltonen LA (eds) Squamous cell carcinoma of the esophagus, IARC Press, Lyon, pp 11–19

29. Engel LS, Chow WH, Vaughan TL, Gammon MD, Risch HA, Stanford JL, Schoenberg JB, Mayne ST, Dubrow R, Rotterdam H, West AB, Blaser M, Blot WJ, Gail MH, Fraumeni JF Jr (2003) Population attributable risks of esophageal and gastric cancers. J Natl Cancer Inst 95:1404–1413

30. Shimizu Y, Omori T, Yokoyama A, Yoshida T, Hirota J, Ono Y, Yamamoto J, Kato M, Asaka M (2008) Endoscopic diagnosis of early squamous neoplasia of the esophagus with iodine staining: high-grade intra-epithelial neoplasia turns pink within a few minutes. J Gastroenterol Hepatol 23:546–550

31. Dowlatshahi K, Skinner DB, DeMeester TR, Zachary L, Bibbo M, Wied GL (1985) Evaluation of brush cytology as an independent technique for detection of esophageal carcinoma. J Thorac Cardiovasc Surg 89:848–851

32. Shimizu M, Nagata K, Yamaguchi H, Kita H (2009) Squamous intraepithelial neoplasia of the esophagus: past, present, and future. J Gastroenterol 44:103–112

33. Sepe PS, Moparty B, Pitman MB, Saltzman JR, Brugge WR (2009) EUS-guided FNA for the diagnosis of GI stromal cell tumors: sensitivity and cytologic yield. Gastrointest Endosc 70:254–261

34. Hoda KM, Rodriguez SA, Faigel DO (2009) EUS-guided sampling of suspected GI stromal tumors. Gastrointest Endosc 69:1218–1223

35. Cover TL, Blaser MJ (2009) Helicobacter pylori in health and disease. Gastroenterology 136:1863–1873

36. Mostaghni AA, Afarid M, Eghbali S, Kumar P (2008) Evaluation of brushing cytology in the diagnosis of Helicobacter pylori gastritis. Acta Cytol 52:597–601

37. Sherman ME, Anderson C, Herman LM, Ludwig ME, Erozan YS (1994) Utility of gastric brushing in the diagnosis of malignant lymphoma. Acta Cytol 38:169–174

38. Laine L, Cohen H, Sloane R, Marin-Sorensen M, Weinstein WM (1995) Interobserver agreement and predictive value of endoscopic findings for H. pylori and gastritis in normal volunteers. Gastrointest Endosc 42:420–423

39. Park do Y, Lauwers GY (2008) Gastric polyps: classification and management. Arch Pathol Lab Med 132:633–640

40. Morais DJ, Yamanaka A, Zeitune JM, Andreollo NA (2007) Gastric polyps: a retrospective analysis of 26,000 digestive endoscopies. Arq Gastroenterol 44:14–17

41. Ginsberg GG, Al-Kawas FH, Fleischer DE, Reilly HF, Benjamin SB (1996) Gastric polyps: relationship of size and histology to cancer risk. Am J Gastroenterol 91:714–717
42. Fenoglio-Preiser C, Carneiro F, Correa P, Guilford P, Lambert R, Megraud F, Munoz N, Powell SM, Rugge M, Sasako M, Stolte M, Watanabe H (2000) World health organization classification of tumors: Pathology and Genetics: Tumors of the digestive system. In: Hamilton SR, Aaltonen LA (eds) Gastric carcinoma, IARC Press, Lyon, pp 39–52
43. Ahn HS, Lee HJ, Yoo MW, Kim SG, Im JP, Kim SH, Kim WH, Lee KU, Yang HK (2009) Diagnostic accuracy of T and N stages with endoscopy, stomach protocol CT, and endoscopic ultrasonography in early gastric cancer. J Surg Oncol 99:20–27
44. Tatsuta M, Iishi H, Nakaizumi A, Okuda S, Taniguchi H, Hiyama T, Tsukuma H, Oshima A (1993) Fundal atrophic gastritis as a risk factor for gastric cancer. Int J Cancer 53:70–74
45. Fuchs CS, Mayer RJ (1995) Gastric carcinoma. N Engl J Med 333:32–41
46. Wotherspon A, Chott A, Gascoyne RD, Muller-Hermelink HK (2000) World health organization classification of tumors: Pathology and Genetics: Tumors of the digestive system. In: Hamilton SR, Aaltonen LA (eds) Lymphoma of the stomach, IARC Press, Lyon, pp 57–61
47. Pavlovic AR, Krstic M, Tomic D, Bjelovic M, Jesic R, Suvajdzic N (2005) Endoscopic ultrasound (EUS) in initial assessment and follow-up of patients with MALT lymphoma treated drug therapy. Acta Chir Iugosl 52:83–89
48. Arantes V, Logrono R, Faruqi S, Ahmed I, Waxman I, Bhutani MS (2004) Endoscopic sonographically guided fine-needle aspiration yield in submucosal tumors of the gastrointestinal tract. J Ultrasound Med 23:1141–1150
49. Murphy BA, Meda BA, Buss DH, Geisinger KR (2003) Marginal zone and mantle cell lymphomas: assessment of cytomorphology in subtyping small B-cell lymphomas. Diagn Cytopathol 28:126–130
50. Tsang RW, Gospodarowicz MK, Pintilie M, Bezjak A, Wells W, Hodgson DC, Crump M (2001) Stage I and II MALT lymphoma: results of treatment with radiotherapy. Int J Radiat Oncol Biol Phys 50:1258–1264
51. Capella C, Solcia E, Sobin LH, Arnold R (2000) World health organization classification of tumors: Pathology and Genetics: Tumors of the digestive system. In: Hamilton SR, Aaltonen LA (eds) Endocrine tumors of the stomach, IARC Press, Lyon, pp 53–57
52. Meittinen M, Blay JY, Sobin LH (2000) World health organization classification of tumors: Pathology and Genetics: Tumors of the digestive system. In: Hamilton SR, Aaltonen LA (eds) Mesenchymal tumors of the stomach, IARC Press, Lyon, pp 62–65
53. Chatzipantelis P, Salla C, Karoumpalis I, Apessou D, Sakellariou S, Doumani I, Papaliodi E, Konstantinou P (2008) Endoscopic ultrasound-guided fine needle aspiration biopsy in the diagnosis of gastrointestinal stromal tumors of the stomach. A study of 17 cases. J Gastrointestin Liver Dis 17:15–20
54. Palazzo L, Landi B, Cellier C, Cuillerier E, Roseau G, Barbier JP (2000) Endosonographic features predictive of benign and malignant gastrointestinal stromal cell tumours. Gut 46:88–92
55. Sheehan MM, Fraser A, Ravindran R, McAteer D (2007) Bile duct brushings cytology–improving sensitivity of diagnosis using the ThinPrep technique: a review of 113 cases. Cytopathology 18:225–233
56. Shen J, Brugge WR, Dimaio CJ, Pitman MB (2009) Molecular analysis of pancreatic cyst fluid: a comparative analysis with current practice of diagnosis. Cancer Cytopathol 117:217–227
57. Garcea G, Ong SL, Rajesh A, Neal CP, Pollard CA, Berry DP, Dennison AR (2008) Cystic lesions of the pancreas: a diagnostic and management dilemma. Pancreatology 8:236–251
58. Brugge WR, Lewandrowski K, Lee-Lewandrowski E, Centeno BA, Szydlo T, Regan S, del Castillo CF, Warshaw AL (2004) Diagnosis of pancreatic cystic neoplasms: a report of the cooperative pancreatic cyst study. Gastroenterology 126:1330–1336

59. Adsay NV, Hasteh F, Cheng JD, Klimstra DS (2000) Squamous-lined cysts of the pancreas: lymphoepithelial cysts, dermoid cysts (teratomas), and accessory-splenic epidermoid cysts. Semin Diagn Pathol 17:56–65

60. Jian B, Kimbrell HZ, Sepulveda A, Yu G (2008) Lymphoepithelial cysts of the pancreas: endosonography-guided fine needle aspiration. Diagn Cytopathol 36:662–665

61. Liu J, Shin HJ, Rubenchik I, Lang E, Lahoti S, Staerkel GA (1999) Cytologic features of lymphoepithelial cyst of the pancreas: two preoperatively diagnosed cases based on fine-needle aspiration. Diagn Cytopathol 21:346–350

62. Kosmahl M, Egawa N, Schroder S, Carneiro F, Luttges J, Kloppel G (2002) Mucinous nonneoplastic cyst of the pancreas: a novel nonneoplastic cystic change? Mod Pathol 15:154–158

63. Capella C, Solcia E, Kloppel G, Hruban RH (2000) World health organization classification of tumors: Pathology and Genetics: Tumors of the digestive system. In: Hamilton SR, Aaltonen LA (eds) Serous cystic neoplasms of the pancreas, IARC Press, Lyon, pp 231–233

64. Belsley NA, Pitman MB, Lauwers GY, Brugge WR, Deshpande V (2008) Serous cystadenoma of the pancreas: limitations and pitfalls of endoscopic ultrasound-guided fine-needle aspiration biopsy. Cancer 114:102–110

65. Le Borgne J, de Calan L, Partensky C (1999) Cystadenomas and cystadenocarcinomas of the pancreas: a multiinstitutional retrospective study of 398 cases french surgical association. Ann Surg 230:152–161

66. Lal A, Bourtsos EP, DeFrias DV, Nemcek AA, Nayar R (2004) Microcystic adenoma of the pancreas: clinical, radiologic, and cytologic features. Cancer 102:288–294

67. Huang P, Staerkel G, Sneige N, Gong Y (2006) Fine-needle aspiration of pancreatic serous cystadenoma: cytologic features and diagnostic pitfalls. Cancer 108:239–249

68. Silverman JF, Zhu B, Liu Y, Lin X (2009) Distinctive immunohistochemical profile of mucinous cystic neoplasms of pancreas, ovary and lung. Histol Histopathol 24:77–82

69. Singh M, Maitra A (2007) Precursor lesions of pancreatic cancer: molecular pathology and clinical implications. Pancreatology 7:9–19

70. Tanaka M, Chari S, Adsay V, Fernandez-del Castillo C, Falconi M, Shimizu M, Yamaguchi K, Yamao K, Matsuno S (2006) International consensus guidelines for management of intraductal papillary mucinous neoplasms and mucinous cystic neoplasms of the pancreas. Pancreatology 6:17–32

71. Salla C, Chatzipantelis P, Konstantinou P, Karoumpalis I, Sakellariou S, Pantazopoulou A, Manika Z (2007) Endoscopic ultrasound-guided fine-needle aspiration cytology in the diagnosis of intraductal papillary mucinous neoplasms of the pancreas. A study of 8 cases. Jop 8:715-724

72. Adsay NV, Merati K, Basturk O, Iacobuzio-Donahue C, Levi E, Cheng JD, Sarkar FH, Hruban RH, Klimstra DS (2004) Pathologically and biologically distinct types of epithelium in intraductal papillary mucinous neoplasms: delineation of an "intestinal" pathway of carcinogenesis in the pancreas. Am J Surg Pathol 28:839–848

73. Satoh K, Kaneko K, Hirota M, Toyota T, Shimosegawa T (2000) The pattern of CPP32/caspase-3 expression reflects the biological behavior of the human pancreatic duct cell tumors. Pancreas 21:352–357

74. Khalid A, Brugge W (2007) ACG practice guidelines for the diagnosis and management of neoplastic pancreatic cysts. Am J Gastroenterol 102:2339–2349

75. Kloppel G, Hruban RH, Longnecker DS (2000) World health organization classification of tumors: Pathology and Genetics: Tumors of the digestive system. In: Hamilton SR, Aaltonen LA (eds) Ductal adenocarcinoma of the pancreas, IARC Press, Lyon, pp 221–230

76. Mertz HR, Sechopoulos P, Delbeke D, Leach SD (2000) EUS PET, and CT scanning for evaluation of pancreatic adenocarcinoma. Gastrointest Endosc 52:367–371

77. Krishna NB, LaBundy JL, Saripalli S, Safdar R, Agarwal B (2009) Diagnostic value of EUS-FNA in patients suspected of having pancreatic cancer with a focal lesion on CT scan/MRI but without obstructive jaundice. Pancreas 38:625–630

78. Erickson RA, Sayage-Rabie L, Beissner RS (2000) Factors predicting the number of EUS-guided fine-needle passes for diagnosis of pancreatic malignancies. Gastrointest Endosc 51:184–190

79. Chang KJ, Nguyen P, Erickson RA, Durbin TE, Katz KD (1997) The clinical utility of endoscopic ultrasound-guided fine-needle aspiration in the diagnosis and staging of pancreatic carcinoma. Gastrointest Endosc 45:387–393

80. Rosch T, Lightdale CJ, Botet JF, Boyce GA, Sivak MV Jr, Yasuda K, Heyder N, Palazzo L, Dancygier H, Schusdziarra V et al (1992) Localization of pancreatic endocrine tumors by endoscopic ultrasonography. N Engl J Med 326:1721–1726

81. Figueiredo FA, Giovannini M, Monges G, Charfi S, Bories E, Pesenti C, Caillol F, Delpero JR (2009) Pancreatic endocrine tumors: a large single-center experience. Pancreas 38:936–940

82. Kloppel G, Luttges J, Klimstra D, Hruban R, Kern S, Aldler G (2000) World health organization classification of tumors: Pathology and Genetics: Tumors of the digestive system. In: Hamilton SR, Aaltonen LA (eds) Solid-pseudopapillary neoplasm, IARC Press, Lyon, pp 246–248

83. Jani N, Dewitt J, Eloubeidi M, Varadarajulu S, Appalaneni V, Hoffman B, Brugge W, Lee K, Khalid A, McGrath K (2008) Endoscopic ultrasound-guided fine-needle aspiration for diagnosis of solid pseudopapillary tumors of the pancreas: a multicenter experience. Endoscopy 40:200–203

84. Jhala N, Siegal GP, Jhala D (2008) Large, clear cytoplasmic vacuolation: an under-recognized cytologic clue to distinguish solid pseudopapillary neoplasms of the pancreas from pancreatic endocrine neoplasms on fine-needle aspiration. Cancer 114:249–254

85. Bardales RH, Centeno B, Mallery JS, Lai R, Pochapin M, Guiter G, Stanley MW (2004) Endoscopic ultrasound-guided fine-needle aspiration cytology diagnosis of solid-pseudopapillary tumor of the pancreas: a rare neoplasm of elusive origin but characteristic cytomorphologic features. Am J Clin Pathol 121:654–662

86. Klimstra DS, Longnecker D (2000) World health organization classification of tumors: Pathology and Genetics: Tumors of the digestive system. In: Hamilton SR, Aaltonen LA (eds) Acinar cell carcinoma, IARC Press, Lyon, pp 241–243

87. Peng HQ, Darwin P, Papadimitriou JC, Drachenberg CB (2006) Liver metastases of pancreatic acinar cell carcinoma with marked nuclear atypia and pleomorphism diagnosed by EUS FNA cytology: a case report with emphasis on FNA cytological findings. Cytojournal 3:29

88. Stelow EB, Bardales RH, Shami VM, Woon C, Presley A, Mallery S, Lai R, Stanley MW (2006) Cytology of pancreatic acinar cell carcinoma. Diagn Cytopathol 34:367–372

89. Kurzawinski TR, Deery A, Dooley JS, Dick R, Hobbs KE, Davidson BR (1993) A prospective study of biliary cytology in 100 patients with bile duct strictures. Hepatology 18:1399–1403

90. Siqueira E, Schoen RE, Silverman W, Martin J, Rabinovitz M, Weissfeld JL, Abu-Elmaagd K, Madariaga JR, Slivka A (2002) Detecting cholangiocarcinoma in patients with primary sclerosing cholangitis. Gastrointest Endosc 56:40–47

91. Nakeeb A, Pitt HA, Sohn TA, Coleman J, Abrams RA, Piantadosi S, Hruban RH, Lillemoe KD, Yeo CJ, Cameron JL (1996) Cholangiocarcinoma. A spectrum of intrahepatic, perihilar, and distal tumors. Ann Surg 224:463–473 (discussion 473–465)

92. Burke EC, Jarnagin WR, Hochwald SN, Pisters PW, Fong Y, Blumgart LH (1998) Hilar cholangiocarcinoma: patterns of spread, the importance of hepatic resection for curative operation, and a presurgical clinical staging system. Ann Surg 228:385–394

Chapter 7
Genitourinary Cytopathology (Kidney and Urinary Tract)

Güliz A. Barkan and Eva M. Wojcik

7.1 Renal Cytology

7.1.1 Introduction

Fine needle aspiration (FNA) of kidney masses has been performed for the diagnosis of mass lesions, confirmation of advanced neoplasia and metastases, staging of tumors, and rarely as a therapeutic measure for cystic lesions [1]. In the past, the decision of whether to perform a nephrectomy used to be based on radiographic features and size, precluding the use of FNA [2]. Today, where treatment is not limited to surgery alone the indications for renal FNA have expanded.

7.1.2 The Indications of FNA in Solid Renal Masses

1. Patients with presumed malignant lesions who are not candidates for resection. These include patients with unresectable primary tumors, patients with metastatic disease, patients with other primary tumors and patients with other comorbidities precluding the surgical approach.
2. To decide on the approach for surgery, especially, in smaller masses and masses located close to the renal pelvis. For example, a small renal cell carcinoma could be treated with laparoscopic morcellation, however, no matter how small an

G. A. Barkan (✉) · E. M. Wojcik
Department of Pathology, Loyola University Medical Center, 2160 South First Ave,
Maywood, IL 60153, USA
e-mail: gbarkan@lumc.edu

E. M. Wojcik
e-mail: ewojcik@lumc.edu

R. Nayar (ed.), *Cytopathology in Oncology*,
Cancer Treatment and Research 160, DOI: 10.1007/978-3-642-38850-7_7,
© Springer-Verlag Berlin Heidelberg 2014

urothelial carcinoma is, most of the time the treatment is radical nephrectomy with staging and intraoperative frozen sections.

3. In situations where non-surgical treatment, i.e., minimally invasive methods such as cryotherapy, or radiotherapy are preferred, a pretreatment diagnostic FNA is strongly recommended.
4. In cases where preoperative/neoadjuvant chemotherapy or biological response modifiers, such as immunotherapy are preferred, a pretreatment diagnostic FNA is necessary.
5. In cases where pretreatment molecular/cytogenetic typing of the tumor is recommended to individualize the treatment of choice, a pretreatment diagnostic FNA is strongly recommended. This is more of a futuristic indication for advanced stage renal neoplasms in which targeted therapy modalities could be used.

7.1.3 The Indications for FNA in Cystic Renal Masses

1. Simple cysts for therapeutic aspiration. This is more of an indication of the past; today most simple cysts are just followed up clinically and radiologically.
2. When dealing with radiologically indeterminate cystic lesions (Bosniak Category II–III) in patients with other comorbidities where surgery is not a viable option.

7.1.4 Patient Assessment Prior to FNA

Screening for bleeding diathesis is generally recommended in all patients irrespective of bleeding history. In a survey of radiologists in the USA, 81 % ordered prothrombin time, 78 % ordered partial thromboplastin time, and 58 % ordered platelet count prior to the FNA [3]. In general, a platelet count of >70,000/ml is required. Patients on aspirin and nonsteroidal anti-inflammatory drugs are advised to stop taking them at least 5 days prior to the FNA. Similarly, patients on warfarin are advised to stop taking it in order to establish an acceptable international normalized ratio, which usually requires 3–5 days. Continuous heparin should be stopped 4 h prior to the procedure.

7.1.5 Technique for Renal FNA

The FNA is performed under conscious sedation in addition to local anesthesia with parenteral sedatives and analgesics. Usually, the patient is placed in a prone/ semiprone or lateral decubitus position depending on the location of the mass. FNA and/or core biopsies are generally performed under computed tomography

(CT) and/or ultrasonography (US) guidance (Fig. 7.1 shows a CT with needle placement for FNA). Magnetic resonance imaging (MRI) is not frequently used because of limited availability, the higher cost, and the need for nonferromagnetic biopsy needles. The US has the advantages of portability, it is multiplanar and allows for real-time imaging, in addition to a lower cost. US-guided FNAs can be performed freehand or with a guide. However, US-guided FNA is highly operator-dependent, requiring a steep learning curve. The advantages of CT guidance are: (1) improved visibility over the US, (2) good spatial resolution, (3) better needle visualization, and (4) better sampling since heterogeneous areas of the tumor can be visualized. The disadvantages of CT guidance are: (1) higher cost, (2) exposure to ionizing radiation, and (3) lack of real-time monitoring during the needle insertion.

The FNA is performed with a 20–25 gauge needle (spinal or Chiba) through a coaxial guide or cannula under image guidance. The usage of a guiding cannula allows multiple needle passes and or core biopsies. Since the cannula traverses through normal tissues only once its usage reduces the risk of needle tract seeding [3].

7.1.6 Complications of Renal FNA

The complications of renal FNA are very rare and include: perirenal hemorrhage, pneumothorax, infection, A-V fistula, and urinoma. To date there are very rare (6) reports of needle tract seeding reported between 1977 and 1992. [4–9] It appears

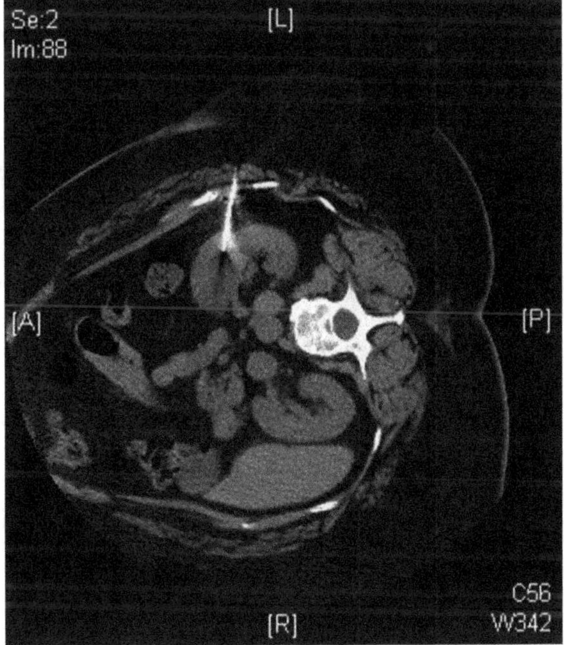

Fig. 7.1 CT scan of a left lower pole renal mass with needle placement. Patient is in the right lateral decubitus position. The needle is visualized by repeat CT imaging to document placement prior to aspiration

that rather than the size of the needle used, the remote possibility of seeding may increase with the number of passes, lack of a guiding cannula, and with the use of noncutting needles. [6] That said, the overall estimated risk reported by Wunderlich et al. is >0.01 % [10]. Although extremely unlikely, death has also been reported as a complication of renal FNA. In a large review of more than 16,000 intraabdominal (not only renal) FNA's Smith et al. reported an overall mortality rate of 0.031 % [11]. Also, in these reported very rare cases, it is somehow not clear what exactly was the underlying cause of death and how strongly it was related to FNA.

7.1.7 Role of Immediate Assessment

After the specimen is obtained the aspirate material is smeared on several slides, some of which are air dried, some are fixed in an alcohol-based fixative. The air-dried smears are stained with a modified Diff Quik stain and the alcohol-fixed smears are stained with the Papanicolaou method. The immediate cytological assessment of the specimen is performed by a cytopathologist or a cytotechnologist, usually on the Diff Quik-stained slide. If necessary, extra passes are performed to produce a cell block and/or core biopsy on which additional studies such as immunohistochemical stains can be performed. We recommend collecting the aspirate material in RPMI or PBS in the event that, cytogenetics, FISH, flow cytometry (FCM), other molecular studies or electron microscopy can be performed later if needed. If a core biopsy is being performed at the same session, we recommend that specimen adequacy to be assessed by touch imprints of the core biopsy.

7.1.8 Renal FNA Statistics and the Definition of Adequacy

The accuracy of FNA of kidney in diagnosing tumors ranges from 73 to 94 %. Similarly, the sensitivity ranges from 50 to 90 %, and the specificity ranges from 50 to 93 %. The diagnostic yield quoted in earlier papers ranges from a low of 40 %, however with the newer imaging techniques, and increased expertise in the fields of the interventional radiology and cytopathology, it has risen to up to 95 % [12–18]. Nevertheless, there are several challenges in diagnoses like recognizing normal renal elements, identifying well-differentiated renal cell carcinomas, differentiating between oncocytoma and chromophobe renal cell carcinomas, and differentiating between high grade papillary renal cell carcinoma, urothelial carcinoma, collecting duct carcinoma and metastatic carcinomas. Other potential problems are necrotic, hemorrhagic, or cystic tumors, which may lead to a false negative diagnosis. Currently, there is no consensus on adequacy criteria, however, Troung et al. [13] have suggested that the FNA performed on a solid mass be considered unsatisfactory if (1) the aspirate shows soft tissue and/or normal kidney elements only, or (2) there are only peripheral blood elements with or without necrotic cellular debris, or (3) if there are very few well-preserved cells. According to the same study, a specimen is deemed "satisfactory for evaluation" if "technically acceptable and representative" which is somewhat elusive. In practice, a sample is deemed satisfactory if it is sufficiently cellular to conjure a differential diagnosis and to render a specific diagnosis—that admittedly is somewhat subjective. Cystic lesions, on the other hand, are even more challenging. Even though abundant fluid is aspirated the smear could be acellular; or more likely it could be composed of macrophages only. These findings do not necessarily exclude the possibility of an undersampled malignancy with cystic degeneration. However, currently, the only criterion to deem an aspirate from a cystic renal mass satisfactory is the aspiration of fluid, regardless of cellularity (also suggested by Truoung et al.) [13].

7.1.9 Approach to Cystic Lesions

The majority of renal mass lesions (70–85 %) are cysts; [19, 20] and they are mostly benign, acquired, and solitary. Renal cysts are classified radiologically according to the likelihood of the cyst being benign/malignant (Bosniak System) [21] Category I being benign, IV being most likely malignant, II and III indeterminate. It is controversial whether or not to perform FNA on simple cysts (Bosniak I), however, it is becoming a common practice to opt for FNA when there in any concern for malignancy (Bosniak II–IV). The incidence of a cyst harboring renal cell carcinoma ranges between 1 and 25 % [22–24], and the negative predictive value of a renal cyst FNA is low. In case of multiple cysts, the differential diagnosis includes cysts due to long term dialysis or transplantation (these have a 9 % chance of developing renal cell carcinoma) [25], and autosomal dominant (adult type) polycystic disease of the kidney. As described above, under the adequacy section, FNA of most simple cysts, including the cases with multiple cysts, yield clear, pale straw-colored fluid, which shows a few foamy macrophages and usually no epithelial elements (Fig. 7.2 is an FNA from a cystic renal lesion showing macrophages only).

7.1.10 Normal Kidney Cytology

Glomeruli. Formed of cellular lobular/papillary structures with prominent capillary loops (Fig. 7.3) which show normal renal elements with glomeruli, proximal tubular (single arrow) and distal tubular cells (double arrow)). Differential diagnosis: Papillary renal cell carcinoma in which case both cellular atypia and true fibrovascular cores are identified.

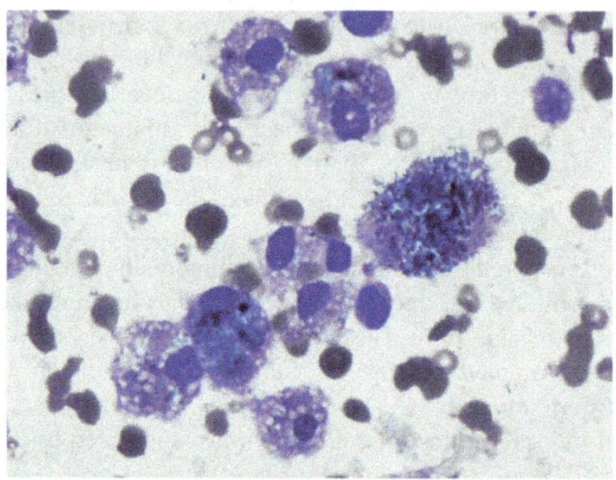

Fig. 7.2 Benign renal cyst (High power, Diff Quik stain). Groups of single cells (macrophages) a vacuolated cytoplasm, eccentrically located bean shaped nucleus. Some cells also have intracytoplasmic hemosiderin pigment

Proximal convoluted tubules. Rare cells with indistinct cytoplasmic borders, abundant granular cytoplasm, and low nuclear cytoplasmic ratio. Differential diagnosis: Oncocytoma, chromophobe renal cell carcinoma. Both have sharply defined cell borders.

Distal convoluted tubules. Rare groups of small cells with clear or granular cytoplasm with well-defined cell borders and inconspicuous nucleoli. These are smaller, flatter epithelial cells compared to the proximal tubular cells. Differential diagnosis: Clear cell renal cell carcinoma shows cytoplasmic vacuolization and nuclear atypia in higher grades, papillary renal cell carcinoma shows atypia and papillae.

Collecting ducts. Small, tight clusters of cells with scanty cytoplasm, high nuclear cytoplasmic ratio, indistinct cellular borders, and inconspicuous nucleoli. Differential diagnosis: High grade papillary carcinoma, collecting duct carcinoma,

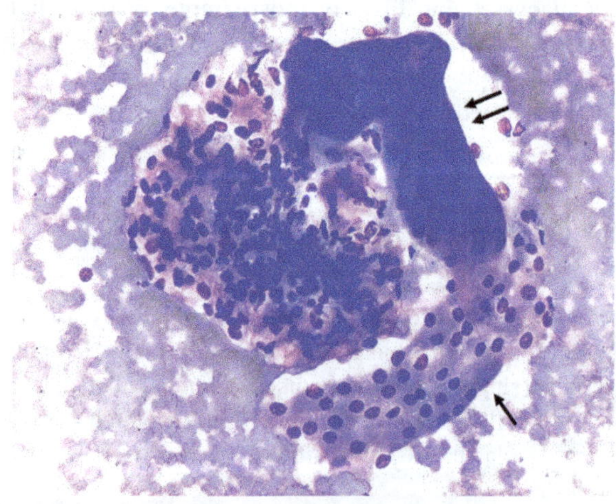

Fig. 7.3 Normal cytologic elements of kidney (High power, Diff Quik stain). Centrally located is the glomerulus formed of loops of round to ovoid cells. Next to the glomerulus are proximal tubular cells (*single arrow*) with granular cytoplasm; and distal tubular cells—formed of a group of smaller cells in a tight cluster (*double arrow*)

metastatic adenocarcinoma. All these entities show more cellular atypia and have more conspicuous nucleoli.

7.1.11 Nonneoplastic Entities

7.1.11.1 Xanthogranulomatous Pyelonephritis

Inflammatory sequela of chronic suppurative renal infection (usually Proteus or *Escherichia coli*), often associated with an obstruction. Cytology shows a cellular aspirate with foamy histiocytes singly and in clusters, multinucleated giant cells, and neutrophils [26]. Differential diagnosis: clinically, radiographically, and pathologically can be confused with renal cell carcinoma. Renal cell carcinoma has a round nucleus compared to the kidney-bean shaped histiocytic nuclei in xanthogranulomatous pyelonephritis. A panel of immunohistochemical stains and histochemical stains can differentiate reliably between the two: Xanthogranulomatous pyelonephritis: PAS, Low molecular weight cytokeratin, Epithelial membrane antigen (–) and CD 68 (+).

7.1.11.2 Renal Abscess

The aspirate is cloudy, white to yellow. Cytology shows acute inflammatory cells. Gram negative organisms are the most common agent.

7.1.11.3 Renal Infarct

Radiographically, they present as a wedge-shaped lesion. Cytology shows necrotic glomeruli and tubules. Rarely atypia, cytoplasmic vacuolation, prominent nucleoli can be seen [27]. Differential diagnosis: Renal cell carcinoma where atypia is more pronounced.

7.1.12 Benign Neoplasms

7.1.12.1 Angiomyolipoma

Composed of smooth muscle, adipose tissue, and vessels. About 20 % of cases are associated with tuberous sclerosis complex. Owing to high vascularity it may be confused with renal cell carcinoma on angiogram. In imaging studies, cases where the adipose component is less prominent than the other components the diagnosis may be difficult. The aspirate smears usually have high cellularity with spindled to epithelioid cells found singly and in clusters. Stromal cells have round to oval nuclei with fine chromatin, and inconspicuous nucleoli. Rare intranuclear inclusions can be seen. Pleomorphism, mitotic figures, and necrosis are exceedingly rare (Fig. 7.4 shows the spindle cell component of angiomyolipoma). Since angiomyolipoma is a member of the PEComa (tumors originating from the perivascular epithelioid cell) family the spindled cells express both melanocytic [HMB45, Melan A (+)] markers and smooth muscle actin (+).

7.1.12.2 Oncocytoma

These neoplasms account for 3–5 % of renal masses. The smears show loosely cohesive small groups and isolated cells with abundant eosinophilic, granular cytoplasm with distinct cell borders, round nuclei with fine chromatin and occasional binucleation (Fig. 7.5). However, nuclear atypia, pleomorphism, and prominent nucleoli can be seen, making it difficult to differentiate from renal cell carcinoma. Differential diagnosis:

(a) Proximal tubular cells: the granules of the cytoplasm spill out in benign tubular cells and the cytoplasmic membranes are indistinct
(b) Hepatocytes: have a polygonal cytoplasm and are HepPar1 (+)
(c) Chromophobe renal cell carcinoma (see below for detailed discussion)
(d) Clear cell renal cell carcinoma: unlike clear cell renal cell carcinoma, oncocytoma is pancytokeratin (+), vimentin (–), CD10 (–).

In case of ascant cellular specimen where further studies such as immunohistochemistry, electron microscopy cannot be done the lesion is better classified as an 'oncocytic neoplasm' on cytology.

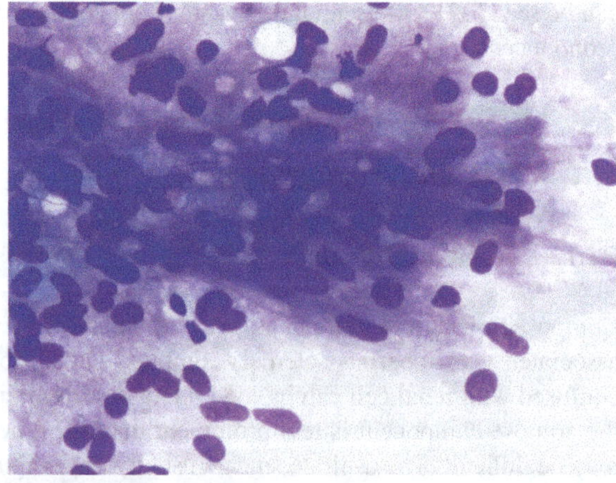

Fig. 7.4 Angiomyolipoma (High power, Diff Quik stain). Cellular smear with ovoid to spindled cells. Clear-cut cytoplasmic borders are not seen. There is no pleomorphism or cytologic atypia. Small fat droplets can be seen in the background

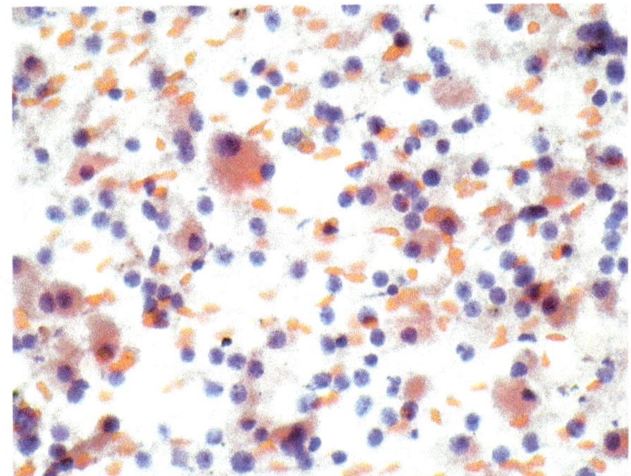

Fig. 7.5 Oncocytoma (High power, Papanicolaou stain). Scattered loosely cohesive cells and single cells with abundant granular cytoplasm. Some cells have lost their cytoplasm and have only naked nuclei. Note some of the cells have prominent nucleoli

7.1.13 Malignant Lesions

7.1.13.1 Renal Cell Carcinoma

This is the most common tumor of the kidney. It is most prevalent in males in the 5–7th decades. It is important to distinguish between types of renal cell carcinoma since they have different prognostic and therapeutic implications.

Clear cell renal cell carcinoma. Approximately 75 % of renal cell carcinomas are clear cell type, and they are associated with chromosome 3p deletions. The cytological features are of a cellular aspirate composed of large clusters and sheets of cells with abundant and vacuolated cytoplasm, low nuclear cytoplasmic ratio, and eccentrically located nuclei (Fig. 7.6). Differential diagnosis: Tubular cells, macrophages, adrenal, hepatocytes—because of the bland nature of low grade renal cell carcinoma it could be mistaken for benign elements. However, benign tubular cells and macrophages are usually not found in large clusters. Hepatocytes have a more granular and polygonal cytoplasm.

Papillary renal cell carcinoma. Approximately 15 % of renal cell carcinomas are papillary, and are associated with trisomy chromosome 7, 16, and 17. These tumors are usually small and peripheral. They could be multifocal and associated with cortical adenomas. The prognosis is better than of the clear cell type. Cytology shows a cellular aspirate with the malignant cells arranged in a papillary configuration around fibrovascular cores. The cells can have a granular or vacuolated cytoplasm with rare intracytoplasmic hemosiderin deposits. nuclear cytoplasmic ratio is high, the nuclei are uniform; and rarely intranuclear grooves may be identified. Occasional foamy macrophages and rare psammoma bodies can also be seen (Fig. 7.7). Differential diagnosis: Benign distal tubular cells, clear cell renal cell carcinoma, urothelial carcinoma, collecting duct carcinoma, and metastatic carcinomas. Like other renal cell carcinomas, the tumor cells are positive for EMA, low molecular weight keratin, and negative for mucin and carcinoembryonic

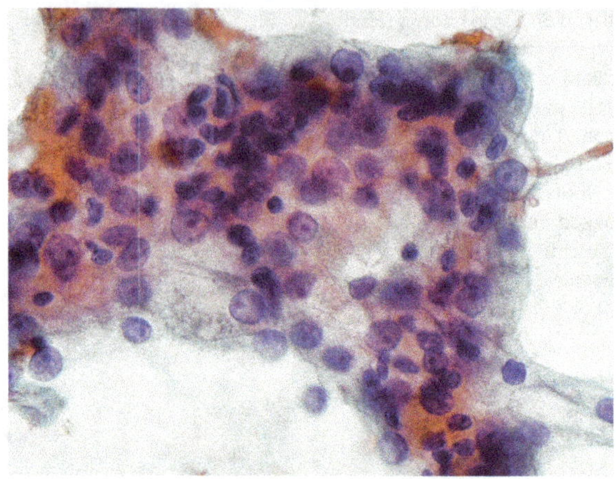

Fig. 7.6 Renal cell carcinoma, clear cell type (High power, Papanicolaou stain). Cellular smear composed of cells with indistinct cytoplasmic borders, finely vacuolated/granular cytoplasm, and prominent nucleoli

antigen; unlike other renal cell carcinoma CK7 positive; unlike collecting duct carcinoma high molecular weight keratin (K903) negative.

Chromophobe renal cell carcinoma. Only 3–5 % of renal cell carcinoma are of chromophobe type and are associated with multiple chromosomal deletions. These tumors also have a better prognosis than clear cell renal cell carcinoma. The aspirates are cellular, composed of broad ribbons and loosely cohesive groups of cells with fluffy/flocculent to granular cytoplasm with focal vacuolization and distinct cell borders. There is frequent binucleation and nuclear size variation (Fig. 7.8). Diff Quik stain shows a perivascular, reticulated zone. Differential diagnosis: Oncocytoma and clear cell renal cell carcinoma. Due to morphologic, molecular, and antigenic similarities, such as c-kit (+) [28] in both tumors it is thought that these tumors could be of similar descent, i.e., different expressions of the same morphologic spectrum, but detailed studies are still needed to verify this theory. A variety of immunohistochemical stains have been reported to be able to

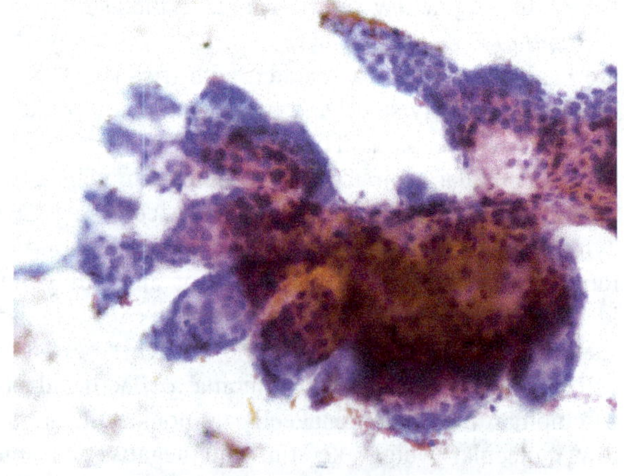

Fig. 7.7 Renal cell carcinoma, papillary type (High power, Papanicolaou stain). Cellular smear with uniform cells, high nuclear cytoplasmic ratio, forming papillary structures. Within some of the papillae macrophages can be identified

differentiate between chromophobe renal cell carcinoma and oncocytoma: ks-cadherin (±) [29], caveolin 1 (±) [30], CD 3 (∓) [31], CD63 (diffuse +/apical or polar +) [32] although to this date the gold standard still electron microscopy where oncocytoma shows abundant cytoplasmic mitochondria and chromophobe renal cell carcinoma shows cytoplasmic microvesicles.

Sarcomatoid renal cell carcinoma. These neoplasms account for 3–5 % of all renal cell carcinomas. The tumors are defined by the presence of a high grade spindle cell component, with or without epithelioid differentiation. If the epithelial component is not seen, cytokeratin (+) cells are necessary for diagnosis. This is not a distinct subtype for renal cell carcinoma; it rather represents dedifferentiation of any type of renal cell carcinoma. The prognosis of this neoplasm is bad with a median survival of 6 months. The aspirate smears show malignant high grade spindle cell component in a background of renal cell carcinoma. Undersampling could fail to detect the sarcomatoid component thus if there is a radiologic suspicion for sarcomatoid differentiation, i.e., areas with different echogenicity it is important to ask for additional samples for an accurate diagnosis. Differential diagnosis: Metastatic high grade sarcoma. Tumor cells in sarcomatoid renal cell carcinoma are EMA, cytokeratin (+), smooth muscle actin (±), vimentin (+).

Collecting duct carcinoma. This is a very rare adenocarcinoma arising from the collecting duct epithelium. The aspirate smears show cells arranged in small clusters, papillary configuration or single cells with scant dense to vacuolated cytoplasm, high nuclear cytoplasmic ratio, hyperchromatic nuclei, and prominent nucleoli. Differential diagnosis: High grade renal cell carcinoma, high grade urothelial carcinoma, and metastatic carcinomas. Cytology alone cannot

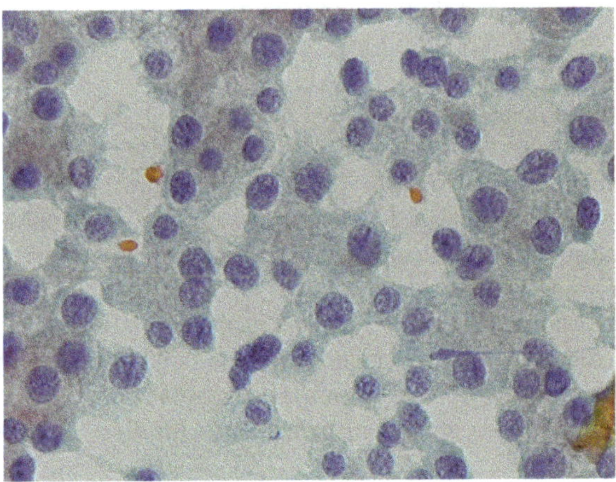

Fig. 7.8 Renal cell carcinoma, chromophobe type (High power, Papanicolaou stain). Sheets of uniform cells with granular cytoplasm, eccentric nuclei, inconspicuous nucleoli. Some cells have a slightly prominent cytoplasmic membrane. Such a picture may be difficult to distinguish from oncocytoma, especially in the absence of supportive ancillary stains, and therefore the diagnosis of oncocytic neoplasm may be made

distinguish these entities. Immunohistochemical stains show that the tumor cells are positive for *ulex* agglutinin, high molecular weight cytokeratin, CK 7, mucin (+); CD 10 (−).

Renal medullary carcinoma. This entity is mostly seen in young black men with sickle cell trait. The aspirate smears reveal cohesive cellular groups with vacuolated cytoplasm, indented nuclei, irregular membranes, and coarse or vesicular chromatin [33]. Differential diagnosis: High grade urothelial carcinoma, metastatic carcinoma.

7.1.13.2 Urothelial Carcinoma

This is the most common tumor of the renal pelvis, accounting for 10 % of all malignant renal tumors. It is most commonly seen in men in 7th decade [1, 34]. There is a significant association with synchronous or metachronous urothelial tumors in other sites so the surgical approach is different than for renal cell carcinoma therefore differentiation of urothelial carcinoma and renal cell carcinoma on cytology is important. The low grade tumors cytologically reveal sheets and papillae composed of cells with dense, nonvacuolated cytoplasm with large hyperchromatic nuclei. High grade tumors reveal single or small clusters of cells with scanty dense to wispy cytoplasm, high nuclear cytoplasmic ratio, with large hyperchromatic nuclei, and cercariform cells. Differential diagnosis of low grade urothelial carcinoma: papillary renal cell carcinoma. Differential diagnosis of high grade urothelial carcinoma: collecting duct carcinomas, metastatic papillary neoplasms (e.g. lung, thyroid) and papillary renal cell carcinoma (history and immunohistochemistry helps in accurate diagnosis). Urothelial carcinomas are CK 7, CK 20, uroplakin III, and thrombomodulin (+).

7.1.13.3 Metastatic Neoplasms

The most common primary sources for carcinomas are breast, lung, intestine, opposite kidney, and stomach [35]. Metastatic tumors of the kidney are often bilateral and multifocal. The history of a previous primary lesion and an immunohistochemistry aid in the diagnosis.

Other Rare Lesions

Lymphoma (secondary involvement of diffuse large B-cell lymphoma is the most common), sarcoma (leiomyosarcoma is the most common type).

Table 7.1 summarizes immunohistochemical profiles of common renal neoplasms.

Table 7.1 Summary of immunohistochemical profiles of common renal neoplasms

	CK7	CD10	EMA	LMW CK	HMW CK	Vimentin	Ulex	CEA	Mucin	Hale's CI
UC	+	−	+	+	+	−	−	±	−	−
PRC	+	+	+	+	−	+	−	−	−	−
CDC	+	−	+	+	+	+	+	+	+	−
RCC	−	+	+	−	−	+	−	−	−	−
CRCC	−	−	+	−	−	−	−	−	−	+
Oncocytoma	−	−	+	−	−	−	−	−	−	±

UC Urothelial carcinoma, *PRCC* Papillary renal cell carcinoma, *CDC* Collecting duct carcinoma, *RCC* Renal cell carcinoma, *CRCC* Chromophobe renal cell carcinoma, *CK 7* cytokeratin 7, *LMW* low molecular weight, *HMW* high molecular weight, *CEA* carcinoembryonic antigen

7.2 Urine Cytology

7.2.1 Introduction

The earliest attempts at microscopic evaluation of the urinary sediment date back to mid 19th century when Lambl [36] and Sanders [37] independently described the abnormal cells in the urine in the Czech and English literatures, respectively. However, the modern era of urinary cytology did not begin until Papanicolaou and Marshall described the cytologic evaluation of urine sediment in a group of 83 patients in 1945 [38]. Today urinary cytology is used primarily to detect recurrent high grade neoplasms of the urinary tract in patients with a history of urothelial carcinoma, although it can also be used as a screening test for high risk populations and as a diagnostic test in symptomatic patients along with cystoscopic evaluation and biopsy follow-up. As Koss eloquently explained, urine cytology is highly effective in detection and diagnosis of high grade malignant tumors, especially carcinoma in situ; however, it is unrealistic to expect urine cytology to diagnose low grade papillary tumors and be able to distinguish it from other space occupying lesions [39]. To date, despite many attempts to identify a magic test that has a high sensitivity and specificity urine cytology still remains to be gold standard for bladder cancer screening [40].

7.2.2 Indications for Urinary Tract Cytology

1. As a screening test in high risk populations such as patients with industrial exposure to aryl amines, heavy smokers, patients living in areas where Schistosoma hematobium is endemic
2. As a follow-up tool for potential recurrence in patients with a previous diagnosis of a urothelial carcinoma
3. As an evaluation tool for symptomatic patients and patients present with hematuria

4. To follow up possible metachronous upper tract lesions in patients with known urothelial carcinoma of the bladder.

7.2.3 Adequacy

Although there are no universally accepted guidelines for adequacy criteria in urinary tract cytology studies have suggested that a total number of 1,000–10,000 urothelial cells in urine specimens are sufficient for evaluation. Suboptimal specimens have been defined as having one or more of the following deficiencies: >15 intermediate or basal urothelial cells, obscuring blood/inflammation, or poor cellular preservation [41, 42].

7.2.4 Types of Urinary Tract Specimens

Table 7.2 summarizes pros and cons of different types of specimens.

1. *Voided urine.* This is the most convenient and easily obtained specimen. However, since urine normally has an acidic pH, it causes degeneration of the urothelial cells that are shed. Also, since it is not a direct sampling method, contamination from external genitalia and vagina can be seen, which on rare occasion comes in handy in diagnosing a dysplastic/neoplastic lesion originating in the external genital tract. The most cellularity is seen in the first morning urine; however, it is also where the most degenerative changes are seen. For that reason, the second morning urine is considered the best sample. In addition, three samples obtained on three consecutive days are considered the most optimal approach when specimen type is considered.
2. *Catheterized urine.* The specimen is collected with a catheter hence requires instrumentation. These specimens are more cellular compared to that of voided urine and may contain pseudopapillary urothelial fragments. However, there is less contamination from the genital tract.
3. *Urinary bladder washing/barbotage.* This method requires cystoscopy and hence the sample is more cellular, cells are preserved better, and there is no contamination from the external genitalia. However, instrumentation effect is seen such as monolayer sheets, pseudopapillary fragments, and columnar-shaped urothelial cells.
4. *Ileal conduit.* Depending on the type of conduit, instrumentation may be required. The specimens are almost always hypercellular with degenerated columnar/glandular cells of ileal epithelium in a dirty background of mucus and bacteria. Degenerated urothelial cells with cytoplasmic inclusions are also seen (Fig. 7.9). However, this is one of the best methods to evaluate recurrence following cystectomy and the upper tract for metachronous lesions.

Table 7.2 Types of urinary tract specimens—pros and cons

	Pros	Cons
Voided urine	Noninvasive	Cellular degeneration due to poor preservation
	Easy to obtain	Genital system contamination
	No instrumentation artifact	Low cellularity
Catheterized urine	Higher cellularity	Requires catheterization, invasive
		Cellular degeneration
		Cytologic changes due to instrumentation
Bladder washing/barbotage	High cellularity	Invasive
	Good cellular preservation	Higher cost
		Cytologic changes due to instrumentation
Ileal conduit urine	Allows follow up of urothelial carcinoma patients	Very high cellularity
	Allows screening and diagnosis of metachronous tumors of the upper urothelial tract	Poor cellular preservation
		May be invasive depending on the type of conduit
Upper tract washing	High cellularity	Invasive
	Good cellular preservation	Cytologic changes due to instrumentation
	Direct sampling enabling Lateralization	Since it samples a larger area is mostly superior to surgical biopsy
Upper tract brushing	High cellularity	Invasive
	Good cellular preservation	Cytologic changes due to instrumentation
	Direct sampling enabling lateralization	Since it samples a larger area is mostly superior to surgical biopsy
		If it does not get fixed immediately air dry artifact could be seen

7.2.5 Specimen Preparation and Evaluation

Regardless of the way a specimen is obtained, it is prepared the same way. The sample is centrifuged and the button is fixed in an ethanol or methanol-based fixative. Some laboratories also add 2 % carbowax in the fixative. A monolayer preparation is made using ThinPrep (Hologic, Bedford, MA) or Surepath (BD Diagnostics–Tripath, Burlington, NC), and stained with the Papanicolaou method. Alternatively, a cytospin preparation could be used also stained with the Papanicolaou method. Studies have compared the use of ThinPrep liquid-based technology with other preparatory techniques including SurePath PREP (BD Diagnostics–Tripath, Burlington, NC), Shandon Cytospin (Thermo Electron, Waltham, MA), nitrocellulose membrane filtration (Magna MCE nitrocellulose filter, BioBlock Scientific, Illkirch, France), and Monoprep (Monogen, Lincolnshire, IL) for the processing of urine cytologic specimens [43–45]. Most previously published studies suggest the utilization of ThinPrep method over other methods since there are fewer obscuring inflammatory cells, less background proteinaceous debris, and improved cytomorphologic features.

7.2.6 Approach to Upper Tract Lesions

Urothelial neoplasms of the renal pelvis and ureter are infrequent, accounting for approximately 5 % of urothelial malignancies in the USA [46]. Although the approach to urothelial malignancies in the upper tract is the same as in the bladder, due to technical difficulties ureteroscopic biopsies are much smaller than cystoscopic biopsies, and therefore could be challenging to interpret. In a study by Tavora et al. [47] in 25 % of the upper urothelial lesions a definitive diagnosis could not be made due to small sample size and lack of proper tissue orientation. Upper tract cytological samples are prepared in the same way as lower tract

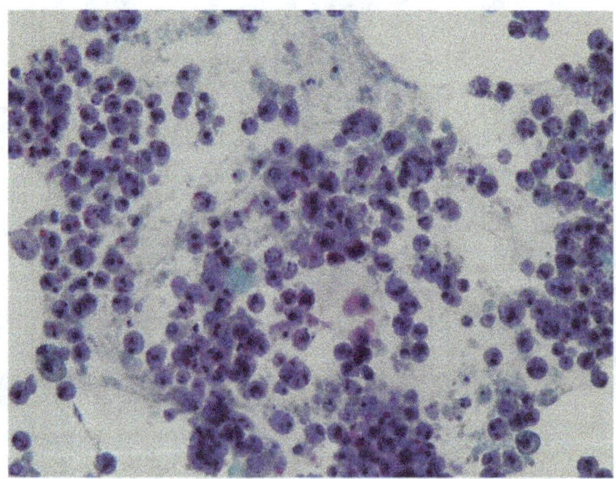

Fig. 7.9 Ileal Conduit (Urine, ThinPrep, High power, Papanicolaou stain). Very cellular specimen showing degenerated glandular and urothelial cells. It is not uncommon to see neutrophils in these specimens as well

samples are prepared. If there are tissue fragments floating in the sample, a cell block preparation with Hematoxylen and Eosin sections are also recommended.

A study reported in 1984 showed that cytology is 78 % accurate in diagnosing upper urothelial lesions, and the remaining 22 % inaccuracy is partly due to sampling error (16 %) and partly due to interpretive error (6 %). The interpretive error in this study is due to false positive diagnosis in patients with urolithiasis and chronic inflammation. However, this study does not compare cytologic and surgical samples [48]. In a study we conducted at our institution, we compared surgical biopsies and cytologic samples (ureteral and renal pelvis washing and brushing) and found that using surgical resection as the gold standard, cytologic sampling of the upper genitourinary tract had an overall sensitivity of 95 % and a specificity of 87 %. Surgical biopsy of the upper genitourinary tract showed an overall sensitivity of only 69 %, though the specificity was 100 % [49]. The reason for this is taking a surgical biopsy large enough for adequate evaluation is technically challenging. However, performing a washing or a brushing is relatively easier and the area sampled is much larger, thus, more material is obtained, reducing errors due to sampling. Therefore, we strongly recommend evaluating/following up upper tract lesions with cytologic samples only or with combined cytologic/surgical samples.

7.2.7 Elements of Normal Urine

Normal urine is mainly composed of urothelial cells, i.e., basal cells, intermediate cells, superficial (umbrella) cells, and squamous cells (contaminant from the external genitalia, cells from trigone, and squamous metaplasia) (Fig. 7.10). Other cells that can be found in normal urine include:

(a) glandular cells from the prostate, endometrium, cystitis glandularis in the bladder, and cells from paraurethral glands
(b) renal tubular cells
(c) peripheral blood elements (leukocytes, lymphocytes, and red blood cells)
(d) seminal vesicle cells and sperm.

Non-cellular elements of urine include crystals, casts, corpora amylacea, lubricant material (seen especially in instrumented specimens), mucus, fibrin, and pollen contaminants.

7.2.8 Benign Conditions

7.2.9 Infectious/Inflammatory Conditions

(*Viruses.* Polyomavirus, Herpes, Cytomegalovirus, Bacteria, Fungi: Candida, Parasite: Trichomonas, Schistosomiasis):

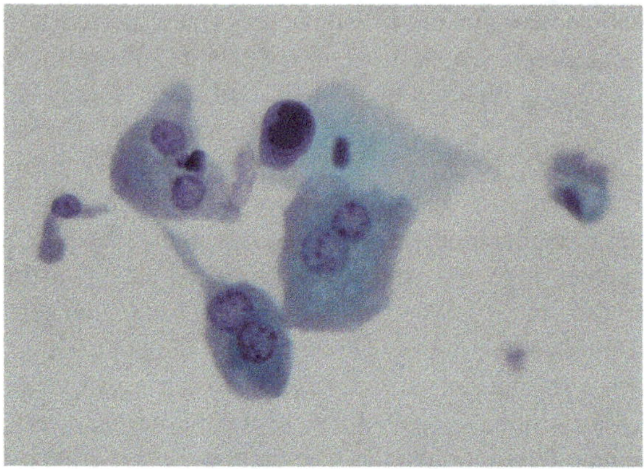

Fig. 7.10 Normal urine—umbrella cells and basal cells (Urine, Bladder Washing, ThinPrep, High power, Papanicolaou stain). Large cells with abundant cytoplasm are superficial (or umbrella cells). These cells can be mono, bi, or multinucleated. Smaller cells are intermediate and basal cells

Discussion of all infectious/inflammatory conditions are beyond the scope of this chapter however Polyomavirus deserves a special recognition in urinary tract cytology.

Polyomavirus. The primary infection occurs during childhood and is usually subclinical. Most adults are seropositive for viral antibodies. The virus generally remains latent in the kidney, but intermittent viruria is demonstrable in 0.3 % of healthy adults. The infection is reactivated in individuals with immunological deficits such as transplant patients, patients on chemotherapy, or AIDS patients.

Cytologically, the polyoma virus-infected cells are characterized by the presence of a single, large, homogenous, basophilic inclusion occupying most of an enlarged nuclear area (Fig. 7.11). The cytological resemblance to high grade urothelial carcinoma cells have resulted in the commonly used nickname "decoy cells". The infected cells have also been called "empty cells" due to the ground glass appearance of the nuclear inclusion. Of note, urothelial cells affected by the virus have an abnormal DNA content demonstrated by various authors on DNA Ploidy analysis [50–54].

7.2.10 Urolithiasis

The patients present with pain radiating to the inguinal region and gross hematuria, which warrants a clinical work up, since the differential diagnosis includes neoplastic lesions. Depending on the size of the stone, a filling defect may be seen on the intravenous pyelogram. The samples are usually cellular. Cytologically, three-dimensional papillary fragments composed of cells exhibiting nuclear enlargement may be seen. The papillary fragments have a smooth contour, with a cytoplasmic collaret. The presence of pseudopapillary clusters has lead to false positive diagnosis, especially that of low grade carcinoma. Therefore, providing the clinical

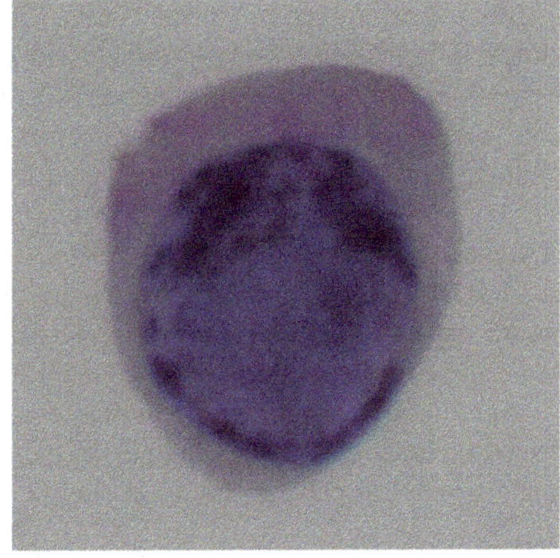

Fig. 7.11 Polyoma virus (Urine, Bladder Washing, ThinPrep, High power, Papanicolaou stain). Single cell with large basophilic homogenous, ground glass nuclear inclusion occupying almost the entire nucleus

history and adherence to the well-defined cytologic criteria is crucial to avoid a false positive diagnosis [55, 56] (Fig. 7.12).

7.2.11 Treatment-Related Changes

Treatment-related changes include intravesical Bacillus Calmette Guérin (BCG), chemotherapy as well as parenteral chemotherapy and radiotherapy, all of which have various effects on the urothelium observed in cytological preparations. Some of these effects can be mistaken for malignancy, especially if the clinical history is not known. The detailed effects of individual therapeutic modalities are beyond the scope of this chapter, however, the following is a brief description of the effects of the most common agents.

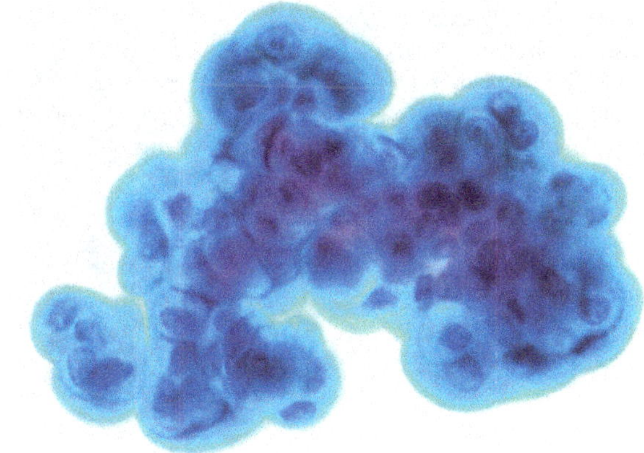

Fig. 7.12 Urolithiasis, reactive changes (Urine, Bladder Washing, ThinPrep, High power, Papanicolaou stain). Group of papillary cells, with minimal cytologic atypia, smooth borders, cytoplasmic collaret, centrally placed nuclei, and finely granular chromatin. Hyperchromasia, pleomorphism, and severe atypia are conspicuously absent

BCG, the most common intravesical immunomodulation agent causes granulomas, inflammation, and multinucleated giant cells that can be seen in the urine samples as a result of its immunomodulant effect [57] (Fig. 7.13).

Cyclophosphamide (cytoxan, endoxan), a widely used chemotherapeutic and immunosuppressive agent alters the urothelial cells to have high nuclear cytoplasmic ratio, large nuclei, hyperchromasia and degenerative changes, that mimick malignancy [58].

Mitomycin and thiotepa are both intravesical chemotherapeutic agents, most commonly effecting umbrella cells, causing nuclear enlargement, multinucleation, and hyperchromatic, granular chromatin [59].

Radiotherapy regardless of the targeted area has similar effects on epithelium. These include cytomegaly, nucleomegaly, multinucleation, polychromasia, and nuclear and cytoplasmic vacuolization [39].

7.2.12 *Malignant Neoplasms*

7.2.12.1 Urothelial Carcinoma

The American Cancer Society predicts that approximately 72,570 new cases of bladder cancer will be diagnosed in 2013 in the USA and approximately 15,210 people will die of the disease. Of these new cases only about 50 % are detected by routine cytologic examination. The majority of bladder cancers (75 %) are superficial in nature at presentation. Approximately 50–70 % of these superficial tumors recur and 10–20 % progress to be invasive at least into muscularis propria. This natural history of bladder cancer results in a very high overall disease prevalence.

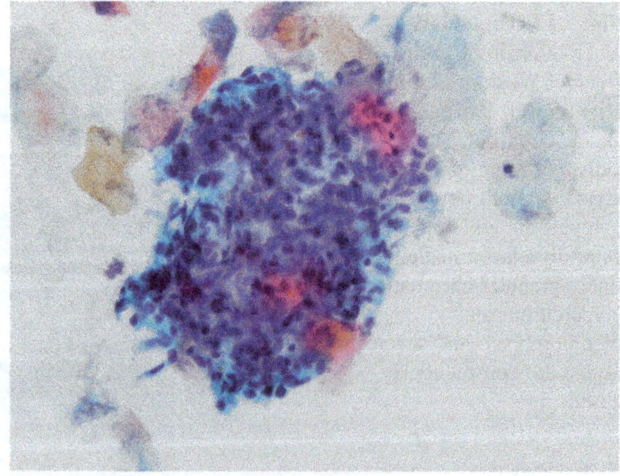

Fig. 7.13 BCG-related changes (Urine, Bladder Washing, ThinPrep, High power, Papanicolaou stain). Granuloma composed of epithelioid histiocytes and lymphocytes in a background of anucleated squamous cells in a patient with known urothelial carcinoma and recent intravesical BCG treatment

The main purpose of urine cytology is to detect lesions that can be difficult to detect cystoscopically and to detect high grade urothelial lesions that are at a greater risk of developing into invasive carcinoma. Papillary low grade urothelial neoplasms are easily seen cystoscopically and therefore unlikely to be missed by the urologist, except those that occur in the upper urinary tract. Therefore, for practical purposes, high grade urothelial carcinoma is diagnosed on cytology, and unless a true papillary fragment with a discernible true fibrovascular core lined by atypical urothelial cells is seen on a cytology sample, a diagnosis of low grade urothelial carcinoma should not be rendered.

With that in mind, the following discussed mostly pertains to diagnosing high grade urothelial carcinoma.

In practice, very much like an abbreviated version of the Bethesda system for reporting cervical cytopathology [60] a four-tiered system is used for diagnosing urinary tract specimens:

1. Normal
2. Atypical urothelial cells identified
3. Suspicious for urothelial carcinoma
4. Urothelial carcinoma

1. *Normal or negative for malignancy.* Meaning the sample is composed of benign urothelial cells and that cells that could remotely raise the suspicion of carcinoma are conspicuously absent. The clinical approach should be to proceed with the next regularly scheduled follow-up.
2. *Atypical urothelial cells present.* This is the category that causes the most controversy among pathologists and clinicians. There are several reasons for this; first of all urothelial atypia is not as well defined in the literature and thus it is in the eye of the beholder. Renshaw [61] attempted to categorize atypical urine specimens based on cytomorphologic features and the risk associated with the different groups, however this is still a very difficult category to define, and one that is associated with considerable difference of opinion. Therefore, there is a wide range of the percentage of atypia ranging between 2 and 30 %. In a study performed at our institution, we looked at the rate of atypical diagnosis in over 5,000 urine specimens composed of both voided urine and bladder barbotage samples and we analyzed the outcome using surgical biopsies as a gold standard [62]. A diagnosis of atypia was rendered in 6.9 % of the voided urine specimens and in 7.9 % of the instrumented specimens. A malignant follow-up diagnosis was observed in 32.7 % cases in the instrumented group and in 46.6 % cases in the voided group. Therefore, we concluded that an atypical diagnosis is more predictive of a subsequent malignant biopsy diagnosis in voided urine specimens compared with instrumented urines. In a similar study investigating the outcome of discrepancies in urine specimens, Raab et al. [63] reported an atypia rate of 10.1 % in voided urine specimens. However, Bhatia et al. [64], in a retrospective analysis of atypical urine specimens, reported an atypia rate of only 1.9 %.

Although there is not a universally defined benchmark for the atypia rate, it is prudent to keep the atypia rate low to keep it more meaningful. This important category should be used by the pathologist to convey concern and recognize the difficulty in interpretation of specimens that may require close clinical follow-up. In cases where atypia is considered, a comment including limitations (degeneration, too few cells, well-preserved cells that are qualitatively insufficient to be able to distinguish from reactive cells, etc.) and the differential of lesions to be considered (high grade carcinoma, viral inclusions, therapy-related changes, etc.) should be added.

In addition, a subset of patients with a history of high grade urothelial carcinoma and a negative follow-up could have a lesion in the upper tract that was not biopsied. In these patients with a previous diagnosis of urothelial carcinoma, there is a higher likelihood of a subsequent malignant diagnosis after an atypical specimen [65].

Currently, the overall yield for a diagnosis of atypia is so low that most urologists pay little attention to it and most of the time follow the patient up as if it were a "negative" diagnosis. However, in cases where there is good communication between the pathologist and the urologist, the laboratories rate of atypia is low (<10 %), the patient has had a previously documented urothelial carcinoma, there is increased clinical suspicion for malignancy, or if the diagnosis comes with a qualifier "highly atypical", the patient should be followed up closely, and the specimen should be triaged using ancillary tests such fluorescence in situ hybridization, microsatellite analysis, or other markers for the detection of urothelial carcinoma.

3. *Suspicious for Urothelial carcinoma.* Meaning the pathologist sees very rare cells with features that are compatible with urothelial carcinoma, or there are only some features of malignancy; however, either the paucity of these cells or insufficiently fulfilled malignancy criteria preclude a definitive diagnosis of malignancy. In general, if this diagnosis is rendered the patients should be followed up with surgical biopsies.

4. *Urothelial carcinoma.* Meaning there is an undeniable presence of tumor cells fitting the criteria for urothelial carcinoma as outlined. At this point, a surgical biopsy is warranted to determine the presence/depth of invasion, hence the stage of the neoplasm.

Cytologic features of high grade urothelial carcinoma are: increased cellularity, presence of loose clusters and single cells, moderate to marked pleomorphism, eccentric, enlarged, pleomorphic nuclei, irregular nuclear membrane, and coarse chromatin. Prominent nucleoli as well as squamous or glandular differentiation can also been seen (Fig. 7.14).

The differential diagnosis includes: (1) Polyoma virus infection: single, large, homogenous, basophilic inclusions occupying most of an enlarged nuclear area, "decoy cells". Like urothelial carcinoma, cells affected by polyoma virus also have an abnormal DNA content [54]. (2) Seminal vesicle cells: Bizarre cells, with greatly

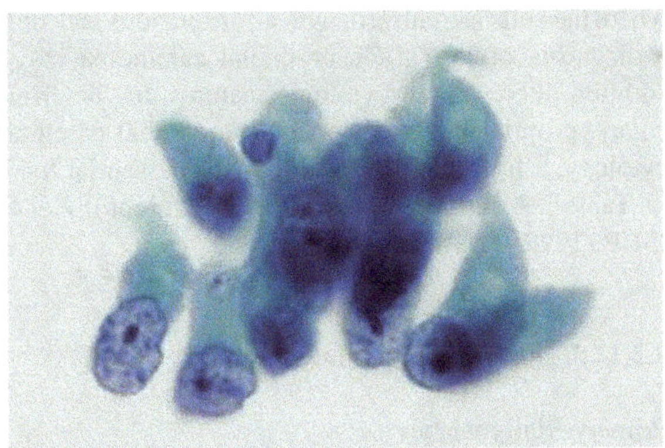

Fig. 7.14 High grade urothelial carcinoma (Urine, Bladder Washing, ThinPrep, High power, Papanicolaou stain). Urothelial cells with high nuclear cytoplasmic ratio, eccentrically located nucleus, and hyperchromasia—classic features of urothelial carcinoma

enlarged nuclei and foamy, fragmented cytoplasm. The chromatin is hyperchromatic, degenerated, and smudgy. In contrast, the chromatin of malignant cells is coarse. Golden-brown lipofuscin pigment and often, spermatozoa accompany seminal vesicle cells. These cells also have an abnormal DNA content [70]. (3) Karyomegalic Interstitial Nephritis [66]—a rare cause of progressive renal failure, which may be familial, and is frequently associated with a history of recurrent respiratory infections. The urine may contain large, pleomorphic cells, mimicking carcinoma. However, the clinical scenario is different from that of urothelial carcinoma.

In Box 1 the WHO/ISUP (1998) consensus classification of the Urothelial Neoplasms of the Urinary Bladder is outlined [67], however to reiterate, since cytologically a diagnosis of papilloma, papillary urothelial neoplasm of low malignant potential, and low grade papillary urothelial carcinoma cannot be reliably made, this terminology is not used in reporting urine cytology. Rarely there are cases where clear-cut papillary fragments are seen with distinct fibrovascular cores,

---

Box 1. WHO/ISUP (1998) consensus classification of the Urothelial Neoplasms of the Urinary Bladder

- Papillary Neoplasms

  - Papilloma
  - Inverted papilloma
  - Papillary urothelial neoplasm of low malignant potential (PUNLMP)
  - Papillary urothelial carcinoma, low grade
  - Papillary urothelial carcinoma, high grade.

- Invasive neoplasms

  - Lamina propria invasion (superficial urothelial carcinoma)
  - Muscularis propria (detrusor muscle) invasion.

where the cells are uniform with a conspicuous lack of pleomorphism. In such cases, a diagnosis of low grade urothelial carcinoma may be rendered (Fig. 7.15). In addition, there are no cytologic features that determine the invasion of the muscularis propria; therefore, once an urothelial carcinoma diagnosis is rendered on cytology, a follow-up surgical biopsy is essential for further evaluation.

Table 7.3 outlines comparison of terminology of the WHO (1974) and WHO/ISUP (1998) classification.

7.2.12.2 Nonurothelial Malignancies

Primary Malignancies

Squamous Cell Carcinoma
This is only rarely encountered in the USA, accounting for >5 % of all bladder carcinomas. It is more common in the African counties, particularly in Egypt where it is endemic, and is associated with schistosomiasis. Outside Africa it is mostly associated with chronic inflammation and urolithiasis.

Cytologically, well-differentiated squamous cell carcinoma shows cells with dense cytoplasm, cytoplasmic orangophilia if keratinizing, and hyperchromatic small nuclei. Poorly differentiated carcinomas, on the other hand, have pleomorphic, hyperchromatic cells with high nuclear cytoplasmic ratio, prominent nucleoli, and necrotic background.

Morphologically, squamous cell carcinoma and its precursors arising in the genital tract can not be distinguished from squamous cell carcinoma arising in the bladder. Therefore, when dysplastic squamous cells are seen in the urine specimen, a differential diagnosis of urothelial carcinoma with squamous differentiation,

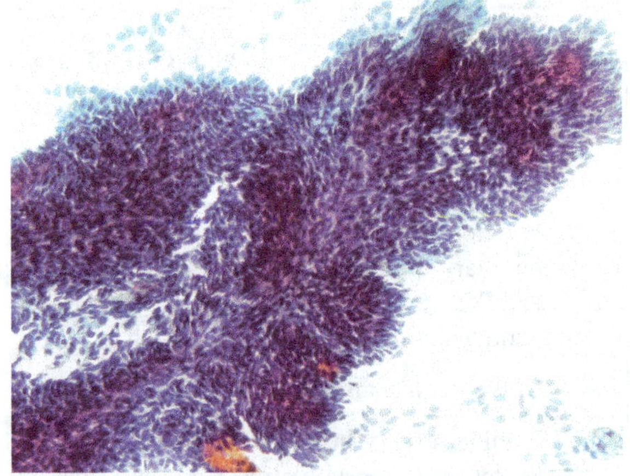

Fig. 7.15 Low grade urothelial carcinoma (Renal Pelvis Washing, ThinPrep, High power, Papanicolaou stain). Monomorphic, uniform urothelial cells forming a cohesive papillary group with a central fibrovascular core. Pleomorphism is conspicuously absent

Table 7.3 Comparison of terminology of the WHO (1974) and WHO/ISUP (1998) classification

WHO (1974)	WHO/ISUP (1998)
Papilloma	Papilloma
TCC I	Low malignant potential/low grade UC
TCC II	Low grade UC/high grade UC
TCC III	High grade UC

squamous cell carcinoma of the bladder, and dysplastic cells arising in the genital tract should be raised. Although squamous cell carcinomas of the genital tract are more likely to be HPV-related, the differentiation of these two entities is mostly based on clinical findings.

Adenocarcinoma

This is also a rare neoplasm, accounting for <2 % of all bladder carcinomas. It may arise in the bladder or urachus.

Cytologically, well-differentiated adenocarcinoma forms glandular structures, and is composed of cells with hyperchromatic nuclei and finely vacuolated cytoplasm. In poorly differentiated carcinomas, signet ring cells may also be seen. Immunohistochemistry could be performed to differentiate primary adenocarcinoma from metastasis (Cytokeratin 20+positive, Cytokeratin 7–negative, CDX-2 and villin (+/–)).

Small Cell Carcinoma

This is a highly aggressive malignancy, accounting for <1 % of the bladder carcinomas. Majority of small cell carcinomas are seen in combination with urothelial carcinoma. As small cell carcinomas elsewhere in the body, these tumors may present with paraneoplastic syndromes.

Cytologically, they are composed of small round to oval cells, with high nuclear cytoplasmic ratio, scant cytoplasm, hyperchromatic nucleus with coarse—'salt and pepper' chromatin, and nuclear molding. Occasional mitotic figures can also be identified.

The cells are usually positive for at least one of the three most commonly used neuroendocrine markers: chromogranin, synaptophysin, and CD 56. However, neither the morphology nor the positivity of the markers aid in defining the site of origin for this carcinoma. Small cell carcinomas arising in the bladder, prostate as well as elsewhere in the body are morphologically identical, and thus far reliable organ specific markers are not reported. Regardless of the location, small cell carcinoma has a poor prognosis.

Secondary Malignancies in the Bladder

Less than 10 % of bladder tumors represent secondary neoplasms, most of which are direct invasion from prostate, cervix, uterus, or GI tract. The most common distant metastases are malignant melanoma, carcinomas of stomach, breast, kidney, and lung.

7.2.13 Ancillary Tests Used in Urine Cytology

7.2.13.1 DNA Ploidy

The evaluation of DNA ploidy in urinary specimens is an adjunct test used for both diagnostic and prognostic purposes. In general, low grade urothelial carcinomas are diploid and high grade tumors are aneuploid. As a result, aneuploidy is a strong indicator of high grade malignancy as well as carcinoma in situ. Also aneuploidy in conjunction with suspicious cytology is highly predictive of tumor recurrence. In addition, it has been shown that DNA ploidy analysis provides independent prognostic information.

Diploid   Normal (2c or 2 N) amount of DNA corresponding to 46 chromosomes
Aneuploid   Abnormal (increased or decreased) amount of DNA
Tetraploid   Double amount of DNA (4c or 4 N DNA)
Hyperploid   DNA content >5c.

7.2.13.2 DNA Ploidy: FCM

FCM was first applied to study bladder washings from patients with urinary carcinomas [68]. It has been documented that flow cytometric DNA ploidy results correlate well with cystoscopic and cytologic findings. When FCM and urine cytology were used together, an improved diagnostic ability was observed. However, recent reports did not confirm these early findings. In addition, FCM requires numerous cells, therefore only bladder washes are suitable specimens.

7.2.13.3 DNA Ploidy: Image Analysis

This technology has been used for decades to evaluate DNA ploidy in urine specimens. Image analysis (IA) is a broad term, encompassing morphometry, densitometry and even neural networks. Typically, the term is used to describe an integrated, interactive computer-based system in which measurements of specific cellular features, including the amount of DNA, are analyzed [69]. In this method, cells (100–200) are visually selected by operator. All urine specimens are suitable for analysis. Nuclear DNA ploidy is evaluated on Feulgen-stained slides.

7.2.13.4 DNA Ploidy: Laser Scanning Cytometer

The Laser Scanning Cytometer (LSC) is highly suited for DNA ploidy analysis, combining features of both flow and image cytometry and is capable of measuring multicolor fluorescence, light scatter and location of cells fixed to a microscopic slide. It is capable of rapid and automatic measurements of a large number of cells. In addition, cell location is recorded so the cells of interest can be relocated for a morphologic examination and classification. The problem with DNA Ploidy as previously eluded, is the potential false positivity that could be seen in superficial cells, Polyoma virus-infected cells, and seminal vesicle cells [54, 70–72].

7.2.13.5 Morphometry

Morphometry has been defined as the "quantitative description of a structure". In practice, this term is usually applied to quantitative techniques that measure the features of size, shape, and texture in two dimensions and/or spatial relationships from cells or other tissue structures. The need for measurement comes from the recognition that interobserver and intraobserver diagnostic decisions are poorly reproducible. Morphometry has several advantages over conventional visual assessment: objectivity, reproducibility, and the ability to detect changes too subtle to be visually appreciated in individual cells. Therefore, morphologic diagnostic accuracy and precision can be improved by applying this technique.

7.2.13.6 Fluorescence in situ Hybridization

A number of studies aimed at defining loss of heterozygosity have shown a general chromosomal instability in urothelial carcinoma with loss of parts of chromosome 9 at early stages and of chromosomes 3, 4, 8, 11, 13, 17, and 18 during further development of the tumor. It has been postulated that two different tumor suppressor gene loci on chromosome 9 are involved as tumorigenic events in bladder cancer. It was also postulated that loss of heterozygosity of 9p might be associated with the development of tumors with more aggressive behavior.

Fluorescence in situ hybridization (FISH) has been demonstrated as a viable method for determination of chromosome specific anomalies in cells obtained from urine specimens for early tumor detection or recurrence. Currently a commercially available multi-color FISH Probe Mixture designed for interphase cell analysis for detection and quantification of chromosome 3, 7, 17, and the 9p21 region (UroVysion ™ Multi-color FISH Probe Mixture, Abbott) is being used. The sample should contain at least 25 cells to be deemed satisfactory for evaluation. A count of only four or more cells with polysomy (gains of three or more copies of at least two of the probes) and/or 12 cells for no signal for chromosome ip21 is considered a positive result. In a recent metaanalysis of UroVysion performance the reported sensitivity ranged between 39 and 93 % (mean 72 %) and specificity ranged between 53 and 100 % (mean 83 %) [73].

7.2.13.7 Urothelial Tumor Markers

Lewis X. The only blood group antigen with potential prognostic application. This test has a relatively high reported sensitivity (83 %) and specificity (85 %). However, it is not intensely investigated and its expression on the umbrella cells may interfere with the results of the assay [74].

ImmunoCyt/uCyt. ImmunoCyt/uCyt (Diagno- Cure Inc., Quebec, QC, Canada) has been developed by Fradet and Lockhart and was aimed at improving the low sensitivity of cytology. This test obtained FDA clearance in 2000. This fluorescence test combines three monoclonal antibodies- M344 and LDQ10, labeled with fluorescein, a green fluorescence, have been raised against mucin-like antigens. 19A211, labeled with Texas red, recognizes a high molecular form of carcinoembryonic antigen [75]. Although this test cannot be performed in a physician's office, it was not aimed to be performed in large centralized laboratories. The major disadvantages are that the test is largely operator-dependent and time-consuming and requires at least 500 cells to call a case negative, and only one cell to call the case positive. Furthermore, this test requires on site training, significant experience and regular quality controls by the company. Sensitivity of Immuno-Cyt/uCytt ranges from 53 to 100 % (average 90 %) and specificity ranges from 64 to 95 % (74 %) [76].

Cytokeratin 20. Cytokeratin 20 by immunocytochemistry provides sensitivity and a specificity of 65 and 90 %, respectively, but the sensitivity is lower for low-grade tumors [77]. However, with the RT-PCR method sensitivity is raised to 91 %.

Telomerase. Telomerase activity is measured using a telomeric repeat amplification protocol (TRAP). This method requires a minimum 30 ml of urine. The reported sensitivity ranges from 29 to 66 % (mean 39 %) [74].

BTA stat and BTA TRAK. (Polymedco, Cortlandt Manor, NY) Antibodies detecting proteins (complement factor H-related protein) present in urine and can be used at a physician's office [78]. Both tests are FDA approved. BTA stat is an immunoassay. BTA TRAK is a standard ELISA, which quantitatively measures the amounts of complement factor H-related protein. The BTA Stat shows an improved sensitivity and specificity as compared to the original BTA test. The sensitivity of both tests ranges from 17 to 89 % and is dependent on tumor grade, stage and size [76]. However, although these tests may improve the sensitivity of cytology, such improvement remains modest for low-grade, low-stage tumors [78].

At this moment, despite numerous controversial reports, most authors would agree that this test could be utilized only as an adjunct to cytology, particularly for the detection of recurrent tumors.

NMP ^{TM}. NMP-22 (Matritech, Cambridge, MA, USA) is a nuclear matrix protein involved in proper distribution of chromatin during replication. NMP-22 levels are usually low in normal cells whereas they are 25-fold or greater in patients with bladder cancer. This is a quantitative sandwich ELISA test using two antibodies, which recognize two different epitopes. The antibodies in this assay recognize two domains of the nuclear mitotic apparatus protein. This quantitative assay has a recommended cut off point of 10 IU/ml. The sensitivity is around 50–70 % and specificity reaches 60–90 % [79–81]. This test is FDA approved. However, the reliability of the test is questionable because of the heterogeneity in the diagnostic performance among populations from different institutions [82].

BLCA-4 and BLCA-1. These are nuclear matrix proteins identified by proteomic analyses. Both have a high sensitivity and specificity. The analysis is a sandwich ELISA and uses two monoclonal antibodies. Both are potentially useful markers for the detection of bladder cancer [83].

HA-HAse. This ELISA-like test combines the analysis of hyaluronic acid and hyaluronidase. HA-HAse is expressed by tumors and involved in angiogenesis, tumor growth, and invasion. The test has a high sensitivity to detect low and high grade and stage tumors. In one study, HA-HAse was reported with a sensitivity of 83 % and a specificity of 78 % [84].

Survivin. This is an antiapoptotic protein. The test is being performed by BioDot microfiltration detection system. There is only limited data published to date. However, it appears to be a promising marker with relatively high sensitivity and specificity [83].

CYFRA 21-1. CYFRA 21-1 (CIS Bio International, Gif-Sur Yvette, France) is ELISA test. The assay uses two monoclonal antibodies, BM 19-21 and KS19-1, to recognize cytokeratin 19 fragments. Reported sensitivity and specificity of this test in a metaanalysis is between 75 and 88 % (mean 85 %), and 73–95 % (mean 82 %), respectively [74].

In the age of reflex testing, and synchronous testing of cytology as well as ancillary techniques there is no surprise that there would be situations where one of the tests might be reported positive while the other is negative. So what should be the follow-up protocol in such cases?

How do we handle a positive UroVysion FISH test in light of a negative cytology?

As reported by Soloway [85] although the FISH test is sensitive, it can produce false positive results, which may need to an "unnecessary" set of biopsies. To date the UroVysion FISH test is FDA approved for voided urine cytology only, but bladder washing/barbotage samples are tested with this method as well. Barbotage samples notoriously have more umbrella cells (superficial cells) compared to voided specimens. It has been shown that umbrella cells contain abnormal amount of DNA [72], therefore should be excluded from DNA evaluation to avoid a false positive disgnosis. Similarly, especially in hypercellular samples, cell aggregates could be interpreted as one cell also leading to a false positive diagnosis. The UroVysion test is a costly test, therefore in cases where there is a disagreement between cytology and the FISH test, a follow-up routine cytology is recommended over follow-up with either FISH test or surgical biopsies.

How do we handle a negative UroVysion FISH test in light of a positive cytology?

If the urinary cytology has been diagnosed as "positive for carcinoma," however, a concomitant UroVysion test is negative this may represent a couple of scenarios: (1) Sampling error, meaning the carcinoma cells present in the urine cytology are not present in the FISH sample. (2) Interpretive error in either test, or (3) the presence of a nonurothelial carcinoma such as small cell carcinoma or adenocarcinoma that may lead to a negative FISH result. Therefore in the scenario where cytology is positive but the concomitant FISH test is negative clinical follow-up with surgical biopsies are recommended.

7.3 Summary

FNA of kidney masses have been performed for the diagnosis of mass lesions, confirmation of advanced neoplasia and metastases, and staging of tumors. In the past, the decision of whether to perform a nephrectomy used to be based on radiographic features and size, precluding the use of FNA. Today, where treatment is not limited to surgery alone, the indications for renal FNA have expanded. Most small renal masses are asymptomatic and are detected incidentally due to improved imaging techniques. Although most urologists agree that the standard of care for renal masses is surgery, if the patient is an elderly individual, or has comorbidities a preoperative FNA could be useful in guiding the management. When we look at data from large referral institutions such as Mayo Clinic, Johns Hopkins Medical Institutions, and the Cleveland Clinic approximately 30 % of the renal masses are benign [86–88]. Therefore, as astutely pointed out by Volpe et al. [3], there is a role for precise pretreatment characterization of the renal masses by FNA, which would decrease the unnecessary treatment for benign diseases and reduce the treatment-related mortality and morbidity in addition to reducing patient care costs.

To date, urine cytology remains the gold standard for bladder cancer screening. It has been, and still is, the test against which all new tests are compared when evaluating potential bladder tumor markers. The answer to whether urine cytology possesses the optimal combination of sensitivity and specificity to retain consideration as the best screening device depends on the goals of the practice. Urine cytology has excellent specificity with only few false-positive cases. Its overall sensitivity (including both high grade and low grade lesions) is poor, but this is explained by poor criteria for identifying well-differentiated, low-grade urothelial carcinoma in cytology. The natural history of low grade lesions is that of multiple superficial recurrences in 70 – 80 % of patients, with only a minority (10–15 %)

progressing to muscle invasive or metastatic disease [89]. Patients with low-grade urothelial carcinoma are at low risk for progression, they are monitored primarily for the development of a subsequent high grade tumor [90]. Therefore, as suggested by Koss, detection of new low-grade lesions may be clinically irrelevant as compared to early detection of disease progression [39]. Contrary to the low grade lesions, however, urine cytology often results in the identification of high-grade malignant cells even before a cystoscopically distinguishable gross lesion is present. In the last 20 years, a number of noninvasive test have been developed to detect urothelial carcinoma. Although some have been able to show a better sensitivity compared to cytology, only a few have been close to reaching the sensitivity seen in cytology. Most of these tests have not added much to the diagnostic evaluation. Combining some of the new markers with each other and/or cytologic evaluation may optimize their performance status.

References

1. Katz RL (1997) Kidneys, adrenals and retroperitoneum. In: Bibbo M, Wilbur DC (eds) Comprehensive cytology, 2nd edn. WB Saunders, Philadelphia, pp 781–821
2. Renshaw AA, Granter SR, Cibas E (1997) Fine-needle aspiration of the adult kidney. Cancer Cytopath 81:71–88
3. Volpe A, Kachura JR, Geddie WR, Evans AJ, Gharajeh A, Saravanan A, Jewett M (2007) Techniques, safety and accuracy of sampling of renal tumors by fine needle aspiration and core biopsy. J Urol 178:379–386
4. Gibbons RP, Bush WH Jr, Burnett LL (1977) Needle tract seeding following aspiration of renal cell carcinoma. J Urol 118:865–867
5. Kiser GC, Totonchy M, Barry JM (1986) Needle tract seeding after percutaneous aspiration of renal adenocarcinoma. J Urol 136:1292–1293
6. Shenoy PD, Lakhkar BN, Ghosh MK, Patil UD (1991) Cutaneous seeding of renal carcinoma by Chiba needle aspiration biopsy. Case report. Acta Radiol 32:50
7. Wehle MJ, Grabstald H (1986) Contraindications to needle aspiration of a solid renal mass: tumor dissemination by renal needle aspiration. J Urol 136:446
8. Auvert J, Abbou CC, Lavarenne V (1982) Needle tract seeding following puncture of renal oncocytoma. Prog Clin Biol Res 100:597
9. Abe M, Saitoh M (1992) Selective renal tumour biopsy under ultrasonic guidance. Br J Urol 70:7
10. Wunderlich H, Hindermann W, Al Mustafa AM, Reichelt O, Junker K Schubert J (2005) The accuracy of 250 fine needle biopsies of renal tumors. J Urol 174:44
11. Smith EH (1991) Complications of percutaneous abdominal fine-needle biopsy. Review Radiol. 178:253–258
12. Brierly RD, Thomas PJ, Harrison NW, Fletcher MS, Nawrocki JD, Ashton-Key M (2000) Evaluation of fine-needle aspiration cytology for renal masses. BJU Int 85:14–18
13. Todd LD, Truong TD, Dhurandhar B, Ramzy I (1999) Fine-needle aspiration of renal masses in adults; analysis of results and diagnostic problems in 108 cases. Diagn Cytopathol 20:339–349
14. Campbell SC, Novick AC, Herts B, Fischler DF, Meyer J, Levin HS, Chen RN (1997) Prospective evaluation of fine needle aspiration of small, solid renal masses: accuracy and morbidity. Urology 50:25–29

15. Haubek A, Lundorf E, Lauridsen KN (1991) Diagnostic strategy in renal mass lesions. Scand J Urol Nephrol Suppl 137:35–39
16. Orell SR, Langlois SL, Marshall VR (1985) Fine needle aspiration cytology in the diagnosis of solid renal and adrenal masses. Scand J Urol Nephrol 19:211–216
17. Murphy WM, Zambroni BR, Emerson LD (1985) Aspiration biopsy of the kidney. Cancer 56:200–205
18. Juul N, Torp-Pedersen S, Gronvall S, Holm HH, Koch F, Larsen S (1985) Ultrasonically guided fine needle aspiration biopsy of renal masses. J Urol 133:579–581
19. Lang EK (1987) Renal cyst puncture studies. Urol Clin North Am 14:91–102
20. de Kernion JB, Belldegrun A (1992) Renal tumors. In: Campbell MF, Retik AB, Vaughan ED, Walsh PC (eds) Campbell's Urology, 2nd edn. WB Saunders, Philadelphia, pp 1055–1067
21. Bosniak MA (1991) Difficulties in classifying cystic lesions of the kidney. Urol Radiol 13:91–93
22. Truong LD, Krishnan B, Barrios R et al (1995) Renal neoplasms in acquired cystic disease of the kidney. Am J Kidney Dis 26:1–12
23. Emmet JL, Levine SR, Woolner LB (1963) Co-existence of renal cyst and tumor: incidence of 1007 cases. Br J Urol 35:403–410
24. Khorsand D (1965) Carcinoma within solitary renal cysts. J Urol 93:440–444
25. Hughson M, Hennigar G, McManus J (1980) Atypical cysts, acquired renal cystic disease and renal cell tumors in end stage dialysis kidneys. Lab Invest 42:475–480
26. Nguyen GK, Percutaneous FNA (1987) biopsy cytology of the kidney and adrenal. Pathol Annual 22:163–191
27. Silverman JF, Gurley AM, Harris JP et al (1991) Fine needle aspiration cytology of renal infarcts. Cytomorphologic findings and potential diagnostic pitfalls in two cases. Acta Cytol 35:736–741
28. Kruger S, Sotlar K, Kausch I, Horny HP (2005) Expression of KIT (CD117) in renal cell carcinoma and renal oncocytoma. Oncology 68:269–275
29. Mazal PR, Exner M, Haitel A, Krieger S, Thomson RB, Aronson PS, Susani M (2005) Expression of kidney-specific cadherin distinguishes chromophobe renal cell carcinoma from renal oncocytoma. Hum Pathol 36:22–28
30. Garcia E, Li M (2006) Caveolin-1 immunohistochemical analysis in differentiating chromophobe renal cell carcinoma from renal oncocytoma. Am J Clin Pathol 125:392–398
31. Alroy J, Ucci AA, Azabdoaftari G, Banner BF, Cheville JC (2005) Expression of CD3 antigens in renal tubule epithelium and renal oncocytomas. Pathol Res Pract 201:803–808
32. Mete O, Kilicaslan I, Gulluoglu MG, Uysal V (2005) Can renal oncocytoma be differentiated from its renal mimics? The utility of anti-mitochondrial, caveolin 1, CD63 and cytokeratin 14 antibodies in the differential diagnosis. Virchows Arch 447:938–946
33. Assad L, Resetkova E, Oliveira VL, Sun W, Stewart JM, Katz RL, Caraway NP (2005) Cytologic features of renal medullary carcinoma. Cancer 1051:28–34
34. Santamaria M, Jauregui I, Urtasun F, Bertol A (1995) Fine needle aspiration biopsy in urothelial carcinoma of renal pelvis. Acta Cytol 39:443–448
35. Gattuso P, Ramzy I, Truong LD (1999) Utilization of fine-needle aspiration in the diagnosis of metastatic tumors to the kidney. Diagn Cytopathol 21:35–38
36. Lambl W Uber Harnblasenkrebs. Einbeitag zur mikroskopischen Diagnostic am Krakenbette. Prager Vierteljahreshift f. Heilkunde. 1865;49:1–15
37. Sanders WR (1864) Cancer of the bladder. Fragments forming urethral plugs discharged in urine. Concentric colloid bodies. Edinb Med J 10:273–275
38. Papanicolaou GN, Marshall VF (1945) Urine sediment smears: a diagnostic procedure in cancers of urinary tract. Science 101:519–521
39. Koss L, Melamed M (2005) In: Koss' diagnostic cytology and its histopathologic bases, Koss L, Melamed M eds 5th ed. Philadelphia, PA: Lipincott Williams & Wilkins; 2005:38–846
40. Brown FM (2000) Urine Cytology Is it still the gold standard for screening? Urol Clin North Am 27:25–37

41. Morse N, Melamed MR (1974) Differential counts of cell populations in urinary sediment from patients with primary epidermoid carcinoma of bladder. Acta Cytol 18:312–315

42. Murphy WM, Crabtree WN, Jukkola WN, Soloway MS (1981) The diagnostic value of urine versus bladder washing in patients with bladder cancer. J Urol 126:320–322

43. Wright RG, Halford JA (2001) Evaluation of thin-layer methods in urine cytology. Cytopathology 12:306–313

44. Elsheikh TM, Kirkpatrick JL, Wu HH (2006) Comparison of ThinPrep and Cytospin preparations in the evaluation of exfoliative cytology specimens. Cancer 108:144–149

45. Hwang EC, Park SH, Jung SI (2007) etal. Usefulness of liquid-based preparation in urine cytology. Int J Urol 14:626–629

46. Jemal A, Siegal R, Ward E. et al (2008) Cancer statistics, 2008 CA. Cancer J Clin 58:71–96

47. Tavora F, Fjardo DA et al (2009) Small endoscopic biopsies of the ureter and renal pelvis: pathologic pitfalls. AJSP 33:1540–1546

48. Gittes RF (1984) Retrograde brushing and nephroscopy in the diagnosis of upper tract urothelial cancer. Urol Clin North Am 11:617–622

49. Havens MA, Cabay RJ, Mehrotra S, Kapur U, Wojcik EM, Barkan GA (2009) Upper genitourinary tract cytology: more sensitive than surgical biopsy? Cancer Cytopath 117:371

50. Coleman DV (1975) The cytodiagnosis of human polyoma virus infection. Acta Cytol 19:93–96

51. Kahan AV, Coleman DV, Koss LG (1980) Activation of human polyoma virus infection. Detection by cytologic techniques. Am J Clin Pathol 74:326–332

52. Koss LG, Sherman AB, Eppich E (1984) Image analysis and DNA content of urothelial cells infected with human polyoma virus. Anal Quant Cytol 6:89–94

53. Koss LG (1995) Cytologic manifestation of benign disorders affecting cells of the lower urinary tract. In: Koss LG (ed) Diagnostic cytology of the urinary tract: with histopathologic and clinical correlation, 1st edn. Lippincott Williams & Wilkins, Philadelphia, pp 52–55

54. Wojcik EM, Miller MC, Wright BC, Veltri RW, O'Dowd GJ (1997) Comparative analysis of DNA content in Polyoma Virus infected urothelial cells, urothelial dysplasia and transitional cell carcinoma. Anal Quant Cytol Histol 19:430–436

55. Highman W, Wilson E (1982) Urine cytology in patients with calculi. J Clin Pathol 35:350–356

56. Rubben H, Hering F, Dahm HH, Lutzeyer W (1982) Value of exfoliative urinary cytology for differentiation between uric acid stone and tumor of upper urinary tract. Urology 22:571–573

57. Betz SA, See WA, Cohen MB (1993) Granulomatous inflammation in bladder wash specimens after intravesical Bacillus Calmette-Guerin therapy for transitional cell carcinoma of the bladder. Am J Clin Pathol 99:244–248

58. Forni AM, Koss LG, Geller W (1964) Cytological study of the effect of cyclophosphamide in man. Cancer 17:1348–1355

59. Murphy WM, Soloway MS, Finebaum PJ (1981) Pathological changes associated with topical chemotherapy for superficial bladder cancer. J Urol 126:461–464

60. Solomon D, Nayar R, Davey D, Wilbur D, Kurman R (eds.) (2004) In the bethesda system for reporting cervical cytology: definitions, criteria, and explanatory notes, 2nd edn. Springer, New York, pp 1–188

61. Renshaw AA (2000) Subclassifying atypical urinary cytology specimens. Cancer 90:222–229

62. Kapur U, Venkataraman G, Wojcik EM (2008) Diagnostic significance of 'atypia' in instrumented versus voided urine specimens. Cancer 114:270–274

63. Raab SS, Grzybicki DM, Vrbin CM, Geisenger KR (2007) Urine cytology discrepancies. Am J Clin Pathol 127:946–953

64. Bhatia A, Dey P, Kakkar N, Srinivasan R, Nijhawan R (2006) Malignant atypical cell in urine cytology: a diagnostic dilemma. Cyto journal 3:28–33

65. Deshpande V, McKee GT (2005) Analysis of atypical urine cytology in a tertiary care center. Cancer 105:468–475

66. Palmer D, Lallu S, Matheson P, Bethwaite P, Tompson K (2007) Karyomegalic interstitial nephritis: a pitfall in urine cytology. Diagn Cytopathol 35:179–182
67. Epstein JI, Amin MB, Reuter VR, Mostofi FK et al. (1998) for the bladder consensus conference committee. The World Health Organization/International Society of urological pathology consensus classification of urothelial (transitional cell) neoplasms of the urinary bladder. Am J Surg Pathol 22:1435–1448
68. Badelment RA, Kimmoel M, Gay H, Cibas ES, Whitmore WF Jr, Herr HW, Fair WR, Melamed MR (1987) The sensitivity of flow cytometry compared with conventional cytology in the detection of superficial bladder carcinoma. Cancer 59:2078–2085
69. Danque PO, Chen HB, Patil J, Jagirdar J, Orsatti G, Paronetto F (1993) Image analysis versus flow cytometry for DNA ploidy quantitation of solid tumors: a comparison of six methods of sample preparation. Mod Pathol 6:270–275
70. Wojcik EM, Bassler TJ, Orozco R (1999) DNA ploidy of seminal vesicle cells. A potential diagnostic pitfall in urine cytology. Analyt Quant Cytol Histol 21:29–34
71. Bakhos R, Shankey TV, Fisher S, Flanigan RC, Wojcik EM (2000) Comparative analysis of DNA flow cytometry and cytology of urine barbotages—review of discordant cases. Diagn Cytopathol. 22: 65–69
72. Wojcik EM, Brownlie RJ, Bassler TJ, Miller MC (2000) Superficial urothelial cells (umbrella cells)—a potential cause of abnormal DNA ploidy results in urine specimens. Analyt Quant Cytol Histol 22:411–415
73. Hajdinjak T (2008) UroVysion FISH test for detecting urothelial cancers: meta-analysis of diagnostic accuracy and comparison with urinary cytology testing. Urol Oncol 26:646–651
74. van Rhijn BW, van der Poel HG, van der Kwast TH (2005) Urine markers for bladder cancer surveillance: a systematic review. Eur Urol 47:736–748
75. Fradet Y, Lockhart C (1997) The immunocyt trialists. Performance characteristics of a new monoclonal antibody test for bladder cancer. ImmunocytT M. Can J Urol 4:400–405
76. Tetu B (2009) Diagnosis of urothelial carcinoma. Urine Modern Pathol. 22:S53–S59
77. Melissourgos ND, Kastrinakis NG, Skolarikos A et al (2005) Cytokeratin-20 immunocytology in voided urine exhibits greater sensitivity and reliability than standard cytology in the diagnosis of transitional cell carcinoma of the bladder. Urology 66:536–541
78. Lokeshwar VB, Soloway MS (2001) Current bladder tumor tests: does their projected utility fulfill clinical necessity? J Urol 165:1067–1077
79. Grossman HB, Soloway M, Messing E et al (2006) Surveillance for recurrent bladder cancer using a point-of-care proteomic assay. JAMA 295:299–305
80. Serretta V, Pomara G, Rizzo I et al (2000) Urinary BTA-stat, BTA-trak and NMP22 in surveillance after TUR of recurrent superficial transitional cell carcinoma of the bladder. Eur Urol 38:419–425
81. Giannopoulos A, Manousakas T, Mitropoulos D et al (2000) Comparative evaluation of the BTAstat test, NMP22, and voided urine cytology in the detection of primary and recurrent bladder tumors. Urology 55:871–875
82. Shariat SF, Marberger MJ, Lotan Y et al (2006) Variability in the performance of nuclear matrix protein 22 for the detection of bladder cancer. J Urol 176:919–926
83. Lokeshwar VB, Habuchi T, Grossman HB et al (2005) Bladder tumor markers beyond cytology: International consensus panel on bladder tumor markers. Urology 66:35–63
84. Hautmann S, Toma M, Lorenzo GMF et al (2004) Immunocyt and the HA-HAase urine tests for the detection of bladder cancer: a side-by-side comparison. Eur Urol 46:466–471
85. Soloway MS (2008) Possible malignancy after cytology analysis in a 45-year old man. Curr Urol Rep 9:182–184
86. Frank I, Blute ML, Cheville JC, Lohse CM, Weaver AL, Zincke H (2003) Solid renal tumors: an analysis of pathological features related to tumor size. J Urol 170:2217

87. Gill IS, Matin SF, Desai MM, Kaouk JH, Steinberg A, Mascha E et al (2003) Comparative analysis of laparoscopic versus open partial nephrectomy for renal tumors in 200 patients. J Urol 170:64
88. Link RE, Bhayani SB, Allaf ME, Varkarakis I, Inagaki T, Rogers C (2005) Exploring the learning curve, pathological outcomes and perioperative morbidity of laparoscopic partial nephrectomy performed for renal mass. J Urol 173:1690
89. Kroft SH, Oyasu R (1994) Urinary bladder cancer: mechanisms of development and progression. Lab Invest 71:158–174
90. Soloway MS (1999) Editorial: Do we have a prostate specific antigen for bladder cancer? J Urol 161:447–448

Chapter 8
Body Cavity Fluids

Michael J. Thrall

8.1 Introduction

Body cavity fluid specimens come from the mesothelium-lined pleural, peritoneal, and pericardial cavities and have much in common with one another. These specimens can pose unique challenges for the cytologist. Although the specimens are relatively simple to obtain, diagnosis is often rendered difficult by the very abundance of material provided for analysis. Isolating and identifying small numbers of diagnostically critical cells in large volumes of fluid can prove difficult. The frequent presence of abundant inflammation or blood in these fluids compounds the problem. Furthermore, the properties of the cells that normally line serous cavities, the mesothelium, cause many interpretive dilemmas that extend beyond morphology into the realm of immunocytochemistry and other ancillary techniques. Most malignancies in these specimens are adenocarcinomas, but mesothelioma, melanoma, and lymphoid malignancies also occur. When malignancy can be confidently identified, determining the precise source of origin can be very difficult because of the tendency for all epithelioid processes to take on similar appearances when the cells are suspended in fluid. Immunocytochemistry can be extremely useful when determining the origin of the malignancy, but in many cases clinical history and radiological findings render ancillary testing unnecessary. The high clinical stakes involved in diagnoses of malignancy in these fluids also adds to the challenge. Positive body cavity fluids often signal end-stage disease progression and preclude some forms of treatment with curative intent. This fact makes cytologists particularly cautious in their handling of difficult cases to avoid false positive or false negative interpretations that may have a harmful impact on the patient.

M. J. Thrall (✉)
The Methodist Hospital, Houston, TX, USA
e-mail: MJThrall@tmhs.org

M. J. Thrall
Weill Cornell College of Medicine, New York, USA

R. Nayar (ed.), *Cytopathology in Oncology*,
Cancer Treatment and Research 160, DOI: 10.1007/978-3-642-38850-7_8,
© Springer-Verlag Berlin Heidelberg 2014

Although some cases remain challenging in everyday practice, common sources of error are well-known and can usually be avoided. Most cytologists see enough body cavity fluid specimens to become comfortable with the range of normal findings, wide though it is, and provide confident diagnoses in the majority of cases. This chapter will outline the methods used by cytologists to arrive at their diagnoses and explain the potential pitfalls and dilemmas that may create problems for pathologists and, consequently, other care-givers.

8.2 Preparation

8.2.1 Gross Appearance

Prior to any processing, the first task with any pathology specimen, including fluids, is gross examination. The volume, color, and transparency of the fluid are routinely noted and generally appear on final cytology reports. If the fluid is viscous or contains flecks or chunks this information should also be recorded. Odor may also contain some clues to the underlying process. The observations of the laboratory generally match those of the physicians responsible for collecting the specimen. Significant discrepancies between the reported description and the appearance at the time of removal from the patient should raise concern about a specimen misidentification. In general, fluids are very well preserved by refrigeration alone. Sterile collection containers, anticoagulant, and fixatives are not necessary. Indeed, fixatives may interfere with processing, staining, and interpretation of the findings.

The most common "abnormal" finding in body cavity fluid specimens is the presence of blood. Since the traumatic introduction of blood at the time of the extraction procedure is commonplace, a small amount of blood is probably best considered a normal finding. Large amounts of blood, however, may accompany malignant processes, though gross blood by itself has low sensitivity and specificity. The presence of macroscopically detectable pieces of tissue or debris is another gross finding that has been associated with malignancy. Cholesterol crystals may also give a similar gross appearance. A shimmering effect noted upon agitation of the sample may serve as a clue to the presence of crystals.

High viscosity may be seen in cases of pseudomyxoma peritonei. Indeed, the viscosity may be so high as to preclude effective sampling, or effective processing in the cytology laboratory. Inadvertent sampling from a mucinous tumor, such as an ovarian cystic neoplasm, rather than the peritoneum itself may give similar findings. Increased viscosity, though to a lesser degree, may be manifest in some mesothelioma cases in which large amounts of hyaluronic acid are produced by the tumor. Such effusions are often described as having the consistency of honey.

As a general rule, grossly purulent effusions are infectious in origin until proven otherwise. Malignancy may however occur in this setting. Brown-tinged fluid most often results from the presence of hemosiderin-laden macrophages and is indicative of prior bleeding into the space with partial digestion of the heme. Rarely, melanoma within body cavity fluids may produce enough pigment to be grossly visible. Chylous effusions often show a layering effect, with a creamy lipid layer forming at the surface if given time to settle.

8.2.2 Preparatory Techniques

Body cavity fluid specimens are very well preserved by refrigeration at 4 °C, and therefore they can sit overnight or over the weekend with essentially no loss of quality for diagnostic purposes [1]. The fundamental problem in processing body cavity fluids is the separation of the cells of interest from the large volumes of fluid in which they are dispersed. Most laboratories concentrate the cells by use of a machine that spins the sample. One common method uses a cytocentrifuge designed to simultaneously concentrate the cells and distribute them onto a slide. Alternatively, wire-loop cell collection from a cell pellet, followed by smearing on a slide, may be employed. For markedly hypocellular specimens the fluid may be spun through a filter that is stained and directly analyzed. Over the last 15 years the use of liquid-based thin-layer Papanicolaou-stained preparations, for body cavity fluids has gone from experimental to mainstream. Thin-layer preparations yield comparable or higher sensitivity than conventional processing while being simultaneously easier to examine [2–5]. Large-scale interlaboratory comparisons of diagnostic performance on thin-layer body fluid specimens indicate that they perform at least as well as other preparation types [6].

Body cavity fluids typically make good cell blocks, especially in cases where malignancy is suspected, because the specimens are highly cellular with abundant residual material. Cell blocks are useful either to look for additional examples of rare atypical cells or to facilitate immunocytochemical testing. Due to the high cellularity, flow cytometry can often be performed easily on these specimens as well.

8.3 Normal Body Cavity Fluids

8.3.1 Anatomy and Physiology

There are three major serous cavities: pleural, pericardial, and peritoneal. An outpouching of the peritoneal cavity also forms the tunica vaginalis in males, but this structure is of minimal importance in cytology. All of these cavities are lined by mesothelial cells whose primary function is to secrete lubricating serous fluids that allow the organs within each cavity to glide smoothly over the cavity walls or, in the case of the peritoneum, each other. Under normal circumstances these cavities contain only minimal fluid and few cells.

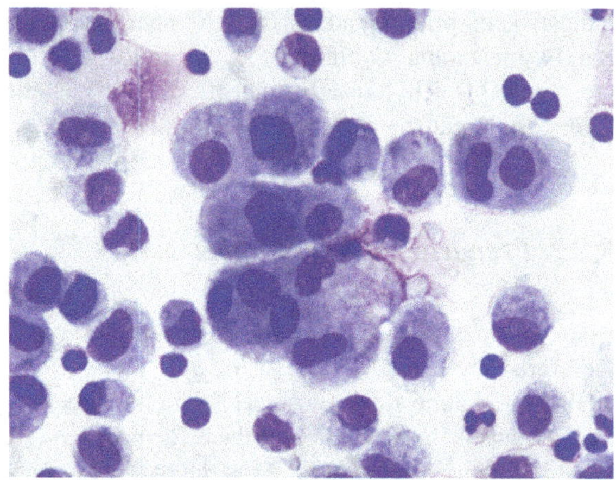

Fig. 8.1 Benign mesothelial cells. The nuclei are centrally located and surrounded by vacuolated cytoplasm. Note the presence of windows between cells and skirts on the outer edges of the cells. There is also binucleation, nuclear enlargement, and nuclear contour irregularity present in an inflammatory background, showing some of the reactive changes often seen in these specimens. (DiffQuik stain, 600× magnification.)

Clinically, increased volumes of fluids are much more readily apparent than hypercellularity in disease states. The important distinction between transudative effusions and exudative effusions can be made on the basis of chemical tests. Indeed, this testing is often the primary driver of fluid collection for analysis. Many times fluid is also removed for symptom relief. In such situations cytology is often just an "add on" test ordered for the sake of completeness. Transudative effusions are usually hypocellular. Exudative effusions commonly contain inflammatory cells but malignancy is only occasionally found in the setting of low clinical suspicion. Generally speaking, these scenarios account for most body cavity fluid specimens in cytology laboratories and lead to few diagnostic problems.

8.3.2 Benign Cells

8.3.2.1 Mesothelial Cells

The most important normal cells present in body cavity fluids are, of course, mesothelial cells (Fig. 8.1). Mesothelium is a specialized type of epithelium derived from mesoderm that exists only along the linings of the serous cavities. It is similar in many ways to other epithelial types, not only in terms of appearance under the microscope but also at the ultrastructural and molecular levels. It is important to keep in mind the fundamental kinship of these cells to understand why they so frequently cause problems for pathologists.

Mesothelial cells differ from typical epithelial cells in that they have numerous very long microvilli. This feature creates diagnostically helpful findings, in the form of gaps between cells ("windows") or attenuated cytoplasm at the edges of cells ("skirts") that can be used by cytologists to confidently identify mesothelial cells in many instances.

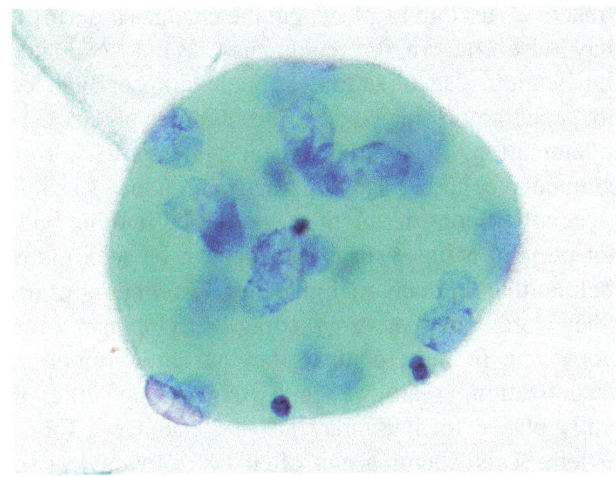

Fig. 8.2 Collagen ball. The cells surround a homogeneous round ball of collagen, with the nuclei seen only on the edge of the structure when examined on high power. The surrounding mesothelial cells are bland with small nuclei that lack atypia or prominent nucleoli. Comparison with Fig. 8.5 shows why these structures might cause confusion with adenocarcinoma at low power. (Papanicolaou stain, 600× magnification.)

Mesothelial cells have additional cellular features that are useful in identifying them. The nuclei are generally centrally placed within the cell, round, and contain noticeable nucleoli. The cytoplasm takes on the appearance of "ground glass" or may be foamy due to many small vacuoles. Individual cell contours tend to be round in tapped fluids. Cells in washings often have a more scale-like squamoid appearance.

At low power, mesothelial cells form up into a number of different patterns. Spontaneously shed cells in effusion specimens are usually present as a mixture of rounded cell clusters of various sizes, chains, and individual cells. This spectrum is reassuring, especially if the nuclei are uniform and bland. The groups are said to resemble florets, due to the tendency for cells on the edge to bulge from the surface like flowers in a bouquet.

In washings, honeycomb sheets are often identified in addition to or instead of spheroid clusters. This reflects the physics of cells in fluids. Cells of any type will tend to round up over time because this is the least energetic conformation due to the minimization of the surface area exposed to charged water molecules. Cell groups in washing specimens often do not have sufficient time to undergo this transformation.

In some instances mesothelial cells may be found in association with a central core of homogenous material, forming a three-dimensional structure known as a collagen ball (Fig. 8.2). These represent fragments of mesothelium still associated with underlying stroma, perhaps due to forceful removal by washing or the detachment of a small papillary tuft with an intact core. Their primary importance lies in the fact that they may mimic malignancy by creating large structures that stand out from the background. The presence of small bland cells around the outside of the ball, in combination with an acellular center, usually dispels concern.

Mesothelial "atypia" is an extremely common problem. Generally the report is worded in such a way as to avoid the loaded term "atypia", often with the word "reactive" used in its place, but the changes are truly atypical in the sense that they may raise concern for malignancy. Whole cell and nuclear enlargement, multinucleation, vacuolization, frequent mitoses, and cell-in-cell configurations are not uncommon in benign mesothelial processes, especially in response to inflammation. These often appear against a backdrop of high cellularity that may compound concern. Such findings may induce suspicion of a more serious process, especially if considering the criteria used in other body sites where mesothelium is not present. Mitoses, in particular, can be seen more frequently in benign mesothelium than in many malignancies. The finding of one cell "hugging" another, in other words completely wrapping its cytoplasm around its neighbor, is also very worrisome in most contexts but has little import in these specimens. Marked vacuolization, creating a single "signet ring"-like central vacuole with a peripherally placed nucleus, may also raise concern for a single-cell adenocarcinoma pattern. This dilemma can often be resolved by comparing the other cytologic features of the "signet ring" cell with adjacent mesothelium. Furthermore, the nucleus is rarely as atypical, or as deeply or irregularly indented by the vacuole, as what is seen in adenocarcinoma.

When analyzing body cavity fluid specimens, the wide range of "normality" in mesothelial cells must be kept in mind. Even in surgical pathology specimens markedly reactive mesothelium cannot be reliably separated from malignancy in the absence of frank invasion [7]. Only with experience can cytologists develop some sense for the full range of "reactive" mesothelial changes that may accompany inflammation or radiation exposure [8].

8.3.2.2 Blood Elements

Blood and blood elements are almost always present in effusion specimens received by laboratories, either due to trauma from the acquisition procedure or the true presence of those cells in the cavity. Red cells are easily recognized as benign but may cause diagnostic difficulty by obscuring other more significant cell types. For this reason, laboratories routinely use techniques designed to lyse red cells so as to remove them from the visual field.

Nucleated cells of hematopoietic origin are always present in body cavity fluid specimens, and are usually of little or no clinical significance, but occasionally may be a key to diagnosis, especially if they are numerous. Some of the most important clinical associations for the different cell types have been listed in Table 8.1.

Lymphocytes are frequently identified in body cavity fluid specimens, but usually have little or no diagnostic importance. Small numbers of such lymphocytes may be physiologic and are usually not mentioned in cytology reports. Differentiating normal B cells from normal T cells is difficult or impossible in these specimens without ancillary studies. For the most part, reactive lymphocytes in effusions are of predominantly T cell lineage, but this is rarely confirmed in clinical practice unless lymphoma is suspected. The term "chronic inflammation"

Table 8.1 The potential implications of the presence of increased numbers of hematopoietic cells in body cavity fluid specimens

Cell type	Major associations
Lymphocytes	Long-standing effusions
	Lymphoma
	Response to solid malignancies
	Tuberculosis
Neutrophils	Bacterial infection
	Infarction of intracavity organs
	Malignancy
	Collagen vascular disease
Eosinophils	Idiopathic
	Air in the body cavity
	Hypersensitivity
	Parasites
	Pulmonary infarct or pneumonia
	Malignancy

may be used in cytology reports for body cavity fluids. Generally, this merely means that significant numbers of benign-appearing lymphocytes are present with no further clinical implications. Cytologists worried about a specific infection or a malignant process should use more definitive terminology.

Neutrophils are also frequently identified in effusion specimens. A true increase in neutrophils in body cavity fluids is indicative of an acute inflammatory process. Cases with abundant neutrophils generally correspond to grossly evident pus and often the diagnosis is already known or suspected clinically. However, the presence of only occasional neutrophils is more difficult to interpret because it may be an artifact of blood contamination. If the red cells have been lysed away, a frequent occurrence, differentiating true inflammation from an incidental finding can be difficult because a comparison of the ratio of neutrophils to red cells is not possible. Many cytologists prefer to report the presence of neutrophils whenever present because it may provide a clue to the presence of spontaneous bacterial peritonitis or some other treatable acute infectious process that might otherwise go undetected. The use of the term "acute inflammation" on a cytology report should be taken to mean that significant numbers of neutrophils are present in the specimen and that the treating physician should be alert to the possibility of bacterial infection of the space. A special type of neutrophil seen in the setting of systemic lupus erythematosus is the so-called "LE cell", which contains homogenized partially degraded nuclear material within a large cytoplasmic vacuole, presumably reflecting phagocytosis of the material (Fig. 8.3).

Eosinophils are not commonly seen in substantial numbers in body cavity fluids, and are outright rare in the peritoneum and pericardium. The cells are easily recognized, when present, by their bilobed nuclei and prominent eosinophilic granules. Trauma/bleeding is the most common cause of eosinophilic effusions. Eosinophilic effusions only occasionally correspond to hypersensitivity or parasitic infections. In many cases no identifiable cause is found. Occasionally, there may

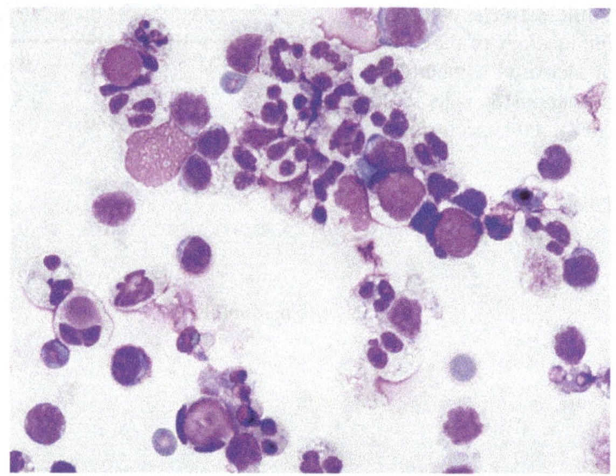

Fig. 8.3 LE cells. Here several "LE cells" can be seen, neutrophils can be seen that contain homogenized engulfed nuclear material within vacuoles. There is an inflammatory background consistent with the history of systemic lupus erythematosus. (DiffQuik stain, 600× magnification.)

be an underlying malignancy [9]. Basophils and mast cells may also be found in effusion specimens but usually make up a minor population and have no diagnostic significance.

Histiocytes, also known as macrophages, often appear in effusion specimens. These cells typically have abundant foamy or lacy cytoplasm and so-called "bean shaped" off-center nuclei. They are not always morphologically distinctive and confusion with benign mesothelial cells or malignancy can occur. The presence of large clear vacuoles or engulfed cells may suggest the possibility of adenocarcinoma. Their presence is not typically reported unless they are very numerous. The finding of histiocytes, in and of itself, has little diagnostic specificity unless they take on elongated and giant forms and are associated with necrotic debris, in which case they are strongly suggestive or even diagnostic of rheumatoid arthritis.

8.3.2.3 Psammoma Bodies

Psammoma bodies are lamellated round calcifications formed from papillary cellular structures. Most psammoma bodies seen in body cavity fluids are found in the context of serous carcinoma. Typically, the malignancy is obvious and psammomatous calcifications are noted as an interesting background phenomenon, often with a ring of obviously malignant viable cells surrounding them. Isolated psammoma bodies, however, create a diagnostic dilemma. In all likelihood, rare psammoma bodies not associated with malignant cells derive from benign processes, but in the context of high clinical suspicion complete dismissal of the finding may not be possible. Reporting of the presence of psammoma bodies without an outright diagnosis of malignancy, therefore, represents an equivocal diagnosis.

8.4 Malignancy in Body Cavity Fluids

8.4.1 Mesothelioma

Mesothelioma attracts interest out of proportion to its frequency due to its unusual risk associations and the socio-legal implications that follow this diagnosis. The link between this disease and prior asbestos exposure, particularly to amphibole subtypes, has made this one of the most feared occupational exposure-related diseases. The grim prognosis of the disease compounds the anxiety of those potentially exposed to asbestos fibers and contributes to the large legal settlements that victims and their families often lay claim to following diagnosis. Asbestos is a mineral that occurs in nature and is, in some areas, a not uncommon component of the rock. The use of asbestos by various industries led to a spike in mesothelioma cases some decades after its introduction, but many countries have now banned it for commercial use since its attendant risks are widely known. Unfortunately, history-taking almost always reveals some possible asbestos exposure, limiting the usefulness of that information. Analysis of body cavity fluids for asbestos bodies has a very low yield.

The diagnosis of mesothelioma by cytology is a daunting challenge. As has been noted, the range of reactive changes in benign mesothelial cells extends very broadly. This means that most "atypia" seen in mesothelial cells or clusters will not represent malignancy. Furthermore, mesothelioma may be extremely bland cytologically, making diagnosis difficult even in extensive surgical pathology specimens. As a general rule, mesothelioma recapitulates the appearance of normal mesothelium with central round nuclei, vacuolated cytoplasm, the presence of windows and skirts, and clusters with a knobby contour. Some features are suggestive of malignant mesothelium in cytology preparations: cellularity and cell size. It has been stated that mesothelioma is best separated from reactive mesothelial cells in body cavity fluids by the presence of "more and bigger cells in more and bigger clusters" (Fig. 8.4). This rule of thumb certainly applies, but suggests the vagaries involved in reaching this diagnosis. Attempts to create objective standards for cell cluster size have not proven successful, since sufficiently stringency to exclude benign changes reduces the sensitivity to a very low level. Cell size evaluation is also subjective. Uniform marked enlargement of mesothelial cells with concomitant nuclear enlargement, chromatin clumping, and prominent nucleoli is suggestive of malignancy. However, cells with these features are not uncommon in benign cases, and drawing a sharp line between positive and negative cannot be reliably done.

Ancillary studies are of no value in distinguishing benign from malignant mesothelium. Electron microscopy shows the same characteristic long cilia that are seen in normal mesothelium. Immunocytochemistry also shows the same patterns of staining in both mesothelioma and benign mesothelium. Molecular studies may in the future find characteristic markers that could distinguish malignant or premalignant processes.

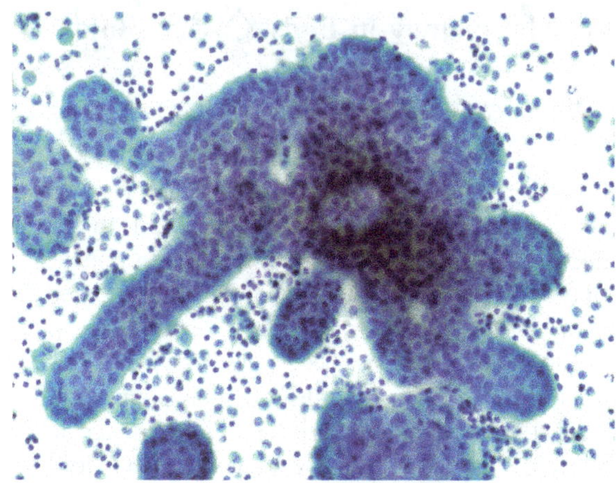

Fig. 8.4 Mesothelioma. There is an enormous and complex cell cluster with large cells as demonstrated by comparison with background inflammatory cells. Individual atypical mesothelial cells can also be seen nearby. Nucleoli and clumpy chromatin can be discerned in many of the cells, even at this power. (Papanicolaou stain, 200× magnification.)

Many cytologists believe that a primary diagnosis of mesothelioma should not be made in body cavity fluid specimens. It should be noted that there are those who do not accept this position [10, 11]. However, the Mesothelioma Reference Panel group has recently recommended that mesothelioma should not be diagnosed unless unequivocal invasive malignancy can be demonstrated on surgical pathology material [7]. As a result, cases where mesothelioma is highly suspected in body cavity fluid cytology are frequently interpreted as "atypical mesothelial proliferation", often with an accompanying comment suggesting additional correlation or follow-up. In patients with an established diagnosis of mesothelioma on surgical pathology material, most cytologists would feel comfortable rendering an outright diagnosis if the findings were compatible.

Even when a diagnosis of mesothelioma has been established, it may not be possible to diagnose persistent or recurrent disease from fluid alone. Many mesotheliomas are predominantly or entirely composed of spindled cells, resembling sarcoma rather than adenocarcinoma. Such tumors virtually never shed diagnostic cells into body cavity fluids.

8.4.2 Other Malignancies

Most effusions containing malignant cells do not derive from the relatively rare mesotheliomas that are primary to the body cavities. Rather, positive body cavity fluids almost always represent involvement of body cavities by malignancy derived from other types of epithelium with secondary spread. Occasionally, nonepithelial malignancies may also appear in fluids: lymphoma/leukemia, melanoma, and sarcomas. Differentiating these various types of malignant process from benign fluids, and from each other, constitutes the primary challenge of cytological body cavity fluid interpretation. Knowledge of patterns of spread can aid in the diagnosis of malignancy in any area of pathology. The different compartments of the thorax have unique patterns of involvement by tumor type. Gender and age are also key considerations.

Malignant effusions are rare in pediatric populations. Body cavity fluid cytology specimens are correspondingly unusual. Most malignancies that are found will be hematologic, especially leukemias [12]. Pediatric solid tumors, including neuroblastoma, Wilms tumor, and others may rarely appear in peritoneal fluid. The diagnosis of such tumors would be a once-in-a-lifetime event for most cytologists.

The frequency of malignancy involving effusions rises through adulthood in accord with the increasing incidence of carcinomas, which make up the predominant causes of positive body cavity fluid specimens in both genders. Among younger adults, melanoma, breast cancer, and gastric cancer are relatively more likely due to the epidemiology of those malignancies.

Older adults, who are the source of most of the positive specimens, have well-defined risks by site (Table 8.2). Peritoneal fluids much more commonly harbor malignancies in women, among whom serous ovarian/primary peritoneal carcinomas and breast carcinomas predominate. Gastrointestinal primaries also involve peritoneal fluid not uncommonly in both genders and are the most important consideration in men. Gastric carcinomas have an especially marked tendency to cause malignant effusions, whereas colon cancer only rarely involves peritoneal fluid. Despite the fact that most hepatocellular carcinoma arises in the setting of cirrhosis, and is therefore associated with ascites, the tumor virtually never enters into the fluid. Attempts to diagnose hepatocellular carcinoma in ascites fluid have a very low yield [13].

In pleural fluid, lung cancer predominates in both genders. Adenocarcinomas make up the vast majority of these, due to their tendency to arise peripherally in the lung and their proclivity to grow through and along the parietal pleura. Squamous and small cell lung carcinomas involve pleural fluid more rarely. Among women, metastatic breast cancer is the most common malignancy in pleural fluid after lung.

Pericardial fluid malignancies are essentially always from distant sites. Lung adenocarcinoma, due to its high frequency and proximity, is the most frequently discovered type. In women, breast carcinoma predominates. Melanoma also has a proclivity to appear in this location.

Of course, more detailed clinical and radiological history provided with the request for examination, or obtained through a careful review of the history at the time of analysis, often provides more precise information that can be of the utmost usefulness. In most instances, malignancy can be suspected prior to submission of the specimen to cytology [14, 15]. History is also extremely useful when dealing with a malignant process that is not "following the rules" such as breast cancer in a male or lung adenocarcinoma in a 25-year old. In such instances, a lack of clinical correlation can lead to serious mistakes. It is the responsibility of the requestors of the test, as well as the pathologists, to make sure that patient history is known in sufficient detail before a final interpretation is rendered. In many instances cytologists struggle to try to interpret a difficult case, perhaps with the

Table 8.2 The most frequently seen malignancies, by gender, in each of the body cavities

Cavity	Females	Males
Peritoneal	Gynecologic tract	Gastrointestinal tract
	Breast	Lung
	Gastrointestinal tract	Lymphoma
	Lung	Melanoma
	Lymphoma	Renal
	Melanoma	Urothelial
	Renal	
Pleural	Lung	Lung
	Breast	Gastrointestinal tract
	Gynecologic tract	Lymphoma
	Gastrointestinal tract	Melanoma
	Lymphoma	
	Melanoma	
Pericardial	Breast	Lung
	Lung	Melanoma
	Melanoma	

aid of expensive and delay-causing tests, only to find out later that the primary care-givers already knew something that would have instantly resolved the difficulty. Electronic medical records and universal access to radiological images via computer have tremendously reduced this problem, but the key remains good communication between pathologists and the rest of the patient care team.

8.4.2.1 Adenocarcinoma

The most frequent malignancies identified in body cavity fluids are adenocarcinomas (Fig. 8.5). They arise from many different body sites, but, insofar as they are all malignant epithelial tumors with glandular differentiation, they have a great deal in common. Indeed, they often resemble one another so much as to make distinguishing them impossible by morphology alone. Adenocarcinomas stand out from background mesothelial cells found in body cavity fluids in two ways: changes related to malignancy and changes related to origin from glandular epithelium. Neither of these is entirely reliable, but when both are present a diagnosis of adenocarcinoma can usually be made with confidence, especially with corroborating history and radiology. A fundamental rule of body cavity cytology is to look for a "two-cell population". This maxim refers to the dimorphic character of body cavity fluid specimens with the most common manifestation of adenocarcinoma: large clusters of obviously malignant cells, with distinctive cytologic features, that stand out from the adjacent normal mesothelial cells.

Adenocarcinomas show a number of cytomorphologic patterns. The nuclei show enlargement with correspondingly large nucleoli. The chromatin becomes clumpy and the nuclear membranes develop grooves and other contour

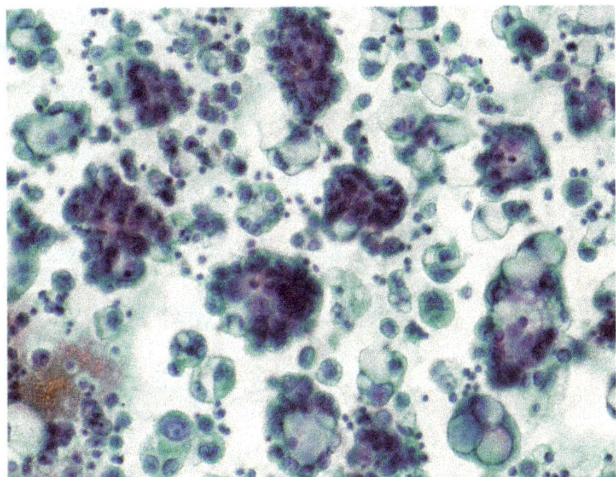

Fig. 8.5 Lung adenocarcinoma. This is a relatively straightforward example of adenocarcinoma that is predominantly composed of obviously malignant cells containing prominent mucin vacuoles and forming large gland-like structures. Comparison with Fig. 8.4 shows some of the similarities between adenocarcinoma and mesothelioma that may cause a diagnostic dilemma: high cellularity, large irregular clusters, atypical nuclei, and prominent nucleoli. (Papanicolaou stain, 400× magnification)

irregularities; however, these features are relatively nonspecific, being common in other malignancies also. This makes sense, because all of these features result from rapid and disordered cell growth and division, common events in all malignant processes. Individual cells typically produce mucin in adenocarcinomas. This may manifest as either a foamy cytoplasm with many small vacuoles or a so-called "signet ring" appearance caused by the presence of a single large vacuole that pushes the nucleus off to one side (Fig. 8.6). Unfortunately, mesothelial cells, whether benign or malignant, also frequently have foamy cytoplasm and may form signet ring-like structures with a large central vacuole. The irregularity and sharp edges of the nuclei in true signet rings of adenocarcinoma may help in distinguishing them from mesothelial imitators, but this may be difficult if only a few such cells are present. In adenocarcinomas, nuclei tend to be off-center even in cells without a dominant vacuole, which also may help in differentiating such cells from mesothelium, which tends to maintain a centrally located nucleus.

Another feature of glands often recapitulated in body fluids is the formation of acinar structures. In fluid cytology, this manifests as a tendency for cells to cling to one another in a tight spherical cluster with a sharp outer border. The presence of many such groups is often the first indication of malignancy in body cavity fluid specimens. In distinguishing adenocarcinoma from mesothelioma, in particular, the presence of smooth outer borders of clusters, as opposed to the "florets" typical of mesothelioma, can be a vital clue. However, as with essentially every other morphologic feature, the finding is not entirely reliable.

Fig. 8.6 Breast
adenocarcinoma with signet
ring morphology. This
adenocarcinoma is composed
of individual malignant cells
rather than clusters. The cells
show a signet ring
configuration with the
nucleus displaced to one side
and indented by mucin
vacuoles. This specimen also
has prominent nuclear
pleomorphism and atypia.
(Papanicolaou stain, 600×
magnification.)

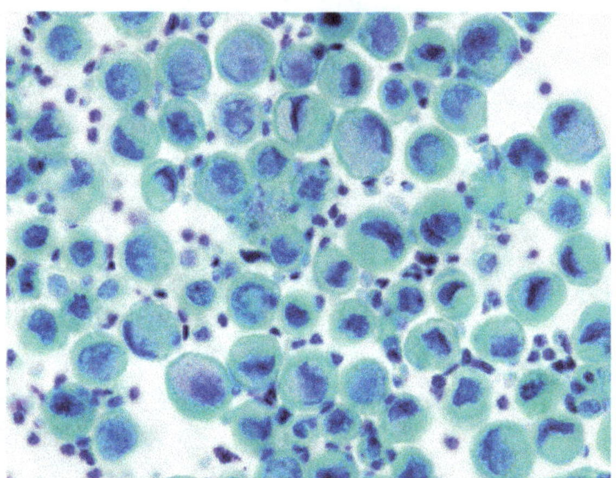

Most adenocarcinomas have overlapping features by cytology. Certain findings discussed below may increase suspicion for one particular type over another, but pathognomonic morphologic findings are rare. Generally, the distinction is not important. The primary tumor is often already known or suspected on the basis of radiological findings or previous biopsy or excision.

Adenocarcinoma of the lung is by far the most common malignancy in pleural fluid and among the most frequent in pericardial and peritoneal fluids as well. Because of the nonspecific cytologic appearance of lung adenocarcinoma, differentiation from reactive mesothelial cells or mesothelioma often requires ancillary techniques. The most common peritoneal adenocarcinoma, serous carcinoma, can also be difficult to differentiate from mesothelioma due to the similarity of its papillary structures to mesothelial proliferations. Differentiating primary peritoneal carcinomas from ovarian or uterine primaries cannot be done by cytology alone. Breast carcinoma, whether manifesting as a signet ring morphology or as more typical clusters of cells, may also pose diagnostic difficulties. One scenario of special concern is in women harboring BRCA mutations, who are prone to both serous and breast carcinomas.

Adenocarcinomas presenting in fluids as single cells, whether showing clear signet ring morphology or not, pose special problems and deserve special attention [16]. These malignancies are as much a pitfall in body cavity fluid cytology as in fine needle aspiration or surgical pathology. The cells tend to be uniform, bland, and infrequent. Even when they are very numerous, their similarity to normal mesothelial cells leads to an absence of the "two-cell population" appearance typical of most adenocarcinomas. Indeed, many such cases appear benign or even normal at low power. Only careful investigation of the cells, often prompted by history, will lead to the correct diagnosis. The danger of false negative body fluid cytology results is high for these specimens, especially when suspicion is low.

8.4.2.2 Other Epithelioid Malignancies

Lung carcinomas other than adenocarcinoma occasionally appear in pleural and, even more rarely, peritoneal or pericardial fluid specimens. Small cell carcinoma, when it does manifest in body cavity fluids, has a distinctive appearance. As the name suggests, the cells are relatively small, composed almost entirely of nucleus, with neuroendocrine features including coarse "salt and pepper" chromatin and inconspicuous or absent nucleoli. The cells are often noted first because they form into characteristic cell rows with nuclear molding, referred to variously as "vertebral columns" or "stacks of coins". When such structures are absent, however, small cell carcinoma may be extremely difficult to detect, especially if carcinoma cells are few or similarly appearing lymphocytes are numerous. Neither scenario is uncommon. Other neuroendocrine carcinomas, including carcinoid tumors, atypical carcinoids, and large cell neuroendocrine tumors may also rarely appear in fluid specimens.

Squamous cell carcinoma also has a distinctive appearance that usually allows for relatively easy identification. The cells typically have a "hard" cytoplasm caused by the accumulation of dense keratins in accordance with the differentiation of the tumor. The cytoplasm takes on a distinctive orange coloration in Papanicolaou stains that can be readily recognized by cytologists, most of whom spend a great deal of time looking for similar cells in cervicovaginal specimens. The presence of "tadpoles" and other bizarre forms caused by keratinization is as diagnostic in body cavity fluids as elsewhere. Unfortunately, not all squamous cell carcinomas announce themselves so clearly. Poorly differentiated examples may be difficult to distinguish from adenocarcinoma, reactive or malignant mesothelium, or other malignancies.

Both squamous cell and neuroendocrine carcinomas may arise in other sites, though even less commonly. This fact needs to be kept in mind when such tumors appear in the absence of a detectable lung mass. Continued searching generally yields a different primary site without too much difficulty. Urothelial carcinomas, in particular, should be kept in mind when squamous or squamous-like cells appear in peritoneal fluid.

Renal cell carcinomas are another unusual tumor type in fluids with a potentially distinctive morphology. Conventional renal cell carcinoma often has a clear cell appearance that can be identified in body cavity fluids. Such cells contain numerous small cytoplasmic vacuoles and often have unusually prominent red nucleoli.

Although not of epithelial derivation, melanoma must always be kept in the differential for epithelioid tumors. Known for their mimicry, melanoma cells can take on a number of appearances. Although formation of large cohesive clusters is very unusual for melanoma, it can imitate just about any other manifestation of epithelial malignancies in body cavity fluids. Occasionally, distinctive features may be present that aid diagnosis. The presence of melanin pigment is pathognomonic but quite unusual. The presence of "double mirror-image nuclei" may also help distinguish melanoma when they are present. Such cells contain paired, prominent nuclei with large red nucleoli, which often bulge the outer nuclear membrane. Prior knowledge of a patient history of melanoma may increase the likelihood of noticing these features, but melanoma is also known for arising in obscure or long-forgotten sites. For these reasons pathologists must constantly remind themselves of the possibility of melanoma.

8.4.3 *Immunocytochemistry for Epithelial Malignancies*

8.4.3.1 Immunocytochemistry in Body Cavity Fluid Specimens

For the most part, immunocytochemistry for body cavity fluid specimens is similar in principle and practice to what is done for other cytology specimen types. Most laboratories attempt to make a cell block from residual fluid for staining. Body cavity fluids are generally very cellular, especially in malignant cases, facilitating the use of this technique. However, there are some cases with low cellularity or limited material that may require other methods. Many laboratories that have a large volume of cytology specimens are proficient in immunostaining thin-layer liquid preparations such as ThinPrep and/or direct smears. Older techniques such as electron microscopy have been almost entirely replaced by immunocytochemistry. Special stains not based on antibody binding continue to have a limited role. In particular, mucicarmine stain is often used to detect mucin production in adenocarcinomas as a part of a broader work-up.

8.4.3.2 Mesothelioma Versus Lung Adenocarcinoma

The predominant differential diagnostic consideration in malignant pleural fluids is the separation of adenocarcinoma of the lung from mesothelioma. This differential is especially difficult because the two tumors resemble one another not only morphologically but also have similar clinical history and radiological findings.

There is consensus that multiple markers for mesothelioma and for adenocarcinoma should always be used because every marker has significant false negative rates and many are also prone to false positives. Expert panels on the diagnosis of mesothelioma have pointedly declined to recommend any particular panel [17]. This is because different laboratories have different degrees of experience and success with the various markers. The belief is that the best results are obtained when pathologists have the freedom to choose a panel tailored to their own laboratories. A great many different markers have been reported to be useful in differentiating mesothelial cells from adenocarcinoma (Table 8.3) [18].

Table 8.3 Immunocytochemical markers used for differentiating mesothelioma from adenocarcinoma, with the most commonly used markers listed nearer to the top

Mesothelioma	Adenocarcinoma
D2-40	MOC-31
Calretinin	Ber-EP4
WT-1	B72.3
Cytokeratin 5/6	CEA
Podoplanin	Leu-M1 (CD 15)
Mesothelin	EMA
HBME-1	E-cadherin
Thrombomodulin	BG-8 (Lewis y)
HMW Cytokeratin	CA 19-9
N-cadherin	
Vimentin	

8.4.3.3 Immunocytochemical Markers for Other Carcinomas Frequently Encountered in Body Cavity Fluid Specimens

For the most part, carcinomas of other types can be more easily differentiated from mesothelioma on clinical and radiological grounds. In some instances a distinctive cytological appearance may also make mesothelioma unlikely. Immunocytochemistry is still useful, however, for those occasional cases where mesothelioma remains in the differential and, more commonly, when carcinoma can be confidently diagnosed but the site of origin remains ambiguous.

For the differentiation of serous carcinoma from mesothelioma, many of the same markers used in the panel for lung adenocarcinoma can be used with similar effectiveness. Important alterations include the replacement of the lung marker TTF-1 with the gynecologic marker PAX-8 and the exclusion of WT-1, which is typically positive in both entities.

Many other tumor types have characteristic markers that can be tested for by immunocytochemistry (Table 8.4). Adenocarcinomas arising from the breast and pancreas pose special problems for immunocytochemistry. Breast prognostic markers can be performed in cytology specimens but have poor sensitivity and specificity for breast origin. Although specific breast markers are available, they are frequently negative and therefore only have value when they stain the cells of interest. No good markers exist for pancreatic adenocarcinomas. Therefore this diagnosis is frequently impossible to make in fluid cytology, though it may be suggested by a lack of staining with specific markers for other frequent carcinomas with a similar appearance.

Squamous cell carcinomas have a less pronounced tendency to involve body cavity fluids than adenocarcinomas. When keratinization can be detected cytologically, the diagnosis poses few problems. However, squamous cell carcinomas involving fluids often are poorly differentiated and may be difficult to recognize by morphology alone. Differentiating squamous cell carcinomas arising from different sites of origin is an essentially impossible task using immunomarkers.

Table 8.4 Commonly used immunocytochemical markers with specificity for particular carcinoma types

Immunomarker	Target Tumor Type(s)	Caveat
BRST-2	Breast	Poor sensitivity
CA-125	Gynecologic	Poor specificity
CDX-2	Gastrointestinal	Poor sensitivity except for colon
Cytokeratin 5/6	Squamous	Also positive in mesothelioma
Estrogen receptor	Breast	Poor sensitivity and specificity
Mammaglobin	Breast	Poor sensitivity
p63	Squamous	Breast carcinomas may be positive
PAX-8	Gynecologic, renal, thyroid	A new marker with limited availability
TTF-1	Lung, thyroid	Negative in squamous lung carcinomas
WT-1	Gynecologic	Also positive in mesothelioma

As a general rule, a good clinical history and knowledge of radiological findings is often much more useful than a panel of immunocytochemical markers for differentiating these different types of adenocarcinoma. Many expensive, time-consuming, and nonconclusive work-ups are performed by pathologists needlessly because of poor communication between patent care-givers. It is the responsibility of all parties to try to avoid this outcome. In most cases, a cytological diagnosis of adenocarcinoma, without any further specification, is entirely sufficient for the purposes of patient care.

8.4.3.4 Immunocytochemistry for Melanoma

Melanoma is frequently considered in the differential diagnosis for malignant epithelioid cells, especially if they are poorly differentiated, dyscohesive, and no site of origin is readily identified. Immunocytochemistry can be extremely useful for ruling out melanoma in body cavity fluids because there are several markers that will almost never stain anything else seen in these specimens: S-100, melan-A (MART-1), HMB-45, and tyrosinase. The less-than-perfect sensitivity of these markers may require the use of several of them, but, in general, they can be used to confidently identify melanoma in most instances.

8.4.3.5 Hematopoietic Malignancies

In hematopoietic malignancies, positive fluid cytology usually represents a late finding. Typically, the cytologist only needs to confirm or refute the presence of malignancy that has already been diagnosed previously. As with carcinoma, however, this may be a more difficult task that it would seem. Lymphomas often cause serous effusions even when malignant cells are not present in the fluid or are present only in minute amounts [19]. Fortunately, flow cytometry provides a very useful tool that enables the confident separation of benign from malignant processes. Body cavity fluid specimens generally work well for flow cytometry and in most cases there is abundant material left for further analysis following the preparation of cytology slides. Flow cytometry is somewhat similar in principle to immunocytochemistry in that it uses antibody binding to determine expression patterns for panels of markers of differential diagnostic usefulness. The small size and dyscohesive nature of lymphocytes, however, makes possible the more sophisticated techniques of flow cytometric analysis that enable much larger panels to be performed on relatively small volumes of material.

8.4.3.6 Small Cell Lymphomas

Lymphomas composed entirely or predominantly of small cells are especially difficult to diagnose in body cavity fluids. The reactive T-lymphocytes characteristically seen in all effusions have nuclear features very similar to those of many lymphomas. Indeed, in the majority of cases of small cell lymphomas the distinction cannot be made with absolute confidence, even if a history of lymphoma is known. One distinctive feature that may offer a clue in cases of small lymphocytic lymphoma is distinct clumping of the chromatin referred to as "cellules grumelees" or "clotted cells". If this finding is present in numerous, monomorphic lymphocytic nuclei, the diagnosis can be strongly suspected. Flow cytometric confirmation would nonetheless be employed in most instances, however. In general, flow cytometry is a useful adjunct whenever a small cell lymphoma is suspected because it considerably improves the sensitivity for diagnosis in these specimens [20].

8.4.3.7 Intermediate and Large Cell Lymphomas

Lymphomas with larger cells are typically more obviously malignant and stand out more distinctly from the background of reactive lymphocytes. The nuclei often show marked pleomorphism, clumpy chromatin, and prominent nucleoli, findings rarely observed in reactive lymphocytes in substantial numbers. The presence of numerous mitoses within enlarged lymphocytes may also serve as a useful clue to malignancy. Lymphocyte apoptosis may manifest as "mercury drop karyorrhexis," the breakdown of nuclear material into multiple very dense and degenerated blobs. This finding is particularly common in cells from processes such as Burkitt lymphoma or diffuse large B cell lymphoma that also show frequent apoptosis in tissue.

As with small cell lymphomas, confirmation of clonality by flow cytometry is of great utility. At times, very ugly large cell lymphomas may raise carcinoma or melanoma as a differential diagnostic possibility. An immunocytochemical panel of CD45 for lymphoma, pan-cytokeratin for carcinoma, and S-100 for melanoma can resolve this problem.

One rare type of lymphoma deserves special attention because of its unique proclivity to manifest in body cavity fluids at presentation: primary effusion lymphoma. This relatively recently described entity is similar in morphology to other large cell lymphomas and is distinguished by its clinical presentation. It essentially always occurs in immune-suppressed individuals, especially AIDS patients. It has been linked to the virus HHV-8, the same herpesvirus responsible for causing Kaposi sarcoma [21]. If the diagnosis is suspected, immunocyto-chemistry can be performed for HHV-8 as a confirmatory step [22].

8.4.3.8 Other Hematopoietic Malignancies

Hodgkin lymphoma, despite being relatively common, very seldom can be diagnosed in body cavity fluids. Reed-Sternberg cells are only rarely seen in fluid cytology specimens. Effusions associated with Hodgkin lymphoma generally only contain nonspecific reactive inflammatory cells.

Plasma cell myeloma is also very rare in effusion specimens. Very infrequently, however, body cavity fluids can be massively involved by malignant plasma cells.

Leukemias may also involve body cavity fluids, though the disease is virtually always diagnosed by other means prior to this presentation. The presence of large numbers of blasts in these specimens is very distinctive and generally does not cause diagnostic problems. Leukemias compose a relatively large share of malignancies in childhood effusions.

Chronic idiopathic myelofibrosis may cause a very interesting finding in body cavity fluid specimens: cells derived from extramedullary hematopoiesis. The presence of mixed blood precursors in effusion specimens, including nucleated red cells, cells of various stages of the myeloid series, and megakaryocytes, is strongly suggestive of this diagnosis.

8.4.4 Sarcomas

Sarcomas are quite rare in body cavity fluid specimens. Bone and soft tissue tumors manifesting in effusions are generally easily recognized as malignant [23]. Distinctive morphologies may be recognizable in some cases, but such findings are of more intellectual than clinical interest. Usually, the underlying tumor has already been diagnosed by other means as involvement of fluids is a late manifestation.

8.5 Intraoperative Body Cavity Washing Specimens

8.5.1 Introduction

Pelvic washings are routinely performed in conjunction with hysterectomy and salpingo-oophorectomy for malignant disease, as well as at the time of second-look procedures. For ovarian primary tumors, the presence of positive cytology will cause an upstage of the disease to FIGO Stage IC or IIC depending on other parameters. Cytology has, up until recently, also been a part of the staging for endometrial carcinomas. In other settings, cytology may not change the official staging but is used to direct treatment decisions. As such, the cytology laboratory plays a key role in the determination of the ultimate treatment course for many of these patients.

Washings are easy and inexpensive to obtain, facilitating studies regarding their utility in surgical settings. So far, body cavity washing cytology has not become a standard procedure outside of gynecologic surgery, but this may change in the future as more studies are performed and more data is gathered regarding the clinical utility of the information such specimens can provide.

8.5.2 Differences between Washing and Effusion Cytology

As has been discussed above, the primary difference between intraoperative washing specimens and effusion specimens is the degree of rounding of the cell clusters. Mesothelial cells usually take on a flat sheet-like configuration in washings, and often form into larger groups than are seen with spontaneously exfoliated mesothelium due to the abrading action of the fluid. Direction of washings toward areas of the peritoneal lining with a gross appearance suspicious for tumor implants often facilitates diagnosis as well. Most positive washings are "loaded" with tumor cells, making their identification straightforward, even for low-grade processes [24]. The opportunity to compare the washing cytology with the appearance of the tumor in simultaneously resected specimens for surgical pathology also facilitates diagnosis.

Directed washings may occasionally, however, cause problems if endometriosis or endosalpingiosis are targeted. The resulting presence of a large number of endometrial or tubal cells, especially, if they have reactive atypia or psammoma bodies, or if the primary tumor is bland and low grade, may lead to a diagnostic dilemma. Immunocytochemistry is of little use in such situations. Comparison with simultaneous surgical pathology specimens can be very helpful.

8.5.3 Controversies in the Use of Cytology for Staging of Endometrial Adenocarcinoma

There has been an ongoing disagreement in the literature about the true prognostic significance of positive cytology alone in the setting of hysterectomy for endometrial adenocarcinoma. Some authors report no difference in recurrence rate or survival in women upstaged by cytology alone from Stage I to Stage III [25, 26].

Others argue that the finding is significant and the practice of intraoperative washings should continue [27–31].

The introduction of less invasive techniques in gynecologic surgery has created additional controversy regarding the value of the pelvic washing specimens from those procedures. Hysteroscopy prior to surgery has been suggested as a cause of positive peritoneal washings [32], but later studies have allayed concern [33]. It has also been argued that more intensive uterine manipulation in laparoscopic procedures may cause tumor spillage from the uterus [34, 35], though not all studies agree [36]. Furthermore, the clinical significance of rare false positives caused by artifactual spillage is far from clear. It may still be better to over-treat a few women rather than under-treat many others who are true positives.

8.5.4 Body Cavity Washings for Non-Gynecologic Tumors

There has been an upsurge in interest in recent years of applying intraoperative washing cytology more broadly outside the pelvis. Numerous studies have been conducted regarding the value of washings following pulmonary [37–43] and gastrointestinal [44–48] surgeries. As a general rule, these studies show that postoperative positive cytology does correspond to a worse prognosis for the patient. However, this finding is often fairly weak or even nonexistent when other staging parameters are controlled for, raising the question of the practical utility of performing washings on a routine basis in clinical practice. Furthermore, lung and gastrointestinal tumors have a fundamentally different biology from gynecologic tumors. They are less likely to spread via implants on serosal surfaces and more likely to recur in the form of distant metastasis. All of these factors mean that the significance of a positive washing cytology for any particular patient is relatively difficult to deduce, precluding broader acceptance of these procedures for clinical practice.

8.6 Fine Needle Aspiration Cytology of the Omentum and Peritoneum

For the most part, directed aspiration cytology of masses occurring in the omentum, or elsewhere in the peritoneum, yield findings similar to effusion or washing cytology. If anything, in these specimens interpretation is made easier by the fact that a defined tumor mass is being heavily sampled with relatively few cells in the background derived from benign processes. These specimens are virtually always taken from gynecologic malignancies and the cytologist only needs to confirm the suspected diagnosis.

8.7 Molecular Pathology of Body Cavity Fluid Specimens

As with every other area of pathology, ancillary molecular techniques are becoming more important in body cavity fluid specimens. A few genetic tests are already being used clinically. The use of body cavity fluid specimens as substrates for EGFR mutation analysis has been demonstrated in multiple studies [49–51]. Similar testing for other cancers, such as colorectal carcinoma, as well as other genes, such as K-RAS, should also be possible. Perhaps more exciting is the prospect of using molecular techniques to aid in diagnosis of problematic cases. Because body cavity fluid specimens are typically highly cellular and leave abundant residual material after routine cytologic processing, they would seem like ideal candidates for research in this area. A number of studies have been published [52, 53], especially, with regard to methylation of DNA as an ancillary marker [54–56]. Although this work shows promise, the findings so far have not been revolutionary. Nevertheless, it seems inevitable that body cavity fluid cytology, like all areas of pathology, will be gradually transformed by molecular insights and techniques.

8.8 Conclusions

Body cavity fluid cytology is a well-established field whose pitfalls and diagnostic dilemmas are widely known and extensively studied. False positive, false negative, and ambiguous results can occur because of the inherent challenges posed by these specimens. The importance of providing pathologists with every possible advantage when making their interpretations, in particular complete patient histories and information about radiological findings, cannot be overstated.

References

1. Manosca F, Schinstine M, Fetsch PA et al (2007) Diagnostic effects of prolonged storage on fresh effusion samples. Diagn Cytopathol 35:6–11
2. Elsheikh TM, Kirkpatrick JL, Wu HH (2006) Comparison of ThinPrep and cytospin preparations in the evaluation of exfoliative cytology specimens. Cancer 108:144–149
3. Gabriel C, Achten R, Drijkoningen M (2004) Use of liquid-based cytology in serous fluids: a comparison with conventional cytopreparatory techniques. Acta Cytol 48:825–835
4. Hoda RS (2007) Non-gynecologic cytology on liquid-based preparations: a morphologic review of facts and artifacts. Diagn Cytopathol 35:621–634
5. Leung CS, Chiu B, Bell V (1997) Comparison of ThinPrep and conventional preparations: nongynecologic cytology evaluation. Diagn Cytopathol 16:368–371
6. Moriarty AT, Schwartz MR, Ducatman BS et al (2008) A liquid concept–do classic preparations of body cavity fluid perform differently than ThinPrep cases? Observations from

the College of American Pathologists Interlaboratory Comparison Program in Nongynecologic Cytology. Arch Pathol Lab Med 132:1716–1718

7. Churg A, Colby TV, Cagle P et al (2000) The separation of benign and malignant mesothelial proliferations. Am J Surg Pathol 24:1183–1200

8. Wojno KJ, Olson JL, Sherman ME (1994) Cytopathology of pleural effusions after radiotherapy. Acta Cytol 38:1–8

9. Ozkara SK, Turan G, Basyigit I (2007) Clinicopathologic significance of eosinophilic pleural effusions in a population with a high prevalence of tuberculosis and cancer. Acta Cytol 51:773–781

10. Patel NP, Taylor CA, Levine EA, Trupiano JK, Geisinger KR (2007) Cytomorphologic features of primary peritoneal mesothelioma in effusion, washing, and fine-needle aspiration biopsy specimens: examination of 49 cases at one institution, including post-intraperitoneal hyperthermic chemotherapy findings. Am J Clin Pathol 128:414–422

11. Naylor B (2008) Pleural, peritoneal, and pericardial effusions. In: Bibbo M, Wilbur DC (eds) Comprehensive cytopathology 3rd edn. Saunders, Philadelphia, pp 515–577

12. Wong JW, Pitlik D, Abdul-Karim FW (1997) Cytology of pleural, peritoneal and pericardial fluids in children. A 40-year summary. Acta Cytol 41:467–473

13. Thrall MJ, Giampoli EJ (2009) Routine review of ascites fluid from patients with cirrhosis or hepatocellular carcinoma is a low-yield procedure: an observational study. Cytojournal 6:16

14. Aleman C, Sanchez L, Alegre J et al (2007) Differentiating between malignant and idiopathic pleural effusions: the value of diagnostic procedures. QJM 100:351–359

15. Ferrer J, Roldan J, Teixidor J, Pallisa E, Gich I, Morell F (2005) Predictors of pleural malignancy in patients with pleural effusion undergoing thoracoscopy. Chest 127:1017–1022

16. Moriarty AT, Stastny J, Volk EE, Hughes JH, Miller TR, Wilbur DC (2004) Fluids–good and bad actors: observations from the College of American Pathologists Interlaboratory Comparison Program in Nongynecologic Cytology. Arch Pathol Lab Med 128:513–518

17. Butnor KJ, Sporn TA, Ordonez NG (2007) Recommendations for the reporting of pleural mesothelioma. Hum Pathol 38:1587–1589

18. Ordonez NG (2005) Immunohistochemical diagnosis of epithelioid mesothelioma: an update. Arch Pathol Lab Med 129:1407–1414

19. Das DK (2006) Serous effusions in malignant lymphomas: a review. Diagn Cytopathol 34:335–347

20. Bangerter M, Hildebrand A, Griesshammer M (2001) Combined cytomorphologic and immunophenotypic analysis in the diagnostic workup of lymphomatous effusions. Acta Cytol 45:307–312

21. Nador RG, Cesarman E, Chadburn A et al (1996) Primary effusion lymphoma: a distinct clinicopathologic entity associated with the Kaposi's sarcoma-associated herpes virus. Blood 88:645–656

22. Brimo F, Michel RP, Khetani K, Auger M (2007) Primary effusion lymphoma: a series of 4 cases and review of the literature with emphasis on cytomorphologic and immunocytochemical differential diagnosis. Cancer 111:224–233

23. Abadi MA, Zakowski MF (1998) Cytologic features of sarcomas in fluids. Cancer 84:71–76

24. Cheng L, Wolf NG, Rose PG, Rodriguez M, Abdul-Karim FW (1998) Peritoneal washing cytology of ovarian tumors of low malignant potential: correlation with surface ovarian involvement and peritoneal implants. Acta Cytol 42:1091–1094

25. Fadare O, Mariappan MR, Hileeto D, Wang S, McAlpine JN, Rimm DL (2005) Upstaging based solely on positive peritoneal washing does not affect outcome in endometrial cancer. Mod Pathol 18:673–680

26. Kasamatsu T, Onda T, Katsumata N et al (2003) Prognostic significance of positive peritoneal cytology in endometrial carcinoma confined to the uterus. Br J Cancer 88:245–250

27. Benevolo M, Mariani L, Vocaturo G, Vasselli S, Natali PG, Mottolese M (2000) Independent prognostic value of peritoneal immunocytodiagnosis in endometrial carcinoma. Am J Surg Pathol 24:241–247

28. Havrilesky LJ, Cragun JM, Calingaert B et al (2007) The prognostic significance of positive peritoneal cytology and adnexal/serosal metastasis in stage IIIA endometrial cancer. Gynecol Oncol 104:401–405
29. Kashimura M, Sugihara K, Toki N et al (1997) The significance of peritoneal cytology in uterine cervix and endometrial cancer. Gynecol Oncol 67:285–290
30. Obermair A, Geramou M, Tripcony L, Nicklin JL, Perrin L, Crandon AJ (2001) Peritoneal cytology: impact on disease-free survival in clinical stage I endometrioid adenocarcinoma of the uterus. Cancer Lett 164:105–110
31. Saga Y, Imai M, Jobo T et al (2006) Is peritoneal cytology a prognostic factor of endometrial cancer confined to the uterus? Gynecol Oncol 103:277–280
32. Egarter C, Krestan C, Kurz C (1996) Abdominal dissemination of malignant cells with hysteroscopy. Gynecol Oncol 63:143–144
33. Biewenga P, de Blok S, Birnie E (2004) Does diagnostic hysteroscopy in patients with stage I endometrial carcinoma cause positive peritoneal washings? Gynecol Oncol 93:194–198
34. Sonoda Y, Zerbe M, Smith A, Lin O, Barakat RR, Hoskins WJ (2001) High incidence of positive peritoneal cytology in low-risk endometrial cancer treated by laparoscopically assisted vaginal hysterectomy. Gynecol Oncol 80:378–382
35. Lim S, Kim HS, Lee KB, Yoo CW, Park SY, Seo SS (2008) Does the use of a uterine manipulator with an intrauterine balloon in total laparoscopic hysterectomy facilitate tumor cell spillage into the peritoneal cavity in patients with endometrial cancer? Int J Gynecol Cancer 18:1145–1149
36. Eltabbakh GH, Mount SL (2006) Laparoscopic surgery does not increase the positive peritoneal cytology among women with endometrial carcinoma. Gynecol Oncol 100:361–364
37. Enatsu S, Yoshida J, Yokose T et al (2006) Pleural lavage cytology before and after lung resection in non-small cell lung cancer patients. Ann Thorac Surg 81:298–304
38. Kotoulas C, Lazopoulos G, Karaiskos T et al (2001) Prognostic significance of pleural lavage cytology after resection for non-small cell lung cancer. Eur J Cardiothorac Surg 20:330–334
39. Lim E, Ali A, Theodorou P, Nicholson AG, Ladas G, Goldstraw P (2004) Intraoperative pleural lavage cytology is an independent prognostic indicator for staging non-small cell lung cancer. J Thorac Cardiovasc Surg 127:1113–1118
40. Nakagawa T, Okumura N, Kokado Y, Miyoshi K, Matsuoka T, Kameyama K (2007) Clinical relevance of intraoperative pleural lavage cytology in non-small cell lung cancer. Ann Thorac Surg 83:204–208
41. Okada M, Sakamoto T, Nishio W, Uchino K, Tsuboshima K, Tsubota N (2003) Pleural lavage cytology in non-small cell lung cancer: lessons from 1000 consecutive resections. J Thorac Cardiovasc Surg 126:1911–1915
42. Shintani Y, Ohta M, Iwasaki T et al (2009) Intraoperative pleural lavage cytology after lung resection as an independent prognostic factor for staging lung cancer. J Thorac Cardiovasc Surg 137:835–839
43. Vicidomini G, Santini M, Fiorello A, Parascandolo V, Calabro B, Pastore V (2005) Intraoperative pleural lavage: is it a valid prognostic factor in lung cancer? Ann Thorac Surg 79:254–257; discussion -7
44. Bando E, Yonemura Y, Takeshita Y et al (1999) Intraoperative lavage for cytological examination in 1,297 patients with gastric carcinoma. Am J Surg 178:256–262
45. Chuwa EW, Khin LW, Chan WH, Ong HS, Wong WK (2005) Prognostic significance of peritoneal lavage cytology in gastric cancer in Singapore. Gastric Cancer 8:228–237
46. Ribeiro U, Jr., Safatle-Ribeiro AV, Zilberstein B et al (2006) Does the intraoperative peritoneal lavage cytology add prognostic information in patients with potentially curative gastric resection? J Gastrointest Surg 10:170–176, discussion 6–7
47. de Manzoni G, Verlato G, Di Leo A et al (2006) Peritoneal cytology does not increase the prognostic information provided by TNM in gastric cancer. World J Surg 30:579–584
48. Nieveen van Dijkum EJ, Sturm PD, de Wit LT, Offerhaus J, Obertop H, Gouma DJ (1998) Cytology of peritoneal lavage performed during staging laparoscopy for gastrointestinal malignancies: is it useful? Ann Surg 228:728–733

49. Cavalli P, Riboli B, Generali D, Passalacqua R, Bosio G (2006) EGFR genotyping in pleural fluid specimens in NSCLC patients. Lung Cancer 54:265–266
50. Kimura H, Fujiwara Y, Sone T et al (2006) EGFR mutation status in tumour-derived DNA from pleural effusion fluid is a practical basis for predicting the response to gefitinib. Br J Cancer 95:1390–1395
51. Zhang X, Zhao Y, Wang M, Yap WS, Chang AY (2008) Detection and comparison of epidermal growth factor receptor mutations in cells and fluid of malignant pleural effusion in non-small cell lung cancer. Lung Cancer 60:175–182
52. Davidson B (2004) Malignant effusions: from diagnosis to biology. Diagn Cytopathol 31:246–254
53. Davidson B, Espina V, Steinberg SM et al (2006) Proteomic analysis of malignant ovarian cancer effusions as a tool for biologic and prognostic profiling. Clin Cancer Res 12:791–799
54. Benlloch S, Galbis-Caravajal JM, Martin C et al (2006) Potential diagnostic value of methylation profile in pleural fluid and serum from cancer patients with pleural effusion. Cancer 107:1859–1865
55. Brock MV, Hooker CM, Yung R et al (2005) Can we improve the cytologic examination of malignant pleural effusions using molecular analysis? Ann Thorac Surg 80:1241–1247
56. Katayama H, Hiraki A, Aoe K et al (2007) Aberrant promoter methylation in pleural fluid DNA for diagnosis of malignant pleural effusion. Int J Cancer 120:2191–2195

Chapter 9
Cytopathology in the Diagnosis of Lymphoma

Yi-Hua Chen and Yun Gong

9.1 Introduction

Fine needle aspiration (FNA) is frequently used as a first-line investigation for lymphadenopathy or mass lesions to evaluate for the underlying pathological processes, such as lymphoma, carcinoma, various infections, or reactive conditions [1–4]. It offers a rapid diagnosis or initial assessment to determine the next step of appropriate work-up. FNA is relatively simple, safe, and cost-effective, and can often be carried out at the bedside or in an outpatient setting for superficial palpable mass. For deep-seated mass, ultrasound or CT-guided FNA is often used to obtain diagnostic material [5–7]. When lymphoma presents as a medical emergency, such as mediastinal obstruction secondary to acute lymphoblastic lymphoma (LBL), a rapid assessment by FNA can be of critical importance for prompt clinical intervention [1]. FNA also plays an important role in the long-term follow-up of patients for recurrence or progression of lymphoma [4, 8–10].

Although FNA has been used for decades in the evaluation of lymphadenopathy, its role in the diagnosis of lymphoma, particularly the primary diagnosis of lymphoma, remains controversial [11–13]. The lack of histological architecture, an important component for morphologic evaluation of lymphoma, is a major obstacle in FNA diagnosis of lymphoma. Another restriction is sampling error associated with small sample size. It is often difficult to know with certainty whether the aspirated sample is representative of the pathologic process in the entire lesion [1, 5, 14, 15]. The difficulty is further compounded by the growing complexity and sophistication in lymphoma classification [16].

Y.-H. Chen (✉)
Department of Pathology, Northwestern University Feinberg School of Medicine, Chicago, IL, USA
e-mail: y-chen5@northwestern.edu

Y. Gong
Department of Pathology, Unit 53, The University of Texas MD Anderson Cancer Center, Houston, TX, USA

R. Nayar (ed.), *Cytopathology in Oncology*,
Cancer Treatment and Research 160, DOI: 10.1007/978-3-642-38850-7_9,
© Springer-Verlag Berlin Heidelberg 2014

The key to enhancing the accuracy of FNA diagnosis of lymphoma is a multiparameter approach in which the cytomorphologic features should be evaluated in correlation with the results of ancillary studies [1, 13, 17–28]. In addition, knowledge of the patient's clinical history and radiological findings is also important for appropriate morphologic interpretation. Due to the inherent limitations of FNA, a negative cytological finding does not exclude the possibility of lymphoma. If clinical suspicion for lymphoma remains, a surgical biopsy should be recommended for further clarification [5]. Therefore, "success in malignant lymphoma diagnosis by FNA is contingent on several factors including skill of the aspirator, proper triaging of the specimen, knowledge of lymphoma nomenclature and biology, and most importantly, collegial interaction between cytopathologist and hematopathologist and between pathologist and clinician [14]."

9.2 Overview of Lymphoma Classification

According to the World Health Organization (WHO) Classification of Tumors of Haematopoietic and Lymphoid Tissues published in 2008, lymphoid neoplasms are classified into five major categories: precursor lymphoid neoplasmsms, mature B-cell neoplasms, mature T- and NK-cell neoplasms, Hodgkin lymphoma (HL), and immunodeficiency-associated lymphoproliferative disorders. Each category is further classified into various subtypes based on their clinical, morphologic, biological, phenotypic and genetic features (Table 9.1). HLs are known to be of B-cell lineage; however, they are classified as a separate entity from other B-cell lymphomas due to their unique clinicopathologic features. Additionally, many subtypes of immunodeficiency-associated lymphoproliferative disorders are similar to those occurring in immunocompetent individuals except for a few entities.

9.3 Specimen Collection

The technical details of FNA have been well described elsewhere and beyond the scope of this chapter [29]. An important first step to success in the FNA diagnosis of lymphoma is an immediate on-site assessment of specimen adequacy and proper triaging for ancillary studies. In general, one smear of the initial aspirated material is stained with Diff-Quik for evaluation of specimen adequacy by a cytopathologist. Samples containing only blood, fibrotic tissue, necrotic debris, or poorly preserved cells are considered inadequate. If lymphoma is suspected in the initial assessment, additional aspirations are required to obtain sufficient cells for ancillary studies [17, 18, 30, 31]. For a primary diagnosis of lymphoma, a concurrent needle core biopsy should be obtained for histologic confirmation and immunohistochemical staining for subclassification of lymphoma [32]. The cytology samples and their applicable studies are summarized in Table 9.2.

Table 9.1 Classification of lymphoid neoplasms[a]

Precursor lymphoid neoplasms
B-lymphoblastic leukemia/lymphoma
T-lymphoblastic leukemia/lymphoma

Mature B-cell neoplasms
Chronic lymphocytic leukemia/small lymphocytic lymphoma
Follicular lymphoma
Mantle cell lymphoma
Marginal zone lymphoma
    Extranodal marginal zone lymphoma of mucosa-associated lymphoid tissue (MALT)
    Nodal marginal zone lymphoma
    Splenic B-cell marginal zone lymphoma
Lymphoplasmacytic lymphoma
Burkitt lymphoma
Plasma cell neoplasms
Diffuse large B-cell lymphoma, not otherwise specified (DLBCL, NOS)
Large B-cell lymphoma subtypes
    T cell/histiocyte-rich large B-cell lymphoma
    Primary DLBCL of the CNS
    Primary cutaneous DLBCL, leg type
    EBV positive DLBCL of the elderly
    Lymphomatoid granulomatosis
    Primary mediastinal large B-cell lymphoma
    Intravascular large B-cell lymphoma
    Plasmablastic lymphoma
    Large B-cell lymphoma arising in HHV8-associated multicentric Castleman disease
    Primary effusion lymphoma
B-cell lymphoma, unclassifiable, with features intermediate between DLBCL and Burkitt
    lymphoma
B-cell lymphoma, unclassifiable, with features intermediate between DLBCL and classical
    Hodgkin Lymphoma

Mature T- and NK-cell neoplasms
Peripheral T-cell lymphoma, NOS
Peripheral T-cell lymphoma subtypes
    Anaplastic large cell lymphoma, ALK positive
    Anaplastic lymphoma, ALK negative
    Angioimmunoblastic T-cell lymphoma
    Enteropathy-associated T-cell lymphoma
    Subcutaneous panniculitis-like T-cell lymphoma
    Hepatosplenic T-cell lymphoma
    Adult T-cell leukemia/lymphoma
    Extranodal NK/T-cell lymphoma, nasal type
    Mycosis fungoides
    Primary cutaneous CD30 positive T-cell lymphoproliferative disorders

(continued)

Table 9.1 (continued)

Hodgkin lymphomas (HL)
Nodular lymphocyte predominant HL
Classical HL
    Nodular sclerosis HL
    Mixed cellularity HL
    Lymphocyte-rich HL
    Lymphocyte-depleted HL

Immunodeficiency-associated lymphoproliferative disorders
Lymphoproliferative diseases associated with primary immune disorders
Lymphoma associated with HIV infection
Post-transplant lymphoproliferative disorders (PTLD)
    Plasmacytic hyperplasia and infectious mononucleosis-like PTLD
    Polymorphic PTLD
    Monomorphic PTLD
    Classical Hodgkin lymphoma type PTLD
Iatrogenic immunodeficiency-associated lymphoproliferative disorders

[a] Based on the WHO Classification of Tumours of Haematopoietic and Lymphoid Tissues (2008). Lymphoid leukemias, subtypes of plasma cell neoplasms and some uncommon entities are not listed

Table 9.2 Cytology sample types and applicable studies

Sample types	Preparations	Applicable studies
Fine needle aspiration	Air-dried smears/cytospin	Morphologic evaluation
		Immunohistochemistry (Cytospin)
		FISH
		PCR
	Cell suspension in RPMI	Flow cytometric analysis
		PCR
Cell block	Paraffin-embedded tissue	Morphologic evaluation
		Immunohistochemistry
		Special stains
		PCR
		FISH
Core biopsy	Paraffin-embedded tissue	Morphologic evaluation
		Immunohistochemistry
		Special stains
		PCR
		FISH
	Touch imprint	Morphologic evaluation
		FISH
		PCR

Table 9.3 Common immunophenotype of small B-cell lymphomas

Lymphoma	CD19	CD20	CD5	CD10	CD23	FMC7	CD79b	Surface immunoglobulin
CLL/SLL	+	Dim+	+	−	+	−	−	Dim+
FL	+	+	−	+	−	+	+	+
MCL	+	+	+	−	−	+	+	+
MZL	+	+	−	−	−	+	+	+
LPL	+	+	−	−	−	+	+	+
BL	+	+	−	+	−	+	+	+

CLL/SLL Chronic lymphocytic leukemia/small lymphocytic lymphoma
FL Follicular lymphoma
MCL Mantle cell lymphoma
MZL Marginal zone lymphoma
LPL Lymphoplasmacytic lymphoma
BL Burkitt lymphoma

9.4 Ancillary Studies

Various ancillary studies have been used to aid in the diagnosis and subclassification of lymphoma. The techniques commonly applied to cytology samples include flow cytometric immunophenotyping, polymerase chain reaction (PCR), and interphase fluorescence in situ hybridization (FISH).

9.4.1 Flow Cytometric Immunophenotyping

Flow cytometric immunophenotyping has become an integral part of FNA diagnosis of lymphoma [13, 17, 18, 21–26, 28]. It is particularly important in the evaluation of small B-cell lymphomas as they often have cytomorphologic features overlapping with each other or with reactive lymphoid hyperplasia [14, 16]. The common immunophenotypes of small B-cell lymphomas are summarized in Table 9.3.

The cytology sample most commonly acquired for flow cytometric analysis is FNA material rinsed in RPMI culture medium. Ideally, at least 1×10^6 cells should be collected. In addition, fresh core biopsies can also be used for flow cytometric analysis. Due to the relatively limited cell quantities in FNA samples, knowledge of the patient's prior lymphoma subtype and the immunophenotype can facilitate designing of an optimal panel for flow cytometric analysis. In patients without a prior history of lymphoma, a limited panel targeting B-cell lymphomas (e.g., CD45, CD3, CD19, CD20, CD5, CD10, κ, λ) is usually used for analysis since more than 90 % of non-Hodgkin lymphomas (NHL) are of B-cell lineage [16]. The immunophenotypic profile not only determines B-cell "clonality" based on the staining pattern for κ and λ, but also provides important information for lymphoma subclassification. For example, CD5 expression is associated with chronic lymphocytic leukemia/small lymphocytic lymphoma (CLL/SLL) lymphocytic lymphoma and mantle cell lymphoma (MCL); CD10 is associated with follicular lymphoma (FL); negativity for both CD5 and CD10 supports a diagnosis of marginal zone lymphoma (MZL). However, it is important to recognize the variations of immunophenotype in small B-cell lymphomas particularly those "key markers" that are commonly used to help with the differential diagnosis [33, 34]. For example, MCLs are occasionally CD5-negative, whereas a small subset of MZL are CD5-positive. Therefore, further investigation by other ancillary studies may be required for an accurate diagnosis. In addition, false-negative results may occur and are more frequently seen in large B-cell lymphoma [19]. The possible explanation is that the large lymphoma cells are more likely to be damaged than small lymphocytes during FNA and/or sample preparation for flow cytometric analysis. In some subtypes of lymphoma, e.g., T cell/histiocyte-rich large B-cell lymphoma, the small number of neoplastic lymphocytes may also lead to a false negative result. If morphologic suspicion for lymphoma remains, a tissue biopsy should be recommended for further investigation.

Immunophenotyping is somewhat less helpful in the diagnosis of T-cell lymphoma. Analysis of T-cell "clonality" by flow cytometry involves a broad array of monoclonal antibodies against various TCR variable region beta (Vß) chains, and these assays have not been widely used in the clinical laboratories [35]. T-cell lymphomas often demonstrate aberrant immunophenotype, and the most common phenotypic abnormality is lost or decreased expression of one or more pan T-cell antigens (CD3, CD2, CD5, and CD7). However, reactive T cells may also demonstrate an atypical phenotype, e.g., decreased expression of CD7 in activated T cells. Thus, correlation with morphologic findings, other ancillary studies and clinical features is important for an accurate diagnosis.

Flow cytometric immunophenotyping is not indicated in the evaluation of HL because the results would reflect the phenotype of the abundant reactive lymphocytes in the background rather than that of the small number of large neoplastic cells. A reliable diagnosis of HL is made on a combination of histologic examination and immunohistochemistry. Therefore, if a HL is suspected in the on-site evaluation, a tissue biopsy is essential, particularly in patients without a prior history of lymphoma.

9.4.2 Molecular Genetic Analysis

PCR and FISH are the most useful tools for molecular genetic analysis of lymphoma. The diagnosis of lymphoma can be substantiated by detecting a clonal immunoglobulin heavy chain (IgH) or T-cell receptor (TCR) gene rearrangement. In addition, several genetic abnormalities are associated with specific lymphoma subtypes, e.g., t(11;14) in MCL and t(14;18) in FL. The fresh material obtained by FNA is well suited for PCR and FISH analysis. FISH can also be performed retrospectively using cell blocks, and air-dried smears or cytospins [27, 30, 31]. It is important to recognize that false negative result may occur due to necrosis or

Table 9.4 Common chromosomal translocations associated with lymphoma subtypes and the detection methods

Lymphoma	Chromosomal translocations	Dysregulated genes	PCR/FISH	Dysregulated protein	Immunohisto-chemistry
FL	t(14;18)(q32;q21)	*BCL-2*	Yes/yes	BCL-2	Yes
MCL	t(11;14)(q13;q32)	*CCND1*	Yes/yes	BCL-1 (Cyclin D1)	Yes
BL	t(8;14)(q24;q32) t(8,22)(q24;q11) t(2;8)(p12;q24)	*C-MYC*	Yes/yes	C-MYC	Yes[a]
ALCL	t(2;5)(p23;q35) t(1;2)(q25;p23) Others	*ALK*	Yes/yes	ALK	Yes

[a] Not used for diagnosis of Burkitt lymphoma
FL Follicular lymphoma
MCL Mantle cell lymphoma
BL Burkitt lymphoma
ALCL Anaplastic large cell lymphoma

low number of neoplastic cells in the sample. On the other hand, a clonal lymphocyte population can occasionally be detected in reactive lymphoid proliferation and therefore is not synonymous with malignancy [36–39]. The common chromosomal translocations associated with lymphoma subtypes and the detection methods are summarized in Table 9.4.

9.5 Diagnosis of Lymphoma by FNA

The lymphoid neoplasms appear to recapitulate the developmental stages of normal lymphocytes including morphology and immunophenotype, and this resemblance is the major basis for lymphoma classification and nomenclature [16]. This chapter focuses on the lymphoid neoplasms that are more commonly encountered in cytopathology. The FNA smear features of various lymphomas are summarized in Table 9.5.

9.5.1 Lymphoblastic Leukemia/Lymphoma

Lymphoblastic leukemia/lymphoma (LPL) is a lymphoid neoplasm derived from the immature, progenitor cells committed to B- or T-cell differentiation. LBL is the nodal or extranodal counterpart of acute lymphblastic leukemia (ALL). T-ALL/LBL more commonly presents as a solid tumor, usually as a rapidly growing mediastinal mass, whereas B-ALL/LBL more frequently involves peripheral blood and bone marrow [16].

Table 9.5 Lymphomas on fine needle aspiration (FNA) smears

FNA smear	Lymphomas
Small lymphocyte predominant	
Monotonous	Follicular lymphoma, low-grade
	Mantle cell lymphoma
	Small lymphocytic lymphoma
	Burkitt lymphoma
Polymorphous with plasmacytoid/plasma cells	Marginal zone lymphoma
	Lymphoplasmacytic lymphoma
	Post-transplant lymphoproliferative disorders
Polymorphous with inflammatory cells	Hodgkin lymphoma
	Peripheral T-cell lymphoma
	T cell/histiocyte-rich large B-cell lymphoma
Large lymphocyte predominant	
Large cells	Diffuse large B-cell lymphoma
	Mantle cell lymphoma, pleomorphic variant
	Peripheral T-cell lymphoma
Anaplastic	Anaplastic large cell lymphoma, ALK positive
	Anaplastic large cell lymphoma, ALK negative
	Diffuse large B-cell lymphoma
Plasmablastic	Plasmablastic plasmacytoma/myeloma
	Plasmablastic lymphoma
	Primary effusion lymphoma (body fluid)
Blastic lymphocytes	Lymphoblastic lymphoma
	Mantle cell lymphoma, blastoid variant

9.5.1.1 Cytomorphology

FNA smears of ALL/LBL are usually cellular and show a monotonous population of small to medium-sized lymphocytes. These lymphocytes have high nuclear to cytoplasmic ratio, fine chromatin, small inconspicuous nucleoli and scant or moderate amount of basophilic cytoplasm; cytoplasmic vacuoles and frequent mitoses may be present [21, 40, 41]. One potential pitfall is to assume the cells are from a low-grade lymphoma because of their small size and the lack of prominent nucleoli [21]. The differential diagnosis of ALL/LBL also includes non-lymphoid malignancies such as thymoma, small cell carcinoma, Ewing's sarcoma or neuroblastoma.

9.5.1.2 Immunophenotype

Most ALL/LBLs are dim CD45-positive and express TdT; the latter is the marker to indicate the precursor nature of ALL/LBL and is expressed in the vast majority of B- and T-ALL/LBL. CD34, another precursor antigen, is positive in a subset of B- or T-ALL/LBL. In addition, CD1a and CD99 are markers for T-ALL/LBL. A subset of B- or T-ALL/LBL express CD10. The lineage of the lymphoblasts can be determined by B- or T-cell associated antigens, such as CD3, CD19 and PAX-5. An aberrant expression of myeloid-associated markers, CD33 and CD13, may be seen in some cases. The markers that differentiate ALL/LBL from mature B-cell lymphoma (TdT, CD34, CD1a, and CD99) can all be assessed by immunohistochemistry.

A major diagnostic pitfall is to mistake thymoma for T-LBL in a mediastinal biopsy. T-LBL and lymphocyte-rich thymoma may show identical morphology and immunophenotype in an aspirated sample or a small core biopsy, including positive staining for TdT, CD1a, and CD99. Correlation with clinical presentation and radiological findings is important for FNA interpretation. A surgical biopsy may be required in some cases for further investigation.

9.5.1.3 Molecular Genetics

Molecular analysis for *IgH* or *TCR* gene rearrangement is not helpful for lineage assignment for ALL/LBL since simultaneous clonal *TCR* gene rearrangement can be found in B-ALL/LBL, and similarly, clonal *IgH* rearrangement can be detected in T-ALL/LBL [16]. Cytogenetic abnormalities are seen in the majority of cases of ALL/LBL. Several recurrent genetic abnormalities identified in B-ALL/LBL have prognostic significance; however, currently no genetic markers can reliably predict the outcome of patients with T-ALL/LBL [16].

9.5.2 Mature B-Cell Lymphomas

Mature B-cell neoplasms comprise over 90 % of lymphoid neoplasms worldwide. Diffuse large B-cell lymphoma (DLBCL) and follicular lymphoma (FL) account for more than 60 % of all B-cell lymphomas exclusive of HL and plasma cell myeloma [42].

9.5.2.1 Chronic Lymphocytic Leukemia/Small Lymphocytic Lymphoma

Chronic lymphocytic leukemia (CLL) is the most common leukemia of adults in Western countries. Small lymphocytic lymphoma (SLL) is the tissue counterpart of the same disease and accounts for approximately 12 % of all B-cell lymphomas [16, 42]. The mean age at diagnosis is 65 years, and the male to female ratio is 1.5–2:1 [16]. Patients with CLL/SLL often present with lymphocytosis, and many patients also have peripheral lymphadenopathy [43–45]. The clinical course of the disease is indolent; however, 2–8 % of patients transform to large B-cell lymphoma (Richter's syndrome), and <1 % develop HL [46–49].

Fig. 9.1 Chronic
lymphocytic leulemia/small
lymphocytic lymphoma
(CLL/SLL). The smear shows
a predominance of small
lymphocytes with round
nuclei, clumped chromatin,
and scant cytoplasm.
Occasional large
lymphocytes with centrally
located prominent nucleoli
are also seen, consistent with
prolymphocytes (**a** Diff-
Quick stain, **b** Papanicolaou
stain. Magnification: ×400)

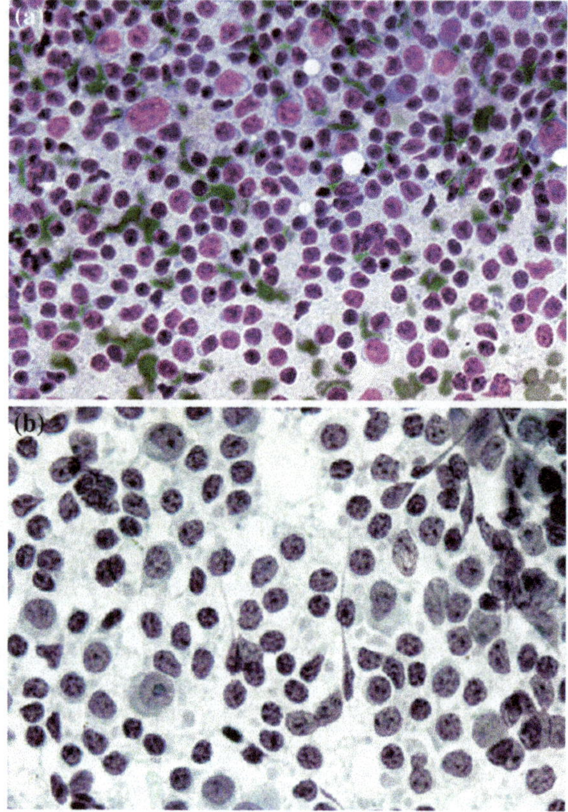

Cytomorphology

FNA smears of CLL/SLL show a monotonous population of small lymphocytes
with round or slightly irregular nuclei, "blocky" chromatin and scant cytoplasm.
The large lymphocytes are often scanty and arranged singly or in small aggregates.
These large cells show round to slightly oval nuclei, moderately condensed
chromatin with a single prominent central nucleolus, corresponding to the
prolymphocytes in the proliferation centers observed in histological sections
(Fig. 9.1).

Immunophenotype

The characteristic immunophenotype of CLL/SLL is the expression of CD5
(virtually all cases) and CD23 (majority of cases). They are negative for CD10,
and the staining for CD20 is usually dim. However, CLL/SLL may show overlapping phenotype with MCL [33, 34]. In addition, MZL can occasionally be

positive for CD5. Therefore, immunohistochemical stain for cyclin D1 should be performed, and a negative result helps to exclude MCL.

Molecular Genetics

Genetic abnormalities are identified in the majority of cases of CLL/SLL, including del13q14, trisomy 13, del11q22-23 (*ATM*) and del17p13 (*TP53*). Although they are not specific for CLL/SLL, detection of these abnormalities by FISH on FNA smears provides evidence of clonality as well as important prognostic information [50].

9.5.2.2 Follicular Lymphoma

Follicular lymphoma (FL) is the second most common NHL in the United States and Western Europe, and accounts for the majority of low-grade lymphomas. FL affects predominantly adults over 60 years of age with slight female predominance. Most patients present with widespread disease involving peripheral and central lymph nodes, bone marrow and spleen. Extranodal sites may also be involved [16, 42].

Cytomorphology

FL derives from the germinal center B cells and recapitulates the normal germinal center cell morphology. The tumor cells in the aspirate smears are composed of small mature-appearing lymphocytes with angulated, elongated, or cleaved nuclei and inconspicuous nucleoli, corresponding to the centrocytes. Large, non-cleaved cells corresponding to the centroblasts are present in varying numbers. Aggregates of neoplastic lymphocytes are frequently found in the direct smears, and tingible body macrophages are usually absent (Fig. 9.2).

FL should be graded on the histologic sections by counting the numbers of centroblasts in 10 neoplastic follicles under a 40× magnification high power field (HPF) [16]. The current WHO classification has grouped grade 1 (0–5 centroblasts per HPF) and grade 2 (6–15 centroblasts per HPF) into "low-grade" FL since there are no significant clinical differences between the two grades. However, distinguishing grade 3 (>15 centroblasts per HPF) from low-grade FL is clinically relevant since patients with grade 3 FL, particularly grade 3b (solid sheets of centroblasts), are often treated according to the protocols for DLBCL. Grading of FL on a FNA sample is not accurate due to the lack of reliable histologic configuration. Although several approaches have been proposed [51], there have been no well-established criteria for grading FL on FNA biopsy.

Fig. 9.2 Follicular lymphoma. **a** The smear shows lymphoid aggregate consisting of a mixture of small to medium-sized cleaved cells (centrocytes) and large non-cleaved cells (centroblasts), recapitulating follicular architecture. (Diff-Quick stain, magnification: ×600). **b** FISH for t(14;18)(q32;q21) performed on the direct FNA smear is positive for *BCL-2* and *IgH* fusion. *Arrows* indicate the yellow fusion signals (Magnification: ×1000)

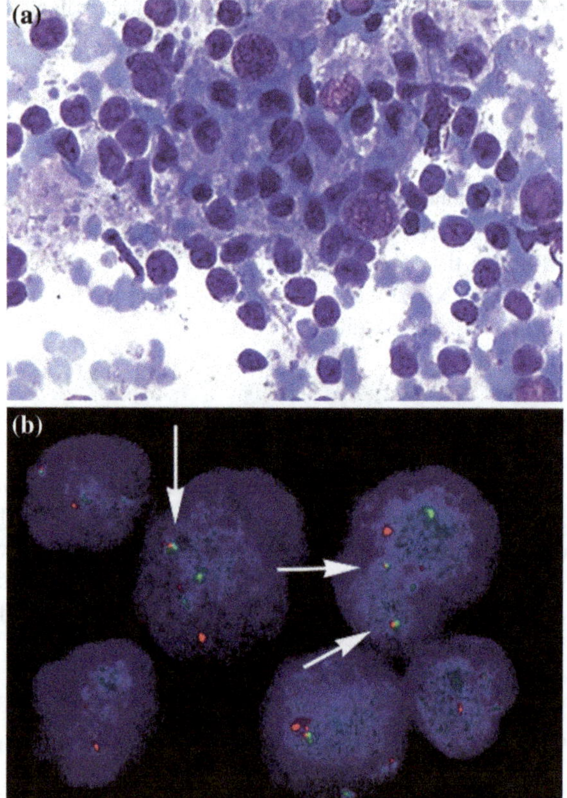

Immunophenotyping

Similar to normal germinal center B cells, the FL cells are characteristically positive for CD10 and BCL-6, and negative for CD5. In contrast to normal germinal center cells, the neoplastic cells overexpress BCL-2 as a consequence of t(14;18) translocation. It is important to recognize that overexpression of BCL-2 is not specific for FL. In fact, the majority of small B-cell lymphomas are positive for BCL-2, such as CLL/SLL, MCL and MZL. Some of these lymphomas may show centrocyte-like cytomorphology; e.g., MCL and MZL. Therefore, a clonal B-cell population with centrocyte morphology and positivity for BCL-2 is not diagnostic for FL. Correlation with other immunophenotype, such as CD10 and BCL-6, will be helpful for an accurate diagnosis.

Molecular Genetics

FL is genetically characterized by chromosomal translocation t(14;18)(q32;q21) resulting in *BCL-2* gene rearrangement and overexpression of BCL-2. FISH analysis for t(14;18) can provide high accuracy in detecting FL on FNA samples, particularly when flow cytometric analysis is unavailable or non-contributory [31, 52] (Fig. 9.2).

9.5.2.3 Mantle Cell Lymphoma

Mantle cell lymphoma (MCL) comprises 3–10 % of NHL and involves middle-aged to older individuals with a male predominance [42]. Most patients present with advanced-stage disease with generalized lymphadenopathy, bone marrow involvement and hepatosplenomegaly. Peripheral blood involvement is common, and extranodal involvement frequently includes Waldeyer's ring and gastrointestinal (GI) tract [16, 53]. Transformation of MCL to large B-cell lymphoma is exceedingly rare, but to the aggressive variants, blastoid or pleomorphic MCL, may occur [16, 54–56].

Cytomorphology

FNA smear of MCL is characterized by a monotonous population of small- to medium-sized lymphoid cells with slightly irregular nuclear contours, finely stippled chromatin and inconspicuous nucleoli. However, the blastoid variant of MCL may resemble lymphoblastic lymphoma, and the pleomorphic variant of MCL may be indistinguishable from large cell lymphoma.

Immunophenotype

The characteristic immunophenotype of MCL is the expression of CD5 and negativity for CD10 and BCL-6. Unlike CLL/SLL, the CD20 staining in MCL is usually brightly positive, and the CD23 is often negative. However, approximately 10–15 % of MCLs are CD5-negative, and rare cases of CD10-positive MCL have also been reported [34]. Thus, immunohistochemical stain for cyclin D1 should be performed, and a positive result supports a diagnosis of MCL.

Molecular Genetics

The genetic hallmark of MCL is chromosomal translocation t(11;14)(q13;q32) which juxtaposes the *CCND1* gene encoding cyclin D1 to the *IgH* gene, leading to the overexpression of cyclin D1. The detection of t(11;14) translocation by FISH is helpful in confirming the diagnosing MCL [30].

9.5.2.4 Marginal Zone Lymphoma

Marginal zone lymphoma (MZL) includes three distinct diseases that arise from the post-germinal center B cells and share a similar immunophenotype. These three entities include extranodal marginal zone B-cell lymphoma of mucosa associated lymphoid tissue (MALT lymphoma), splenic MZL and nodal MZL [16]. MALT lymphoma comprises 7–8 % of all B-cell lymphomas, and commonly involves GI tract, salivary gland and thyroid. Nodal MZL and splenic MZL are rare, each comprising less than 2 % of B-cell lymphomas [42, 57, 58], and they primarily affect adults with an equal sex incidence [42, 59, 60]. Patients with nodal MZL present with localized or generalized lymphadenopathy, whereas patients with splenic MZL rarely have peripheral lymphadenopathy [58–60].

Cytomorphology

MZL is one of the lymphoma subtypes that are difficult to recognize based on cytomorphology alone [14]. FNA smears often show a heterogeneous cell population composed of small lymphocytes, plasmacytoid lymphocytes, plasma cells, and occasional large transformed lymphocytes. Tingible body macrophages may be present, which reflects the common histologic findings of residual normal lymphoid follicles in MZL. These features may be confused with a reactive lymphoid proliferation. In addition, MZL cells may show centrocyte-like morphology mimicking FL, or marked plasmacytic differentiation resembling plasma cell neoplasm [61].

Immunophenotype

Identification of a monotypic B-cell population by flow cytometry is important in differentiating MZL from a reactive lymphoid hyperplasia. The neoplastic B cells are typically negative for CD5 and CD10. In addition, a monotypic plasma cell population with same light chain restriction to the lymphocyte population may be identified by immunohistochemistry. This finding provides additional evidence to support the diagnosis of MZL.

Molecular Genetics

Several balanced chromosomal translocations have been identified in MALT lymphoma including t(11;18)(q21;q21), t(1;14)(p22;q32), t(14;18)(q32;q21), and t(3;14)(p14.1;q32) [16, 62]. Chromosome 7q32 deletion has been found in over 40 % of splenic MZL [63]. However, these genetic abnormalities are not entirely specific for MZL.

9.5.2.5 Lymphoplasmacytic Lymphoma

Lymphoplasmacytic lymphoma (LPL) represents 2–3 % of NHL and primarily occurs in adults with a median age in the 60s and slight male predominance. Most cases involve the bone marrow, but lymph nodes and other extranodal sites may also be involved [16, 42, 57, 64]. Waldenström macroglobulinemia is defined as LPL with bone marrow involvement and an IgM paraprotein of any concentration [16].

Cytomorphology

FNA smears of LPL are characterized by a mixed population of small lymphocytes, plasmacytoid lymphocytes and plasma cells. Dutcher bodies (nuclear inclusion) or Russell bodies (cytoplasmic inclusion) may be observed [21]. The proportion of each cell population may vary significantly. In rare cases, the plasma cells may represent the predominant component that simulate a plasma cell neoplasm. It is difficult to differentiate LPL from MZL on morphologic grounds; correlation with clinical, laboratory and bone marrow findings is helpful in most cases.

Immunophenotype

Similar to MZL, LPL is typically negative for CD5 and CD10. The plasma cell component demonstrates the same light chain restriction as the neoplastic B lymphocytes.

Molecular Genetics

No specific molecular or cytogenetic abnormalities are recognized in LPL.

9.5.2.6 Burkitt Lymphoma

Burkitt lymphoma (BL) is a highly aggressive B-cell lymphoma characterized by chromosomal translocation involving the *C-MYC* gene. It accounts for 30 % of non-endemic pediatric lymphomas and less than 1 % of adult B-cell lymphomas [16, 42, 65]. Patients often present with rapidly growing tumor masses with associated evidence of tumor lysis [66].

Three distinct clinical variants of BL are recognized: endemic, sporadic and immunodeficiency-associated. They share similar histologic features and clinical behavior, but differ in epidemiology, clinical presentation, and genetic features [16, 66]. The endemic form occurs most frequently in children in equatorial Africa. It commonly presents as jaw and other facial bone lesions; breast, ovaries and kidney are also frequently involved. EBV is identified in the majority of endemic cases. The sporadic form of BL is seen worldwide, mainly in children and young adults, and presents most commonly as abdominal masses; EBV is identified in only about 30 % of cases. The immunodeficiency-associated form affects primarily patients with HIV infection. Nodal involvement is most common, and EBV is identified in 25–40 % cases [16, 66].

Cytomorphology

FNA smears of BL show a monotonous population of medium-sized lymphocytes with round or slightly irregular nuclei, deeply basophilic cytoplasm, and prominent cytoplasmic vacuoles. Many background lymphoglandular bodies, frequent mitoses, apoptotic bodies, and tingible body macrophages are often present [67, 68] (Fig. 9.3).

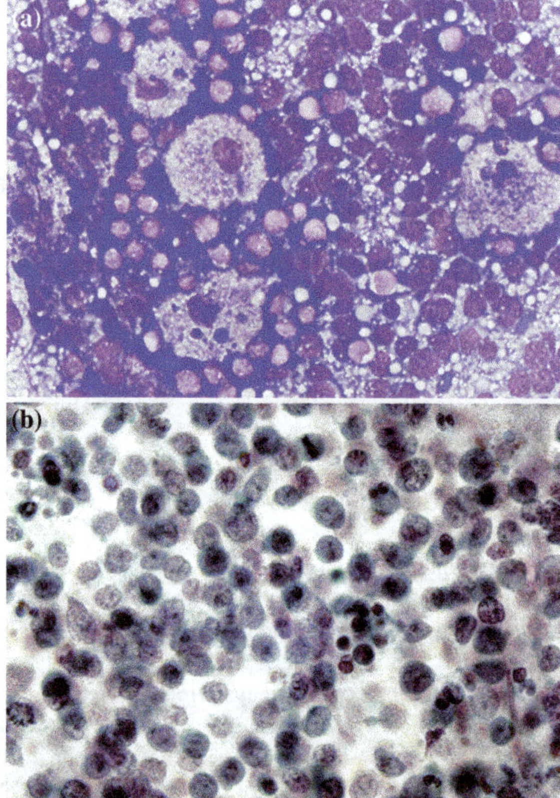

Fig. 9.3 Burkitt lymphoma. The smear shows a monotonous population of medium-sized lymphocytes with round or slightly irregular nuclei, dispersed chromatin, and scant basophilic cytoplasm with multiple cytoplasmic vacuoles. Tingible body macrophages are prominent (**a** Diff-Quick stain, **b** Papanicolaou stain. Magnification: ×600)

Immunophenotype

BL is of germinal center B-cell origin [16, 69]. The neoplastic cells are positive for B-cell-associated antigens as well as CD10 and BCL-6; BCL-2 is negative or only weakly positive [16]. Virtually 100 % of cells are positive for Ki-67. Positivity for EBV is seen in most of the endemic forms, but less frequently in the sporadic or immunodeficiency-associated form [16, 66]. BL is uniformly negative for TdT, which differentiates it from B-lymphoblastic lymphoma.

Molecular Genetics

Virtually all cases of BL have translocation involving the *C-MYC* gene. The most common translocation is t(8;14)(q24;q32) involving the *MYC* gene on chromosome 8 and *IgH* gene on chromosome 14, and less commonly t(2;8)(p12;q24) and t(8,22)(q24;q11) involving the *MYC* gene and *k* light chain gene on chromosome 2 or *λ* light chain gene on chromosome 22 [16] (Table 9.4). FISH analysis for *MYC* gene rearrangement is commonly used to confirm the diagnosis of BL.

9.5.2.7 Diffuse Large B-Cell Lymphoma

Diffuse large B-cell lymphoma (DLBCL) is the most common subtype of B-cell lymphoma and constitutes approximately 37 % of all B cell lymphomas [42, 65]. It is more common in the elderly but may also occur in young adults and children [42, 57, 65]. DLBCL usually arises de novo; some cases may represent progression or transformation of low-grade lymphoma, such as CLL/SLL (Richter's syndrome), FL, MZL or nodular lymphocyte predominant HL (NLPHL) [16, 46, 48, 70, 71]. Both nodal and extranodal sites are commonly involved.

DLBCL is a heterogeneous group of lymphoma in terms of clinical, morphologic and genetic features. A number of clinicopathologically distinct subtypes are recognized, such as T cell/histiocyte-rich LBCL, primary mediastinal LBCL and EBV positive DLBCL of the elderly (Table 9.1). Primary mediastinal large B-cell lymphoma occurs more frequently in young adult females and presents as a localized anterior mediastinal mass; the clinical outcome is better than other DLBCL. A few subtypes of large B-cell lymphoma primarily occur in HIV-infected individuals, such as plasmablastic lymphoma and primary effusion lymphoma.

Cytomorphology

FNA smears of DLBCL usually show numerous abnormal lymphoid cells with nuclear size more than twice the size of normal lymphocytes. The neoplastic lymphocytes may show variable morphology including centroblastic, immunoblastic, or highly pleomorphic. Reed-Sternberg-like cells may also be present. The differential diagnosis of DLBCL includes anaplastic large cell lymphoma (ALCL), HL, as well as non-hematopoietic neoplasms such as carcinoma and melanoma [17, 21].

Several subtypes of DLBCL may potentially be overlooked or misinterpreted in FNA specimens. For example, in T cell/histiocyte-rich LBCL and lymphomatoid granulomatosis, the large neoplastic cells may be obscured by abundant reactive lymphocytes and histiocytes; the Reed-Sternberg-like cells in DLBCL may be a source of confusion with HL [72–75].

Primary mediastinal LBCL have a wide range of cytomorphology. The so-called "compartmentalizing alveolar fibrosis" created by delicate interstitial fibrosis in tissue section cannot be appreciated on FNA specimens.

Plasmablastic lymphoma presents most frequently in the oral cavity; it may also occur in other extranodal sites [16, 76]. The neoplastic cells resemble immunoblasts or plasmablasts. Primary effusion lymphoma typically presents as serous effusion without an identifiable tumor mass; rare cases may present as solid tumor in the extra-cavitary sites without an associated effusion [77, 78]. The neoplastic cells often exhibit large, immunoblastic, plasmablastic, or anaplastic morphology with a variable degree of plasmacytic differentiation (Fig. 9.4).

Immunophenotype

DLBCLs usually express pan B-cell antigens (CD19, CD20, CD22, and CD79a), but negative staining for one or more of these antigens may occur [16]. Restricted expression of surface immunogloulin light chain can be demonstrated by flow cytometry in most, but not all cases. It is important to realize that a negative flow cytometric result does not exclude a diagnosis of DLBCL since the fragility and relative small quantity of the neoplastic cells may lead to a false negative result [19]. In addition, immunohistochemical stain for cyclin D1 should be performed in CD5-positive large cell lymphoma to rule out blastoid or pleomorphic variant of MCL. Rarely the CD5-positive large B-cell lymphomas may represent Richter's transformation of CLL/SLL.

Immunohistochemical stains for CD10, BCL-6, and MUM-1 are utilized to divide DLBCL into two prognostic groups: germinal center B-cell-like (GCB; favorable prognosis) and non-germinal center B-cell-like (non-GCB; unfavorable prognosis) [79].

Primary mediastinal LBCL expresses B-cell antigens but lack the expression of surface immunoglobulins. Approximately 80 % of the cases are positive for CD30. MUM-1 and CD23 are frequently positive, and CD10 expression is less common.

The immunophenotype of plasmablastic lymphomas and primary effusion lymphomas can be confusing because they often lack the expression of B-cell antigens but exhibit a plasma cell phenotype [16]. Neither of the two lymphomas expresses surface immunoglobulins, resulting in a negative staining of surface κ and λ by flow cytometry. The cytoplasmic κ or λ can be detected by immunohistochemistry in 50–70 % of plasmablastic lymphoma but none of the primary

Fig. 9.4 Primary effusion lymphoma. **a** The cytospin of an ascitic fluid sample from a HIV+ patient shows discohesive, large lymphoid cells with plasmablastic or anaplastic appearance. These cells have bizarre nuclei, multiple prominent nucleoli, and abundant deeply basophilic cytoplasm. Some cells show perinuclear clearing, consistent with plasmacytic differentiation (Diff-Quick stain, magnification: x1000). **b** Immunohistochemical stain for human herpesvirus-8 (HHV-8)-encoded latency-associated nuclear antigen (LANA) shows positive, stippled nuclear staining (Magnification: ×1000)

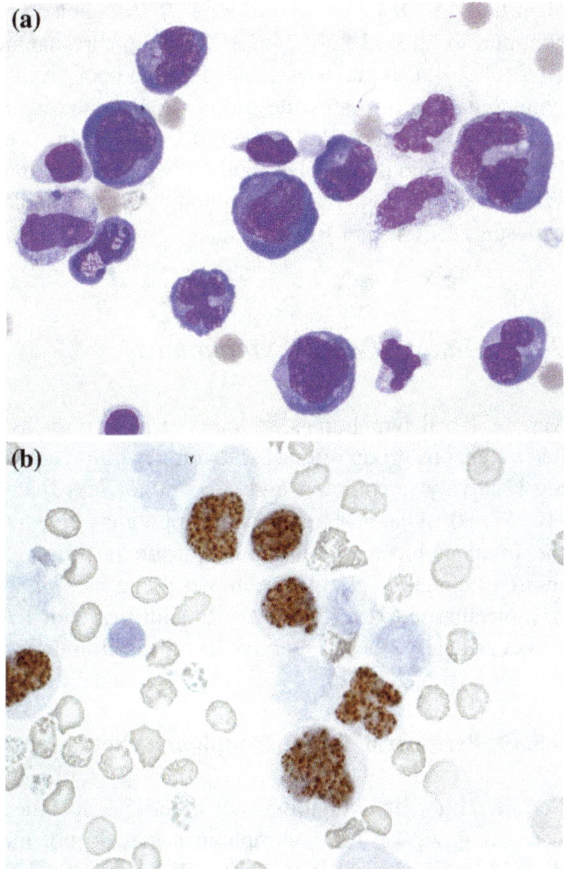

effusion lymphomas. In addition, plasmablastic lymphomas are universally positive for EBV and negative for human herpesvirus-8 (HHV-8), whereas primary effusion lymphomas are universally positive for HHV8 and often co-infected with EBV. Thus, immunohistochemical staining for HHV8-encoded latency-associated nuclear antigen (LANA) is helpful for the diagnosis of primary effusion lymphoma and differentiate it from other DLBCLs (Fig. 9.4). Knowledge of the patient's clinical history and presentation often serves as an initial alert to the diagnosis of the two HIV-associated LBCLs.

Molecular Genetics

Molecular analysis for *IgH* gene rearrangement may provide additional evidence for the diagnosis of certain subtypes of DLBCL, such as T cell/histiocyte-rich LBCL and lymphomatoid granulomatosis. No specific genetic abnormalities are identified in DLBCL. *BCL-6* and *BCL-2* gene rearrangements are relatively common in DLBCL, NOS; *C-MYC* gene rearrangement occurs in approximately 10 % of the cases and is associated with a poor prognosis. A small group of B-cell lymphoma demonstrates the morphologic features of both DLBCL and BL, and carry *C-MYC* and/or *BCL-2* gene rearrangement. These aggressive "gray-zone" lymphomas should be classified into the new provisional entity in the current WHO classification: B-cell lymphoma, unclassifiable, with features intermediate between DLBCL and BL.

9.5.3 *Mature T-Cell Lymphomas*

Mature T-cell lymphomas are derived from post-thymic T cells, and comprise a heterogeneous group of diseases with generally aggressive clinical behavior. They are relatively uncommon and account for less than 15 % of all NHL in adults [16, 57, 80]. Diagnosis of T-cell lymphomas is generally challenging because of the frequent presence of non-neoplastic inflammatory cells, difficulty in determining "clonality" by flow cytometry and lack of specific immunohistochemical or molecular markers [5, 17, 21]. In addition, clonal *TCR* gene rearrangement may be occasionally seen in reactive T-cell proliferation [36, 39].

9.5.3.1 Peripheral T-Cell Lymphoma, Not Otherwise Specified

Peripheral T-cell lymphoma, not otherwise specified (PTCL, NOS) is a heterogeneous group of T-cell lymphomas that do not meet the criteria for the well-defined specific subtypes of T-cell lymphoma. These lymphomas constitute approximately 25–30 % of all PTCLs in Western countries. Most patients are adults and present with generalized lymphadenopathy and systemic B symptoms [80, 81].

Cytomorphology

PTCL, NOS, can show wide variation in cytological features with regard to the proportion of the neoplastic cells to the background non-neoplastic inflammatory cells as well as the degree of atypia of the neoplastic cells [17, 21]. The lymphoma cells may range from small cells indistinguishable from benign lymphocytes to large and highly pleomorphic cells resembling poorly differentiated carcinoma or sarcoma. FNA diagnosis of PTCL with marked inflammatory background can be difficult. When the lymphoma cells exhibit overt malignant features, differential diagnosis often includes B-cell lymphoma, HL or non-hematopoietic neoplasms.

Immunophenotype

Flow cytometric analysis is less helpful in the diagnosis of PTCL as discussed previously. PTCLs usually demonstrate an aberrant T-cell phenotype that is most commonly characterized by lost or decreased expression of CD5 or CD7. However, these atypical phenotypes may occasionally be present in a reactive process.

Molecular Genetics

A clonal *TCR* gene rearrangement is usually, but not always, detected. The majority cases of PTCL, NOS, have cytogenetic abnormalities, but none of them is specific.

9.5.3.2 Anaplastic Large Cell Lymphoma

Anaplastic large cell lymphoma (ALCL), anaplastic lymphoma kinase (ALK)-positive accounts for 10–20 % of childhood lymphomas and 3 % of adult NHL [82]. ALK-negative ALCL tends to occur in older individuals. ALK-positive ALCL has a favorable prognosis compared to ALK-negative ALCL [16, 82–84].

Cytomorphology

FNA smears of ALCL show large pleomorphic cells with convoluted nuclei, prominent nucleoli and abundant cytoplasm. The "hallmark" cells that contain eccentric, kidney-shaped nuclei and abundant amphophilic cytoplasm are often loosely dispersed. The "doughnut" cells (tumor cells containing multilobated nuclei) and multinucleated giant cells with a wreath-like arrangement of nuclei are occasionally found [17, 85]. ALCL shows a broad morphologic spectrum, and approximately 20 % of cases demonstrate atypical morphology such as small cell variant, lymphohistiocytic variant, and Hodgkin-like variant [85–87]. Owing to the diverse morphologic features, the differential diagnosis is often broad and includes DLBCL, HL and non-hematopoietic tumors such as poorly differentiated carcinoma or sarcoma.

Immunophenotype

The tumor cells of ALCL are variably positive for CD45 and T-cell associated antigens, most commonly CD4 and CD2; CD3 is positive in only about 25% of the cases [88, 89]. ALCLs are universally positive for CD30 with strong membranous and Golgi zone staining. By definition, ALK-positive ALCLs are positive for ALK.

ALK-negative ALCL is defined as a CD30-positive T-cell lymphoma morphologically indistinguishable from ALK-positive ALCL. Assessment of a combination of T-cell markers, CD3, CD2, CD5, CD4, and CD7, is important in documenting the T-cell lineage of the neoplastic cells. In addition, the majority of ALCLs are positive for EMA and cytotoxic associated antigens (TIA-1, granzyme B, and/or perforin) [90, 91]. Immunohistochemical stains for these antigens help differentiate ALK-negative ALCL from classical HL (CHL).

Genetic Features

The *TCR* genes are clonally rearranged in 90 % of ALCL. The most specific genetic marker for ALK-positive ALCL is the rearrangement involving *ALK* gene on chromosome 2p23. The most frequent translocation, t(2;5)(p23;q35), involves *ALK* gene and the nucleophosmin (*NPM*) gene on chromosome 5 [16, 82, 83]. Various translocations involving other partner genes also occur. The *ALK* gene rearrangement can be detected by conventional cytogenetics, RT-PCR or interphase FISH analysis [16, 82, 92].

9.5.3.3 Angioimmunoblastic T-Cell Lymphoma

Angioimmunoblastic T-cell lymphoma (AITL) accounts for approximately 15–20 % of all PTCL [81]. AITL is derived from a unique T-cell subset in the germinal center, CD4-positive follicular helper T-cells [16, 93, 94]. Patients with AITL often present with generalized lymphadenopathy, hepatosplenomegaly and systemic symptoms. A pruritic skin rash is common. Clinical features associated with dysregulated immune response are frequently present and include polyclonal hypergammaglobulinemia, positive Coombs' test, positive rheumatoid factor, and circulating immune complex [16, 95–97]. The clinical context is an important consideration in the diagnosis of AITL.

Cytomorphology

FNA diagnosis of AITL is difficult because the cytological features highly mimic those of reactive lymphadenopathy. FNA smears of AITL usually show a polymorphous cell population including small lymphocytes, immunoblasts, plasma cells, eosinophils, and histiocytes; lymphoid tissue fragments containing a scaffold of arborizing small vessels may also be present [98]. In some cases, Reed-Sternberg-like reactive B cells may be present and simulate HL. A definitive diagnosis of AITL should be made on a tissue biopsy sample. However, knowing the cellular composition may help to raise a suspicion for this entity in FNA specimens [98].

Immunophenotype

Similar to its normal counterpart (germinal center T helper cells), AITL expresses CD10, BCL-6, PD-1 and CXCL13 [16, 93, 94, 99, 100]. CD21 staining may demonstrate expanded follicular dendritic cell meshworks. In addition, EBV is positive in approximately 75 % of the cases [16]. However, these features are best appreciated in the tissue biopsy specimens.

Molecular Genetics

Clonal *TCR* gene rearrangement is present in 75–90 % of AITLs [16, 101]. Interestingly, clonal *IgH* gene rearrangement is found in over 30 % of cases, which is likely secondary to the expanded EBV-positive B-cell clones [101]. Many genetic abnormalities have been identified in AILT, but none of them is specific for this entity.

9.5.4 Hodgkin Lymphoma

Hodgkin lymphoma (HL) accounts for approximately 30 % of all lymphomas [16]. It is classified into two major categories: nodular lymphocyte predominant Hodgkin lymphoma (NLPHL) and classical Hodgkin lymphoma (CHL). These two categories differ in clinical features, morphology and immunophenotype [16, 102–105]. CHLs are further subclassified into four subtypes: nodular sclerosis, mixed cellularity, lymphocyte-rich and lymphocyte-depleted. These subtypes of CHL share the same immunophenotype but differ in the clinical features, morphology and frequency of EBV positivity [16]. NLPHL predominantly involves young male patients, and usually presents as localized peripheral lymphadenopathy. CHL has a bimodal age distribution, and often involves cervical lymph nodes and mediastinum. The prognosis of patients with NLPHL is generally good, but multiple relapses do occur. Progression to large B-cell lymphoma has been reported in 3–5 % of cases of NLPHL [16, 70, 102–106].

9.5.4.1 Cytomorphology

FNA smears show a small number of large neoplastic cells in a background of polymorphous inflammatory cells including small lymphocytes, variable numbers of eosinophils, neutrophils, plasma cells and histiocytes. The large neoplastic cells may be mononucleated (Hodgkin cells), or bi-lobed or multilobated (Reed-Sternberg cells) with prominent nucleoli and abundant cytoplasm (Fig. 9.5).

Fig. 9.5 Hodgkin
lymphoma. The smear shows
the presence of
mononucleated Hodgkin cells
in a background of small
lymphocytes, neutrophils,
and eosinophils. Typical
Reed-Sternberg cells are also
present and show bilobed
nuclei with prominent
nucleoli (*inset*) (Wright-
Giemsa stain, magnification:
×600)

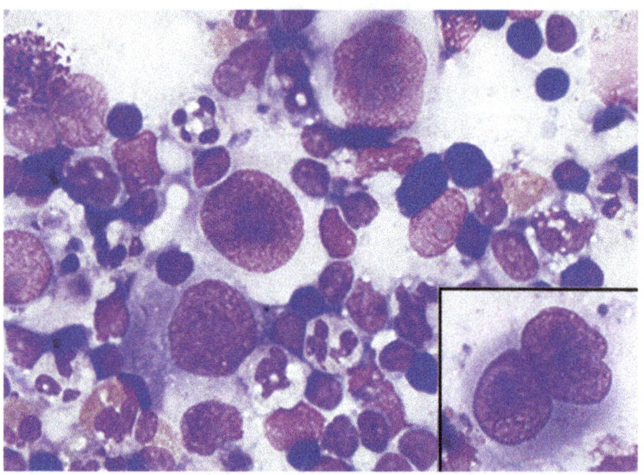

It is possible to make a diagnosis of HL on FNA smears especially for recurrent HL. However, a primary diagnosis and subclassification of HL requires a tissue biopsy [13, 17, 21, 72, 107].

9.5.4.2 Immunophenotype

The neoplastic large cells in NLPHL are positive for CD45, CD20, and CD79a, and negative for both CD30 and CD15; rare cases may show weak CD30 staining. Immunohistochemical stains for CD3, CD57, or PD-1 often show rimming of positive T cells around the large neoplastic cells. In contrast to NLPHL, the neoplastic cells in CHL are negative for CD45, but positive for CD30 (100 %) and CD15 (75–80 %). The majority of CHLs are weakly positive for PAX-5, and up to 40 % of cases show positive CD20 staining in a subset of neoplastic cells with varied intensity [16]. Positive staining for PAX-5 is important to document the B-cell lineage of CHL and differentiate it from T-cell lymphomas such as ALCL. In addition, EBV is positive in a subset of CHL, most frequently in the mixed cellularity subtype (75 %).

9.5.4.3 Molecular Genetics

HL is of B-cell lineage; however, clonal *IgH* gene rearrangement can only be detected in the DNA isolated from neoplastic cells but not from the whole tissue [16]. No recurrent or specific genetic abnormalities are identified in HL.

9.6 Summary

FNA is a simple, safe, and an inexpensive sampling technique that plays an important role in the evaluation of lymphadenopathy. The key to enhancing the accuracy of FNA diagnosis of lymphoma is the multiparameter approach in which the cytomorphologic features are evaluated in correlation with the results of ancillary studies and clinical context. A full understanding of the current lymphoma classification, clinical features associated with each lymphoma subtype and the impact of the diagnosis on patient management is essential in FNA diagnosis of lymphoma. It is also important to recognize the limitations of FNA in the primary diagnosis of some subtypes of lymphoma, and tissue biopsy should be recommended for a definitive diagnosis and subclassification in such cases.

References

1. Buley ID (1998) Fine needle aspiration of lymph nodes. J Clin Pathol 51:881–885
2. Serrano Egea A, Martinez Gonzalez MA, Perez Barrios A, Alberti Masgrau N, de Agustin P (2002) Usefulness of light microscopy in lymph node fine needle aspiration biopsy. Acta Cytol 46:364–368
3. Nasuti JF, Yu G, Boudousquie A, Gupta P (2000) Diagnostic value of lymph node fine needle aspiration cytology: an institutional experience of 387 cases observed over a 5-year period. Cytopathology 11:18–31
4. Kardos TF, Maygarden SJ, Blumberg AK, Wakely PE Jr, Frable WJ (1989) Fine needle aspiration biopsy in the management of children and young adults with peripheral lymphadenopathy. Cancer 63:703–707
5. Sandhaus LM (2000) Fine-needle aspiration cytology in the diagnosis of lymphoma. The next step. Am J Clin Pathol 113:623–627
6. Nakahara O, Yamao K, Bhatia V et al (2009) Usefulness of endoscopic ultrasound-guided fine needle aspiration (EUS-FNA) for undiagnosed intra-abdominal lymphadenopathy. J Gastroenterol 44:562–567
7. Catalano MF, Nayar R, Gress F et al (2002) EUS-guided fine needle aspiration in mediastinal lymphadenopathy of unknown etiology. Gastrointest Endosc 55:863–869
8. Hayder S, Das DK, Bjork O, Lowhagen T (1988) Fine needle aspiration cytology (FNAC) of the testes in childhood acute lymphoblastic leukemia and non-Hodgkin's lymphoma: preliminary report. Pediatr Hematol Oncol 5:29–34
9. de Almeida MM, Chagas M, de Sousa JV, Mendonca ME (1994) Fine-needle aspiration cytology as a tool for the early detection of testicular relapse of acute lymphoblastic leukemia in children. Diagn Cytopathol 10:44–46
10. Russell J, Orell S, Skinner J, Seshadri R (1983) Fine needle aspiration cytology in the management of lymphoma. Aust N Z J Med 13:365–368
11. Hehn ST, Grogan TM, Miller TP (2004) Utility of fine-needle aspiration as a diagnostic technique in lymphoma. J Clin Oncol 22:3046–3052
12. Landgren O, Porwit MacDonald A, Tani E et al (2004) A prospective comparison of fine-needle aspiration cytology and histopathology in the diagnosis and classification of lymphomas. Hematol J 5:69–76
13. Tarantino DR, McHenry CR, Strickland T, Khiyami A (1998) The role of fine-needle aspiration biopsy and flow cytometry in the evaluation of persistent neck adenopathy. Am J Surg 176:413–417

14. Wakely PE Jr (2000) Fine-needle aspiration cytopathology in diagnosis and classification of malignant lymphoma: accurate and reliable? Diagn Cytopathol 22:120–125
15. Das DK (1999) Value and limitations of fine-needle aspiration cytology in diagnosis and classification of lymphomas: a review. Diagn Cytopathol 21:240–249
16. Swerdlow SH CE, Harrie NL, Jaffe ES, Pileri SA, Stein H, Thiele J, Vardiman JW (2008) WHO classification of tumours of Haematopoietic and lymphoid tissues. IARC, Lyon
17. Caraway NP (2005) Strategies to diagnose lymphoproliferative disorders by fine-needle aspiration by using ancillary studies. Cancer 105:432–442
18. Dey P (2006) Role of ancillary techniques in diagnosing and subclassifying non-Hodgkin's lymphomas on fine needle aspiration cytology. Cytopathology 17:275–287
19. Verstovsek G, Chakraborty S, Ramzy I, Jorgensen JL (2002) Large B-cell lymphomas: fine-needle aspiration plays an important role in initial diagnosis of cases which are falsely negative by flow cytometry. Diagn Cytopathol 27:282–285
20. Kocjan G (2005) Best Practice No 185. Cytological and molecular diagnosis of lymphoma. J Clin Pathol 58:561–567
21. Young NA, Al-Saleem T (1999) Diagnosis of lymphoma by fine-needle aspiration cytology using the revised European-American classification of lymphoid neoplasms. Cancer 87:325–345
22. Barroca H, Marques C, Candeias J (2008) Fine needle aspiration cytology diagnosis, flow cytometry immunophenotyping and histology in clinically suspected lymphoproliferative disorder: a comparative study. Acta Cytol 52:124–132
23. Bangerter M, Brudler O, Heinrich B, Griesshamnuer M (2007) Fine needle aspiration cytology and flow cytometry in the diagnosis and subclassification of non-Hodgkin's lymphoma based on the World Health Organization classification. Acta Cytol 51:390–398
24. Mathiot C, Decaudin D, Klijanienko J et al (2006) Fine-needle aspiration cytology combined with flow cytometry immunophenotyping is a rapid and accurate approach for the evaluation of suspicious superficial lymphoid lesions. Diagn Cytopathol 34:472–478
25. Liu K, Stern RC, Rogers RT, Dodd LG, Mann KP (2001) Diagnosis of hematopoietic processes by fine-needle aspiration in conjunction with flow cytometry: a review of 127 cases. Diagn Cytopathol 24:1–10
26. Meda BA, Buss DH, Woodruff RD et al (2000) Diagnosis and subclassification of primary and recurrent lymphoma. The usefulness and limitations of combined fine-needle aspiration cytomorphology and flow cytometry. Am J Clin Pathol 113:688–699
27. Monaco SE, Teot LA, Felgar RE, Surti U, Cai G (2009) Fluorescence in situ hybridization studies on direct smears: an approach to enhance the fine-needle aspiration biopsy diagnosis of B-cell non-Hodgkin lymphomas. Cancer Cytopathol 117:338–348
28. Al-Haddad M, Savabi MS, Sherman S et al (2009) Role of endoscopic ultrasound-guided fine-needle aspiration with flow cytometry to diagnose lymphoma: a single center experience. J Gastroenterol Hepatol 24:1826–1833
29. Geisinger KR, Stanley MW, Raab SS, Silverman JF, Abati A (2003) Modern cytopathology. Churchill Livingstone, Philadelphia
30. Caraway NP, Gu J, Lin P, Romaguera JE, Glassman A, Katz R (2005) The utility of interphase fluorescence in situ hybridization for the detection of the translocation t(11;14)(q13;q32) in the diagnosis of mantle cell lymphoma on fine-needle aspiration specimens. Cancer 105:110–118
31. Gong Y, Caraway N, Gu J et al (2003) Evaluation of interphase fluorescence in situ hybridization for the t(14;18)(q32;q21) translocation in the diagnosis of follicular lymphoma on fine-needle aspirates: a comparison with flow cytometry immunophenotyping. Cancer 99:385–393
32. Gong JZ, Snyder MJ, Lagoo AS et al (2004) Diagnostic impact of core-needle biopsy on fine-needle aspiration of non-Hodgkin lymphoma. Diagn Cytopathol 31:23–30
33. Ho AK, Hill S, Preobrazhensky SN, Miller ME, Chen Z, Bahler DW (2009) Small B-cell neoplasms with typical mantle cell lymphoma immunophenotypes often include chronic lymphocytic leukemias. Am J Clin Pathol 131:27–32

34. Gao J, Peterson L, Nelson B, Goolsby C, Chen YH (2009) Immunophenotypic variations in mantle cell lymphoma. Am J Clin Pathol 132:699–706
35. Beck RC, Stahl S, O'Keefe CL, Maciejewski JP, Theil KS, Hsi ED (2003) Detection of mature T-cell leukemias by flow cytometry using anti-T-cell receptor V beta antibodies. Am J Clin Pathol 120:785–794
36. Collins RD (1997) Is clonality equivalent to malignancy: specifically, is immunoglobulin gene rearrangement diagnostic of malignant lymphoma? Hum Pathol 28:757–759
37. Saxena A, Alport EC, Moshynska O, Kanthan R, Boctor MA (2004) Clonal B cell populations in a minority of patients with Hashimoto's thyroiditis. J Clin Pathol 57:1258–1263
38. Saxena A, Moshynska O, Kanthan R, Bhutani M, Maksymiuk AW, Lukie BE (2000) Distinct B-cell clonal bands in Helicobacter pylori gastritis with lymphoid hyperplasia. J Pathol 190:47–54
39. Witzens M, Mohler T, Willhauck M, Scheibenbogen C, Lee KH, Keilholz U (1997) Detection of clonally rearranged T-cell-receptor gamma chain genes from T-cell malignancies and acute inflammatory rheumatic disease using PCR amplification, PAGE, and automated analysis. Ann Hematol 74:123–130
40. Dunphy CH, Katz RL, Fanning CV, Dalton WT Jr (1989) Leukemic lymphadenopathy: diagnosis by fine needle aspiration. Hematol Pathol 3:35–44
41. Jacobs JC, Katz RL, Shabb N, el-Naggar A, Ordonez NG, Pugh W (1992) Fine needle aspiration of lymphoblastic lymphoma. A multiparameter diagnostic approach. Acta Cytol 36:887–894
42. A clinical evaluation of the International Lymphoma Study Group classification of non-Hodgkin's lymphoma (1997). The Non-Hodgkin's Lymphoma Classification Project. Blood 89:3909–3918
43. Binet JL, Auquier A, Dighiero G et al (1981) A new prognostic classification of chronic lymphocytic leukemia derived from a multivariate survival analysis. Cancer 48:198–206
44. Rai KR, Sawitsky A, Cronkite EP, Chanana AD, Levy RN, Pasternack BS (1975) Clinical staging of chronic lymphocytic leukemia. Blood 46:219–234
45. Hallek M, Cheson BD, Catovsky D et al (2008) Guidelines for the diagnosis and treatment of chronic lymphocytic leukemia: a report from the International Workshop on Chronic Lymphocytic Leukemia updating the National Cancer Institute-Working Group 1996 guidelines. Blood 111:5446–5456
46. Molica S (2010) A systematic review on Richter syndrome: what is the published evidence? Leuk Lymphoma 51:415–421
47. Tsimberidou AM, O'Brien S, Kantarjian HM et al (2006) Hodgkin transformation of chronic lymphocytic leukemia: the M. D. Anderson Cancer Center experience. Cancer 107:1294–1302
48. Tsimberidou AM, Keating MJ (2006) Richter's transformation in chronic lymphocytic leukemia. Semin Oncol 33:250–256
49. Catrina Reading F, Schlette EJ, Stewart JM, Keating MJ, Katz RL, Caraway NP (2007) Fine-needle aspiration biopsy findings in patients with small lymphocytic lymphoma transformed to hodgkin lymphoma. Am J Clin Pathol 128:571–578
50. Caraway NP, Thomas E, Khanna A et al (2008) Chromosomal abnormalities detected by multicolor fluorescence in situ hybridization in fine-needle aspirates from patients with small lymphocytic lymphoma are useful for predicting survival. Cancer 114:315–322
51. Young NA (2006) Grading follicular lymphoma on fine-needle aspiration specimens–a practical approach. Cancer 108:1–9
52. Janikova A, Mayer J, Kren L et al (2009) The persistence of t(14;18)-bearing cells in lymph nodes of patients with follicular lymphoma in complete remission: the evidence for 'a lymphoma stem cell'. Leuk Lymphoma 50:1102–1109
53. Bosch F, Lopez-Guillermo A, Campo E et al (1998) Mantle cell lymphoma: presenting features, response to therapy, and prognostic factors. Cancer 82:567–575

54. Yin CC, Medeiros LJ, Cromwell CC et al (2007) Sequence analysis proves clonal identity in five patients with typical and blastoid mantle cell lymphoma. Mod Pathol 20:1–7

55. Laszlo T, Matolcsy A (1999) Blastic transformation of mantle cell lymphoma: genetic evidence for a clonal link between the two stages of the tumour. Histopathology 35:355–359

56. Norton AJ, Matthews J, Pappa V et al (1995) Mantle cell lymphoma: natural history defined in a serially biopsied population over a 20-year period. Ann Oncol 6:249–256

57. Armitage JO, Weisenburger DD (1998) New approach to classifying non-Hodgkin's lymphomas: clinical features of the major histologic subtypes. Non-Hodgkin's Lymphoma Classification Project. J Clin Oncol 16:2780–2795

58. Nathwani BN, Anderson JR, Armitage JO et al (1999) Marginal zone B-cell lymphoma: a clinical comparison of nodal and mucosa-associated lymphoid tissue types. Non-Hodgkin's Lymphoma Classification Project. J Clin Oncol 17:2486–2492

59. Berger F, Felman P, Thieblemont C et al (2000) Non-MALT marginal zone B-cell lymphomas: a description of clinical presentation and outcome in 124 patients. Blood 95:1950–1956

60. Arcaini L, Paulli M, Burcheri S et al (2007) Primary nodal marginal zone B-cell lymphoma: clinical features and prognostic assessment of a rare disease. Br J Haematol 136:301–304

61. Kaba S, Hirokawa M, Kuma S et al (2009) Cytologic findings of primary thyroid MALT lymphoma with extreme plasma cell differentiation: FNA cytology of two cases. Diagn Cytopathol 37:815–819

62. Remstein ED, Dogan A, Einerson RR et al (2006) The incidence and anatomic site specificity of chromosomal translocations in primary extranodal marginal zone B-cell lymphoma of mucosa-associated lymphoid tissue (MALT lymphoma) in North America. Am J Surg Pathol 30:1546–1553

63. Watkins AJ, Huang Y, Ye H et al (2009) Splenic marginal zone lymphoma: characterization of 7q deletion and its value in diagnosis. J Pathol 220:461–474

64. Pangalis GA, Angelopoulou MK, Vassilakopoulos TP, Siakantaris MP, Kittas C (1999) B-chronic lymphocytic leukemia, small lymphocytic lymphoma, and lymphoplasmacytic lymphoma, including Waldenstrom's macroglobulinemia: a clinical, morphologic, and biologic spectrum of similar disorders. Semin Hematol 36:104–114

65. Morton LM, Wang SS, Devesa SS, Hartge P, Weisenburger DD, Linet MS (2006) Lymphoma incidence patterns by WHO subtype in the United States, 1992–2001. Blood 107:265–276

66. Blum KA, Lozanski G, Byrd JC (2004) Adult Burkitt leukemia and lymphoma. Blood 104:3009–3020

67. Das DK, Gupta SK, Pathak IC, Sharma SC, Datta BN (1987) Burkitt-type lymphoma. Diagnosis by fine needle aspiration cytology. Acta Cytol 31:1–7

68. Stastny JF, Almeida MM, Wakely PE Jr, Kornstein MJ, Frable WJ (1995) Fine-needle aspiration biopsy and imprint cytology of small non-cleaved cell (Burkitt's) lymphoma. Diagn Cytopathol 12:201–207

69. Bellan C, Lazzi S, Hummel M et al (2005) Immunoglobulin gene analysis reveals 2 distinct cells of origin for EBV-positive and EBV-negative Burkitt lymphomas. Blood 106:1031–1036

70. Chittal SM, Alard C, Rossi JF et al (1990) Further phenotypic evidence that nodular, lymphocyte-predominant Hodgkin's disease is a large B-cell lymphoma in evolution. Am J Surg Pathol 14:1024–1035

71. Miettinen M, Franssila KO, Saxen E (1983) Hodgkin's disease, lymphocytic predominance nodular. Increased risk for subsequent non-Hodgkin's lymphomas. Cancer 51:2293–2300

72. Mayall F, Darlington A, Harrison B (2003) Fine needle aspiration cytology in the diagnosis of uncommon types of lymphoma. J Clin Pathol 56:821–825

73. Shahabuddin MD, Raghuveer CV (2003) Reed-Sternberg-like cells in T-cell rich B-cell lymphoma: a diagnostic dilemma. Indian J Pathol Microbiol 46:55–56

74. Tani E, Johansson B, Skoog L (1998) T-cell-rich B-cell lymphoma: fine-needle aspiration cytology and immunocytochemistry. Diagn Cytopathol 18:1–4

75. Galindo LM, Havlioglu N, Grosso LE (1996) Cytologic findings in a case of T-cell rich B-cell lymphoma: potential diagnostic pitfall in FNA of lymph nodes. Diagn Cytopathol 14:253–257; discussion 7–8

76. Delecluse HJ, Anagnostopoulos I, Dallenbach F et al (1997) Plasmablastic lymphomas of the oral cavity: a new entity associated with the human immunodeficiency virus infection. Blood 89:1413–1420

77. Nador RG, Cesarman E, Chadburn A et al (1996) Primary effusion lymphoma: a distinct clinicopathologic entity associated with the Kaposi's sarcoma-associated herpes virus. Blood 88:645–656

78. Chadburn A, Hyjek E, Mathew S, Cesarman E, Said J, Knowles DM (2004) KSHV-positive solid lymphomas represent an extra-cavitary variant of primary effusion lymphoma. Am J Surg Pathol 28:1401–1416

79. Hans CP, Weisenburger DD, Greiner TC et al (2004) Confirmation of the molecular classification of diffuse large B-cell lymphoma by immunohistochemistry using a tissue microarray. Blood 103:275–282

80. Rizvi MA, Evens AM, Tallman MS, Nelson BP, Rosen ST (2006) T-cell non-Hodgkin lymphoma. Blood 107:1255–1264

81. Vose J, Armitage J, Weisenburger D (2008) International peripheral T-cell and natural killer/T-cell lymphoma study: pathology findings and clinical outcomes. J Clin Oncol 26:4124–4130

82. Stein H, Foss HD, Durkop H et al (2000) CD30(+) anaplastic large cell lymphoma: a review of its histopathologic, genetic, and clinical features. Blood 96:3681–3695

83. Falini B (2001) Anaplastic large cell lymphoma: pathological, molecular and clinical features. Br J Haematol 114:741–760

84. Gascoyne RD, Aoun P, Wu D et al (1999) Prognostic significance of anaplastic lymphoma kinase (ALK) protein expression in adults with anaplastic large cell lymphoma. Blood 93:3913–3921

85. Ng WK, Ip P, Choy C, Collins RJ (2003) Cytologic and immunocytochemical findings of anaplastic large cell lymphoma: analysis of ten fine-needle aspiration specimens over a 9-year period. Cancer 99:33–43

86. Kim SE, Kim SH, Lim BJ, Hong SW, Yang WI (2004) Fine needle aspiration cytology of small cell variant of anaplastic large cell lymphoma. A case report. Acta Cytol 48:254–258

87. Aljajeh IA, Das DK, Krajci D (1995) Ki-1-positive anaplastic large cell lymphoma initially diagnosed as Hodgkin's disease by fine needle aspiration (FNA) cytology. Cytopathology 6:226–235

88. Juco J, Holden JT, Mann KP, Kelley LG, Li S (2003) Immunophenotypic analysis of anaplastic large cell lymphoma by flow cytometry. Am J Clin Pathol 119:205–212

89. Muzzafar T, Wei EX, Lin P, Medeiros LJ, Jorgensen JL (2009) Flow cytometric immunophenotyping of anaplastic large cell lymphoma. Arch Pathol Lab Med 133:49–56

90. Foss HD, Demel G, Anagnostopoulos I, Araujo I, Hummel M, Stein H (1997) Uniform expression of cytotoxic molecules in anaplastic large cell lymphoma of null/T cell phenotype and in cell lines derived from anaplastic large cell lymphoma. Pathobiology 65:83–90

91. Krenacs L, Wellmann A, Sorbara L et al (1997) Cytotoxic cell antigen expression in anaplastic large cell lymphomas of T- and null-cell type and Hodgkin's disease: evidence for distinct cellular origin. Blood 89:980–989

92. Shin HJ, Thorson P, Gu J, Katz RL (2003) Detection of a subset of CD30+ anaplastic large cell lymphoma by interphase fluorescence in situ hybridization. Diagn Cytopathol 29:61–66

93. Krenacs L, Schaerli P, Kis G, Bagdi E (2006) Phenotype of neoplastic cells in angioimmunoblastic T-cell lymphoma is consistent with activated follicular B helper T cells. Blood 108:1110–1111

94. de Leval L, Rickman DS, Thielen C et al (2007) The gene expression profile of nodal peripheral T-cell lymphoma demonstrates a molecular link between angioimmunoblastic T-cell lymphoma (AITL) and follicular helper T (TFH) cells. Blood 109:4952–4963

95. Mourad N, Mounier N, Briere J et al (2008) Clinical, biologic, and pathologic features in 157 patients with angioimmunoblastic T-cell lymphoma treated within the Groupe d'Etude des Lymphomes de l'Adulte (GELA) trials. Blood 111:4463–4470

96. Park BB, Ryoo BY, Lee JH et al (2007) Clinical features and treatment outcomes of angioimmunoblastic T-cell lymphoma. Leuk Lymphoma 48:716–722

97. Dogan A, Ngu LS, Ng SH, Cervi PL (2005) Pathology and clinical features of angioimmunoblastic T-cell lymphoma after successful treatment with thalidomide. Leukemia 19:873–875

98. Ng WK, Ip P, Choy C, Collins RJ (2002) Cytologic findings of angioimmunoblastic T-cell lymphoma: analysis of 16 fine-needle aspirates over 9-year period. Cancer 96:166–173

99. Rodriguez-Pinilla SM, Atienza L, Murillo C et al (2008) Peripheral T-cell lymphoma with follicular T-cell markers. Am J Surg Pathol 32:1787–1799

100. Yu H, Shahsafaei A, Dorfman DM (2009) Germinal-center T-helper-cell markers PD-1 and CXCL13 are both expressed by neoplastic cells in angioimmunoblastic T-cell lymphoma. Am J Clin Pathol 131:33–41

101. Tan BT, Warnke RA, Arber DA (2006) The frequency of B- and T-cell gene rearrangements and epstein-barr virus in T-cell lymphomas: a comparison between angioimmunoblastic T-cell lymphoma and peripheral T-cell lymphoma, unspecified with and without associated B-cell proliferations. J Mol Diagn 8:466–475; quiz 527

102. Diehl V, Sextro M, Franklin J et al (1999) Clinical presentation, course, and prognostic factors in lymphocyte-predominant Hodgkin's disease and lymphocyte-rich classical Hodgkin's disease: report from the European Task Force on Lymphoma Project on Lymphocyte-Predominant Hodgkin's Disease. J Clin Oncol 17:776–783

103. Anagnostopoulos I, Hansmann ML, Franssila K et al (2000) European Task Force on Lymphoma project on lymphocyte predominance Hodgkin disease: histologic and immunohistologic analysis of submitted cases reveals 2 types of Hodgkin disease with a nodular growth pattern and abundant lymphocytes. Blood 96:1889–1899

104. Nogova L, Reineke T, Josting A et al (2005) Lymphocyte-predominant and classical Hodgkin's lymphoma–comparison of outcomes. Eur J Haematol Suppl 75:106–110

105. Biasoli I, Stamatoullas A, Meignin V et al (2010) Nodular, lymphocyte-predominant Hodgkin lymphoma: a long-term study and analysis of transformation to diffuse large B-cell lymphoma in a cohort of 164 patients from the Adult Lymphoma Study Group. Cancer 116:631–639

106. Huang JZ, Weisenburger DD, Vose JM et al (2004) Diffuse large B-cell lymphoma arising in nodular lymphocyte predominant Hodgkin lymphoma: a report of 21 cases from the Nebraska Lymphoma Study Group. Leuk Lymphoma 45:1551–1557

107. Das DK, Francis IM, Sharma PN et al (2009) Hodgkin's lymphoma: diagnostic difficulties in fine-needle aspiration cytology. Diagn Cytopathol 37:564–573

Chapter 10
Female Genital Tract

Rosemary Tambouret

10.1 Cervix

10.1.1 Epidemiology of Cervical Cancer

Almost all cervical cancers are associated with persistent infection with high risk human papillomavirus (hrHPV), however, HPV infection is vastly more common than cervical cancer. The lifetime risk of HPV genital infection is high for sexually active women as evidenced by prevalence studies [1, 2]. But of the 40 HPV types known to cause genital infection, less than half are considered high risk, that is, capable of causing a persistent infection with an increased risk of cervical cancer [3]. The majority of hrHPV infections cause low grade cytologic abnormalities that regress spontaneously [4]. The highest risk is associated with hrHPV types 16 and 18 that are associated with 50 and 20 % of cervical cancers, respectively. The estimated number of cases of cervical cancer in the United States in 2012 was 12,170 [5]. According to the population studied, multiple factors influence the epidemiology of cervical cancer including the prevalence of hrHPV, the distribution of the different types of hrHPV, the availability of screening, and treatment for premalignant and malignant lesions of the cervix. The cultural make-up of the population also impacts the rate of cervical cancer in that the number of sexual partners influences the exposure to hrHPV [6]. Finally, in the future, widespread use of HPV vaccines is anticipated to change the prevalence of infection and ultimately, of cervical cancer.

R. Tambouret (✉)
Department of Pathology, Massachusetts General Hospital,
Warren 105/55 Fruit Street, Boston, MA 02114, USA
e-mail: RTAMBOURET@PARTNERS.ORG

R. Nayar (ed.), *Cytopathology in Oncology*,
Cancer Treatment and Research 160, DOI: 10.1007/978-3-642-38850-7_10,
© Springer-Verlag Berlin Heidelberg 2014

10.1.2 Overview of Methods Used to Screen for Cervical Cancer

In many countries, cervical–vaginal cytology (CVC) is the mainstay of cervical cancer screening programs. Approximately, 60 million CVC tests are performed annually in the US [7]. The cytologic method to sample the cervix was first published in a French language medical journal, Presse Medicale, by Babes in 1927, however cervical cytology did not become widely known until publication in the English language in 1934 by George Papanicolaou, after whom the more common name for CVC, the Pap test, is derived [8]. With the institution of Pap test screening programs, the rate of cervical cancer rapidly declined in countries in which it was adopted. Currently, in countries with well established screening programs, more than half of all cases of cervical cancer occur in women who were never screened or who were inadequately screened [9].

However, to this day in many countries the necessary resources to set up screening programs are lacking. For this reason, various international health organizations have promoted other methods for detection of cervical cancer and precursor lesions. The aim is to find a test that is as simple and inexpensive as the Pap test, with similar or superior performance parameters, but which does not demand the highly trained cytotechnologist to read the test. Primary testing for hrHPV is a possibility because of its high sensitivity but the specificity is much lower than that of the Pap test such that many more women would require follow-up testing to identify women with lesions [10]. Also the currently available FDA approved assays for hrHPV testing and/or genotyping are either patented and/or proprietary and thus too expensive for low-resource countries (for example, Digene Hybrid Capture 2, Qiagen, Inc.; Cervista™HPV, Hologic, Inc., Roche's COBAS, Gen-Probe's APTIMA) or although quite inexpensive, are too technically challenging (for example, polymerase chain reaction (PCR) using generic reagents). Until a simplified, accurate, less costly hrHPV test is developed, cytology will remain the most cost effective screening method. Direct visualization of the cervix after application of acetic acid (VIA) has been promoted as a simple test that can be performed by health care workers with little training [11]. If cervical abnormalities are identified, cryotherapy is performed to ablate the transformation zone. One problem with the VIA test is the similarity in appearance of non-precursor inflammatory lesions to cancer precursor lesions (squamous intraepithelial lesions or SIL). Also treatment may distort the cervix such that subsequent examination of the cervix is difficult. Another potential problem is the inadvertent, inadequate treatment of an invasive cancer.

10.2 Cervical Cytology

10.2.1 Collection and Processing

CVC samples are obtained by direct visualization of the cervix after expanding the vagina with a speculum. The goal is to scrap off easily exfoliated cells from the ectocervix, endocervical canal, and the junction between these two regions, the transformation zone, which is the region most susceptible to HPV infection. Sampling devices include the spatula, the brush, and the broom (Fig. 10.1). Wooden or plastic spatulas usually have a double convexity of the tip such that both cervical os and ectocervix can be sampled with a 360° sweep of the cervix; wooden spatulas should not be used with liquid-based preparations. The endocervical sample can be enhanced when the endocervical brush is used to obtain a separate endocervical sample [12]. An abundance of endocervical cells, including large cell groups, is obtained with the friction of the short bristles of the endocervical brush. The brush, introduced into the endocervical canal such that the bristles nearest the examiner are at the level of the external os, is rotated 180°. Use of the endocervical brush before the spatula has been found to be associated with significantly more blood, so order of sampling the endocervix and ectocervix is important. The extended tip spatula has been found to provide optimum samples when used with the endocervical brush [13]. The entire ectocervix and the endocervical canal are sampled simultaneously with the broom, commercially known as the Cervex-brush^{TM} [14]. The bristles on the broom are longest in the center in order to extend into the endocervical canal. The bristles are oriented in such a way that when the device is turned in a clockwise direction, the angled bristles scrape of the superficial epithelial cells. If the broom is turned in a counterclockwise direction, the smooth edge of the bristles will not pick up cells. Cotton swabs should not be used to sample the cervix for cytology because fewer endocervical cells are obtained and SIL is detected less readily [15, 16].

For a conventional smear (CS), the CVC sample is immediately spread as thinly as possible on a glass slide, followed by immediate immersion of the slide in 95 % ethanol or by misting the slide with an ethanol-based spray fixative. The rapid

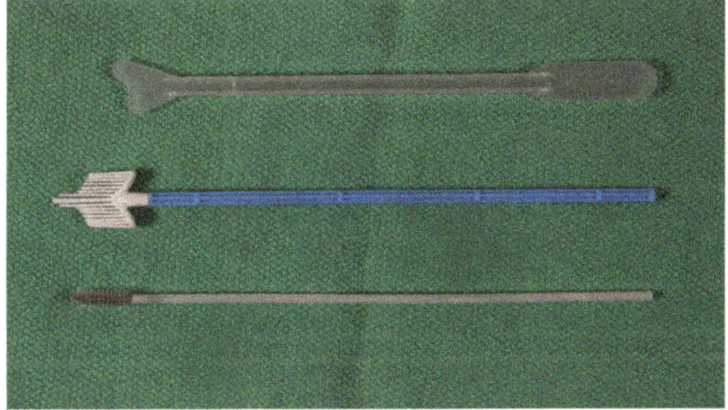

Fig. 10.1 Sampling devices used to obtain cervical-vaginal cytology

fixation is necessary in order to avoid air drying of the cells which leads to distortion of the cellular morphology. Since the late 1990s, an alternative method for preparation of CVC samples, generically known as liquid-based cytology (LBC), has become available. LBC methods were developed in order to facilitate computer assisted screening of cytology slides. Currently in the U.S., two LBC methods are FDA approved: ThinPrep™ (Hologic, Inc) and BD SurePath™ (Becton Dickinson, Inc). Both methods produce a homogenously distributed thin layer of cells restricted to a much smaller area of the slide than the CS (Fig. 10.2). The collection devices for both methods are either a combination of the endo-cervical brush and a plastic spatula or the broom (Cervex-Brush®). ThinPrep (TP) uses a methanol-based fixative into which the collection devices are rinsed and removed. In the case of SurePath (SP), the collection devices have modified scored handles so that the sampling head can be broken off into the ethanol fixative solution to allow for maximum cell recovery by the time the sample is processed. Some clinicians use a combination of the broom and the endocervical brush. This method increases the cost of disposables, but has not been shown to increase cellular yield or to enhance diagnostic utility [17].

Processing of TP entails vortexing to create a uniform suspension of cells followed by vacuum suction of the sample through a fine mesh membrane to which the cells adhere. The cells are transferred by gently pressing the membrane to the glass slide. The SP process entails vortexing and agitation of the sample, followed by centrifugation with a density gradient medium to remove a most of the potentially obscuring erythrocytes and white blood cells. An aliquot of resultant cell pellet is allowed to settle by gravity onto the poly-lysine coated slide.

All CVC samples, both CS and LBC, are stained with the Papanicolaou stain, a mixture of several pigments, designed to provide crisp nuclear staining with hematoxylin and variably colored cytoplasm according to the degree of keratini-zation (Fig. 10.3).

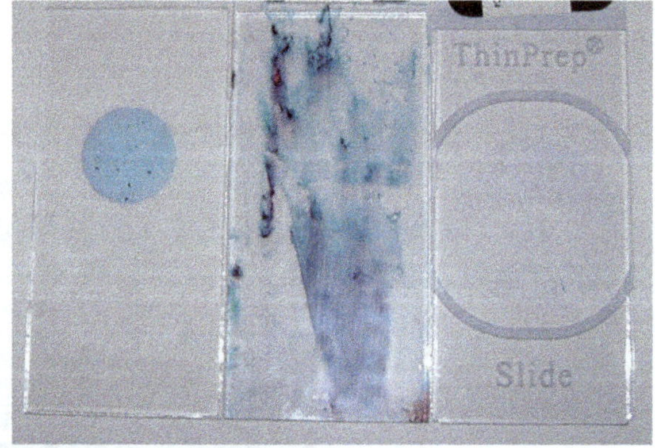

Fig. 10.2 Glass slides from conventional smear, ThinPrep, and SurePrep

Fig. 10.3 Papanicolaou
stained cytology with normal
squamous cells and
endocervical cells designated
as "negative for intra-
epithelial malignancy or
malignancy"

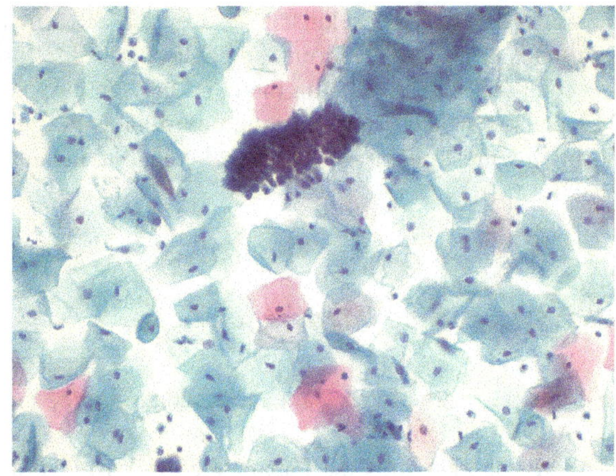

10.2.2 Slide Evaluation and Interpretation

Cervical cytology screening is a high volume test by virtue of the large number of
samples needed to screen the entire adult female population. In most cytology labs,
the screening is done by cytotechnologists (CT) who hold a bachelor's degree and
have 1 year specialized training in cytopathology. The CTs are legally permitted to
result cervical cytology cases deemed negative for intraepithelial lesion or
malignancy (NILM) without further analysis. Any slides found to have abnormal
cells must be passed on to the cytopathologist for review. Depending on the result,
the report will have the name of CT screener and potentially, the cytopathologist.
Although the prevalence of abnormal cervical cytology samples will vary with the
population served, the majority of slides submitted for screening are normal. Thus,
the CTs do the bulk of the work for gynecologic cytology.

Recently, computer assisted screening has been introduced into the cytology lab
and is intended to maintain or increase the sensitivity of the screening process
while easing the manpower shortages affecting the cytotechnology community.
Two types of systems are currently available. Using different approaches, both
systems perform image analysis on CVC slides prior to evaluation of selected
fields of view by the CT. The coordinates of the fields of view are relayed from the
computer to the CT via a hard-wired link to a motorized stage on the microscope.
If no abnormal cells are identified in the computer selected fields of view, the CT
may result the case as NILM. The most widely used machine is the ThinPrep[TM]
imaging system which relies on a proprietary modification of the hematoxylin stain
component of the Papanicolaou stain, such that the nuclei of cells are stained in a
"Feulgen-like" manner. The Feulgen reaction has long been used in image analysis to produce a stoichiometric measurement of the DNA present in cells evaluated by optical density. The ThinPrep[TM] imaging system identifies potentially
abnormal cells in the CVC sample with increased DNA and presents 22 fields of
view, or about one-third of the slide, for evaluation by the CT. The second system,

marketed by Becton–Dickinson for use with SP, relies on a complex algorithm of thousands of images of normal and abnormal cells stored within the computer that are compared to the cells on the cytology sample. No stain modification is used. The computer stores not only the coordinates to localize the fields of view harboring the most potentially abnormal cells but also retains black and white images of these fields of view.

10.2.3 Reporting Terminology

In the early years of cervical cancer screening, the terminology used to report the results of cervical cytology was not standardized. The most commonly used method was known as the Papanicolaou classification system which consisted of five categories or classes ranging from class I, absence of abnormal cells to class V, cytology conclusive for malignancy. However, classes II–IV were not uniformly used. The cytology community recognized the need for a standardized, reproducible system of interpretation and reporting, and so a consensus conference was held in 1987 at the National Cancer Institute. The Bethesda System for Reporting Cervical Cytology, first published in 1988 and subsequently revised in 1991 and 2001, was the result of the NCI meeting. Besides delineation of the required and optional elements of the cervical cytology report, the Bethesda system provided a written discussion of morphologic criteria as well as photographic print and online atlases to illustrate each cellular entity [18]. The atlases have proven to be an invaluable educational tool for CT and cytopathologists. Required elements of the report are listed in Table 10.1. A brief explanation follows herein.

Specimen type is self explanatory, either CS or one of the liquid-based preparations (ThinPrep^{TM} or SurePath^{TM}).

Specimen adequacy is either satisfactory or unsatisfactory. There are two types of unsatisfactory samples. The first type is recognized as unsatisfactory up-front such that the sample is not processed. Examples of reasons for sample rejection include lack of patient identification or an empty specimen container. On the other hand, if the specimen is processed but is found to have too few squamous cells or squamous cells obscured by blood or inflammation, the sample is deemed unsatisfactory. When there are less critical issues with the quality of the sample, the specimen is processed and resulted but the issues, such as absence of endocervical cells, are listed under the subheading of **"quality indicators"**. In the past, lack of endocervical cells was felt to indicate a compromised sample, but more recent studies have not found this to be the case.

Interpretation/Result allows for a variety of options.

The sample will be interpreted as NILM when the epithelial cells appear normal or show "reactive" features (Fig. 10.3). The cause of the reactive changes may be obvious, for example an organism such as *Candida* sp., radiation change, intra-uterine device, but the cause may not be evident. The risk of subsequent epithelial

Table 10.1 Required elements of report

Specimen type	Specimen adequacy	Interpretation	Ancillary testing	Automated review	Educational notes
(1) Conventional smear (2) Liquid-based prep	(1) Satisfactory for evaluation (2) Unsatisfactory for evaluation (a) Specimen not processed (b) Specimen processed	(1) Negative for intraepithelial lesion or malignancy (NILM) (a) Organisms (i) Trichomas vaginalis (ii) c/w Candida spp. (iii) Shift in vaginal flora (iv) c/w Actinomyces spp. (v) c/w Herpes simplex virus (b) Other non-neoplastic findings (i) Reactive cellular changes (ii) Glandular cells post hysterectomy (iii) Atrophy (2) Other (i) Endometrial cells in woman over 40 years of age (3) Epithelial cell abnormalities (a) Squamous cell (i) Atypical squamous cells of un-determined significance(ASCUS) (ii) Cannot exclude HSIL (ASC-H) (iii) LSIL (iv) HSIL (v) Squamous cell carcinoma (b) Glandular cell (i) Atypical (I) Endocervical cells, NOS (II) Endometrial cells, NOS (III) Glandular cells, NOS (IV) Endocervical cells, favor neoplastic (V) Glandular cells, favor neoplastic (ii) Endocervical adenocarcinoma in situ (iii) Adenocarcinoma (I) Specify type or designate NOS (4) Other malignant neoplasms	High risk HPV test results	(1) ThinPrep image analyzer (2) Focal point imager (3) Focal point GS imager	ASCCP guidelines

lesions has been found in small studies of patients with reactive changes to be slightly increased, but not sufficiently increased to warrant closer follow-up or ancillary testing of the sample [19–21]. Other findings that are covered under the NILM category include benign glandular cells identified in a posthysterectomy sample taken from the vaginal vault and changes associated with atrophy. Benign glandular cells in a posthysterectomy sample can result from glandular metaplasia (acquired vaginal adenosis) or if only the uterus has been removed, prolapse of a fallopian tube through the vaginal vault incision [22]. The cytologist must be careful to exclude recurrent tumor if the hysterectomy was performed for an adenocarcinoma.

A special "other" category is used to alert the clinician for the presence of benign appearing exfoliated endometrial cells identified in woman older than 40 years of age (Fig. 10.4). In younger women, shed endometrial cells rarely are associated with underlying abnormalities of the endometrium, but as women approach menopause and beyond, even benign endometrial cells can be a sign of endometrial hyperplasia or adenocarcinoma; it is left to the clinician to see if further investigation is warranted [23–25]. Although debated in the past due to their presence in biopsies of endometrial carcinoma, the presence of foamy histiocytes without accompanying endometrial cells in CVC are not considered to be clinically significant [26, 27]. Providing the laboratory with the date of the last menstrual period (LMP) and patient history is important to put endometrial cells as well as other findings into the correct context and thus the most appropriate Bethesda category.

Epithelial cell abnormalities are divided into squamous and glandular. Squamous abnormalities range from atypical squamous cells to SIL, either low or high grade, to squamous cell carcinoma. The atypical squamous cell category consists of two types: Atypical squamous cells of undetermined significance (ASC-US) and atypical squamous cells, cannot exclude HSIL (ASC-H). The cytologic changes of ASC-US are suggestive of low grade squamous intraepithelial lesion (LSIL) but of

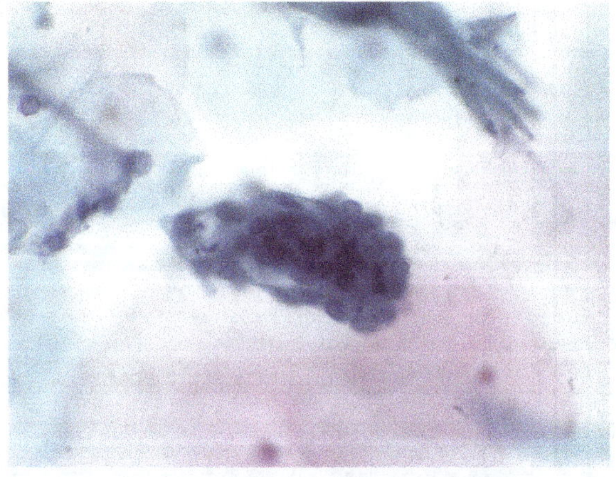

Fig. 10.4 Cluster of shed endometrial cells as may be seen during the first part of the menstrual cycle in reproductive age women

insufficient quantity or quality to warrant the interpretation. Cells designated as ASC-H are smaller cells in the range of immature squamous metaplastic cells. Cytologic features of LSIL consist of HPV cytopathic effects in the nucleus and cytoplasm (koilocytosis) of an intermediate type squamous cell with a modest increase in the nuclear to cytoplasmic ratio (Fig. 10.5). HSIL is identified in generally smaller metaplastic type squamous cells with a significantly increased nuclear to cytoplasmic ratio (Fig. 10.6). Squamous cell carcinoma implies more markedly abnormal cells in greater quantities. Invasion may be suspected if evidence of tissue breakdown, known as "tumor diathesis" (Fig. 10.7). Accurate grading of squamous abnormalities may not be possible if the squamous cells are fully keratinized.

Glandular cell abnormalities imply that the cellular changes are recognized in cells with cytoplasmic features of glandular cells [28]. If possible, the origin of the glandular cells will be indicated, either endocervix or endometrium, but at times,

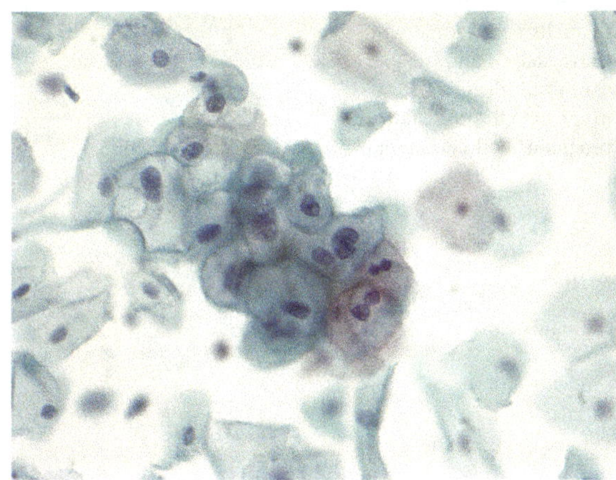

Fig. 10.5 Squamous cells with features of "low grade squamous intraepithelial lesion" as manifested by nuclear enlargement and cytoplasmic cavitation (koilocytosis)

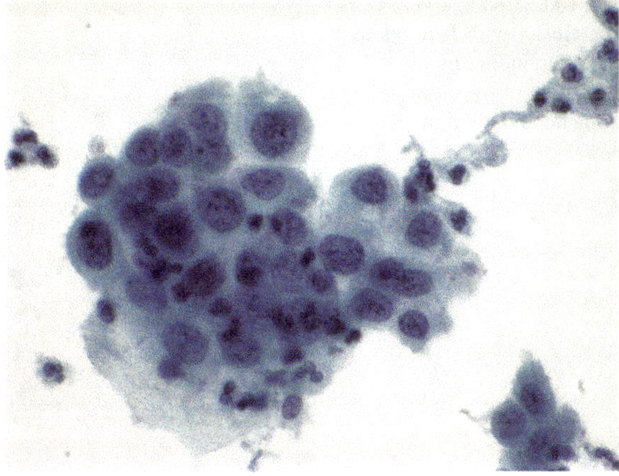

Fig. 10.6 Squamous cells with abnormal, hyperchromatic, irregular nucleus, and scant cytoplasm, features of "high grade squamous intraepithelial lesion"

the abnormal glandular cells cannot be further classified [29, 30]. The degree of abnormality is graded as either "not otherwise specified", to "cannot exclude neoplasia". The cytologic features of endocervical adenocarcinoma-in situ (AIS) are well recognized and permit a precise diagnosis of AIS [31, 32] (Fig. 10.8). AIS must be differentiated from sheets of HSIL cells that mimic AIS [33, 34]. If possible, when invasive adenocarcinoma is identified, the probable site of origin is also indicated [18] (Fig. 10.9). Supracervical or extrauterine origin of adenocarcinoma can also be suspected by the cytomorphology [35] (Fig. 10.10). For instance, cells of serous carcinoma of the adnexa or peritoneum may be shed and transported via the fallopian tube to the endometrial cavity and the endocervical canal to be detected in the CVC sample. An extrauterine origin of the malignancy is often suspected when no or little inflammatory response or tumor diathesis is identified. The malignant cells of serous carcinoma may be accompanied by

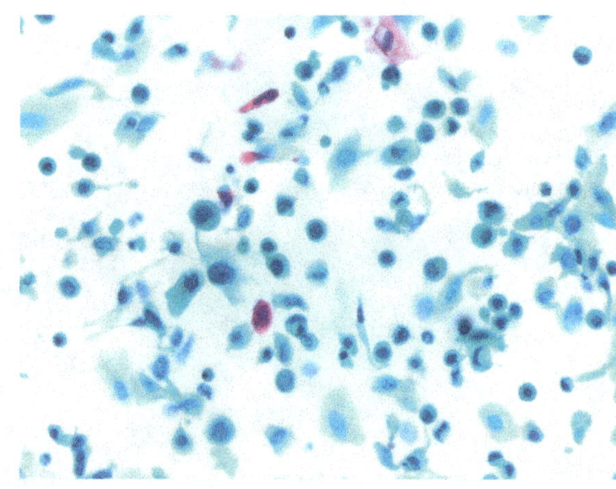

Fig. 10.7 Malignant squamous cells, some with bizarre shapes and keratinized, deeply *red-orange* cytoplasm, features of "squamous cell carcinoma"

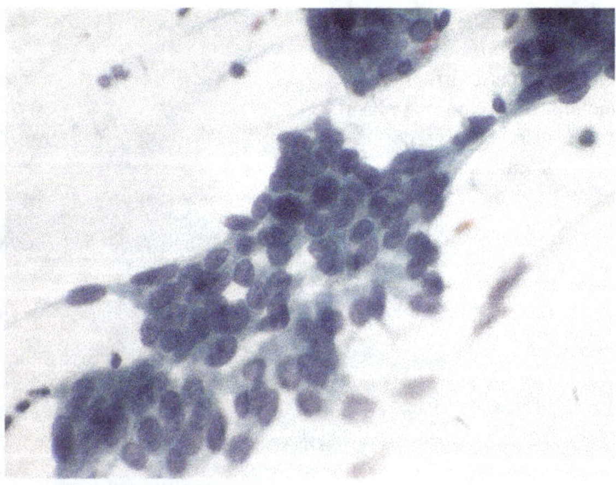

Fig. 10.8 Endocervical cells in a cluster with features of adenocarcinoma-in situ consisting of hyperchromatic, elongate, enlarged nuclei

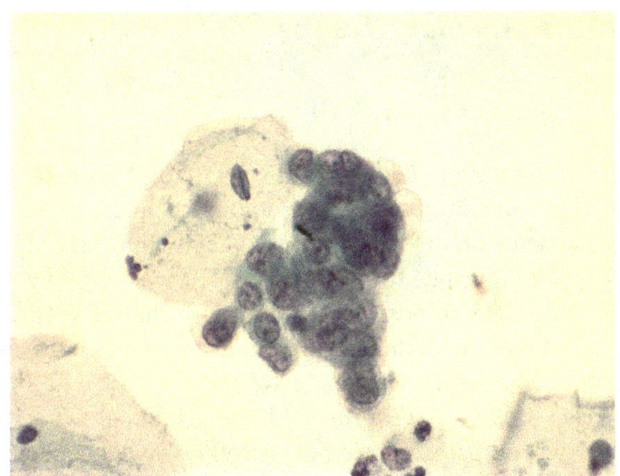

Fig. 10.9 Endocervical cells with large nuclei with irregularly distributed chromatin, large nucleoli, and vacuolated cytoplasm, features of endocervical adenocarcinoma

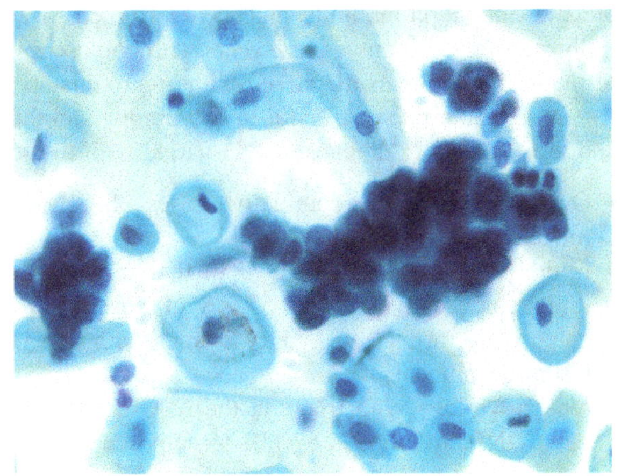

Fig. 10.10 Cluster of tightly aggregated irregular glandular cells with enlarged, irregular nuclei, and focally prominent nucleoli, features of endometrial adenocarcinoma

psammoma bodies, but the presence of psammoma bodies unassociated with glandular cells is most often a benign finding. All methods for preparation of CVC samples perform similarly in regards to detection of glandular abnormalities [36].

Rarely, unusual primary tumors, such as lymphoma, or sarcoma, may be cytologically identified [37, 38]. Likewise, metastatic malignant cells may be found, but in most instances, the primary tumor is known [35]. Initial diagnosis of a malignancy by metastatic tumor cells in the Pap is unusual [39]. Metastatic carcinomas to the cervix can mimic primary cervical adenocarcinoma [40]. **Ancillary testing** currently is high risk HPV testing, but in the future will most certainly include other tests. See the discussion below.

Automated review implies that either the Hologic system or BD system for image analysis is used as the initial screen.

Educational notes and suggestions are optional and refer to published guidelines.

10.2.4 Ancillary Testing

1. Testing for high risk HPV

Following the demonstration in 1976 of HPV as the cause of viral cytopathic effect in abnormal cervical cytology samples, increasingly sensitive tests lead to the conclusion that HPV is associated with nearly all cervical cancers. The results of small published trials suggested cervical cytology interpreted as ASC-US could be triaged to colposcopy according to the HPV test results [41, 42]. Two large studies were undertaken to provide enough data to support a change in management of abnormal cervical cytology [43, 44]. The first study, the ASC-US-LSIL Triage Study (ALTS), funded by the National Cancer Institute, was a randomized trial to compare three types of follow-up management for ASC-US: Immediate colposcopy, triage to colposcopy based on either testing for high risk HPV or by a repeat cervical cytology [44]. The 3,488 enrolled women had an ASC-US interpretation in the community and were assigned to a management arm and then followed every 6 months for 2 years with colposcopy at the last visit. By the end of the trial, CIN3 was diagnosed with approximately equal frequency in all arms (8–9 %) but the rate of referral to colposcopy and the number of additional visits and tests needed to diagnose CIN3 varied with the study arm:

- Only 53.6 % of the cumulative cases of CIN3 were detected at the initial immediate colposcopy;
- in the HPV triage arm, 72.3 % of the cumulative CIN3 were identified at the initial colposcopy, but only 55.6 % of women in the HPV arm were referred to colposcopy; in fact, 92.4 % of women with CIN3 were identified by the HPV test at enrollment;
- repeat cytology with triage at the ASC-US level identified 95.4 % of women with CIN3 but referred 67.1 % to colposcopy and required two visits.

The conclusion of ALTS trial was that reflex testing for HPV from the remaining sample from a liquid-based cervical cytology was the most efficient method for detection of CIN3. The trial also evaluated a separate group of women with LSIL cytology but found that HPV testing did not help in triage since 83 % of the 642 women were high risk HPV positive.

The second large study, begun in 1996 around the same time as the ALTS trial, compared the sensitivity for CIN2+ by reflex HPV testing from LBC to repeat conventional cytology in the triage of 995 women with ASC-US [43]. The sensitivity of HPV testing compared to cytology was 89.2 % versus 75.8 % with a positive predictive value of 15.2 versus 13.0.

In 2001, following these large studies, the American Society for Colposcopy and Cervical Pathology (ASCCP) published guidelines for management of women with cervical cytologic and histologic abnormalities, including HPV testing for women with ASC-US on LBC [45]. In 2007, the ASCCP published revised guidelines for adolescents, incorporation of HPV testing into the work-up algorithm of atypical glandular cells (AGC) and the addition of HPV testing to the cervical cytology screening of women over 30 years of age [46].

Following additional large scale studies that explored the use of hrHPV co-testing with cytology or as a primary screening method [10, 47–50], major revisions to the guidelines were made in 2011 by the U.S. Preventive Services Task Force (USPSTF) [51] and in 2012 jointly by the American Cancer Society (ACS), the ASCCP and the American Society of Clinical Pathology (ASCP) [52].These and other guidelines are discussed in more detail below.

There are several methods used to test for the presence of high risk HPV. The Hybrid Capture 2 (HC2) (Digene) is FDA approved and was the test used in the ALTS trial, thus considerable data support the use of this test [44]. The HC2 is a signal amplification nucleic acid hybridization test for 13 hrHPV types that uses an RNA probe to detect the HPV DNA. The RNA–DNA hybrid is then "captured" by anti-RNA–DNA antibodies fixed to the well of a microtitre plate. Chemilumi-nescent-tagged antibodies attach to the fixed hybrids and the signal is amplified. The result is semi-quantitative but is reported simply as positive or negative. The cutoff for a positive test is 1 pg hrHPV DNA/ml which corresponds to 5,000 DNA copies. Lacking a measure of the number of cells in the test sample, the test cannot be rendered quantitative. In other words, the viral load cannot be accurately determined. The test is sold as a relatively easy to use kit.

The Cervista^{TM} HPV HR test (Hologic, Inc), also FDA approved, is a signal amplified nucleic acid hybridization test that relies on an invader reaction in order to test for 14 high-risk HPV types. The reaction was described in 1993 as the enzymatic cleavage of single stranded DNA by structure, rather than sequence, recognition [53]. The reaction was first used to detect single nucleotide polymor-phisms [54]. In the Cervista test, 14 hrHPV types are detected by three sets of pooled reagents. The probes target 2–3 separate regions of the HPV genome in order to avoid potential false negative tests due to the presence of loss of HPV DNA during integration into the human genome. The test also detects the presence of human DNA as an internal control, so as to provide a semi-quantitative result [55]. Studies have shown the Cervista test to perform comparably to the HC2 [56, 57].

HPV type specific tests will become increasingly important in the era of HPV vaccination and for epidemiological studies. Hologic offers a second separate test, Cervista HPV 16/18, to determine if a positive Cervista test for hrHPV is due to these particularly high risk types. The test result is reported as positive for HPV 16/18. The test has been analytically and clinically validated [58, 59].

Many variations of the PCR exist and many studies of HPV testing to screen for cervical cancer, especially those conducted in Europe have used PCR assays [60, 61]. The Roche Cobas$^{®}$ HPV test, the only FDA approved PCR test, is an almost fully automated real time PCR test using primer pairs to a polymorphic region of the L1 gene to detect 14 hrHPV types (16,18,31,33,35,39,45,51,52,56, 58,59,66,68) and to ß-globin gene. The resultant amplified product(s) are detected by four fluorescent dye labeled probes to HPV16, HPV18, the other 12 HPV types, and the ß-globin gene. Thus the results will indicate the presence of hrHPV with genotyping for HPV16 and HPV18 as well as confirmation of the presence of human cells in the sample (ß-globin). The rationale for genotyping HPV 16 and HPV 18 is their strong association with cervical cancer (HPV 16 in 55–60 % and HPV 18 in 10–15 %) [3, 62, 63]. The test has been analytically and clinically validated [64–66] and has been extensively compared to the HC2 test [67–70]. In addition, a large prospective multicenter clinical trial entitled, Addressing the Need for Advanced HPV Diagnostics (ATHENA) is nearing completion. The study aims to evaluate the performance of the Cobas HPV test as a triage for women with abnormal cytology results (ASC-US), as an adjunctive test in women with negative cytology results and as a primary screening test. A total of 47,208 women aged 21 years and older are enrolled for baseline evaluation including cytology and the cobas HPV test. All women with double negative results, except a subset selected for the follow-up of 3 years longitudinal study with colposcopy, exit the study. All women with any abnormal results are entered into the longitudinal study. Pregnant women are excluded from the longitudinal study. Overall the prevalence of hrHPV was found to be 6.7 % with the prevalence of HPV types 16/18 being 1.2 %. The prevalence of cervical intraepithelial neoplasia 2 or worse ($\geq$CIN2) was 1.2 %. The absolute risk of $\geq$CIN2 in women positive for HPV 16/18 was 11.4 % compared to 6.1 % for other hrHPV types and 0.8 % in women negative for hrHPV [71]. In women with cytology categorized as ASC-US (4.1 %), the Cobas HPV test performed similarly to HC2 in the ALTS trial. HPV 16/18 genotyping was associated with a 24.4 % risk of biopsy proven $\geq$CIN2 as compared to the finding of other hrHPV (14.0 %) or no evidence of hrHPV (0.8 %) [72]. Genotyping was found to be useful in risk assessment by age stratification and when integrated into screening strategies provide more efficient referral to colposcopy [73–75].

The FDA recently approved an alternative type of test for high risk HPV, the Gen-Probe APTIMA test which evaluates the presence of hrHPV mRNA in CVC samples. APTIMA is a qualitative multiplex nuclei acid amplification test for E6/E7 viral mRNA from 14 hrHPV types. The rationale for the test is that biopsy proven $\geq$CIN2 is more likely to be associated with integration of the hrHPV into the human genome with subsequent over expression of the E6/E7 genes that tend to further dysregulate the cell cycle. The idea is that transient innocuous hrHPV infections would not be detected, thus significantly increasing the specificity of the hrHPV test. The APTIMA test has been analytically and clinically validated [76–80]. The test results are reported as positive or negative for the presence of hrHPV E6/E7 mRNA.

2. Other ancillary tests

A number of other tests have been investigated in the hope of increasing the specificity in order to detect the HPV infection most likely to progress to full blown cancer if left untreated.

Tests for human cellular dysregulation include abnormal cell cycle proteins, most notably p16, amplification of human telomerase gene TERC on chromosome 3q, and determination of the methylation status of the human DNA or of the HPV DNA hold promise but larger, more rigorous studies are needed before these tests could be used in screening [81–84]. An immunocytochemical test for p16 and Ki67 (the cell cycle protein detected in actively cycling cells), commercially known as CINtec, is used on CVC samples in Europe and may become available in North America [85–87].

10.2.5 Diagnostic Performance

As a screening test, CVC has been criticized for the variable sensitivity (55–90 %), albeit high specificity (90 %), for SIL [88]. In unscreened populations, well developed precursor lesions are readily picked up by CVC. Treatment of these lesions leads to the rapid decline of cervical cancer as has been demonstrated in many populations. In more well screened populations, such as countries of North America and Western Europe, precursor lesions are less frequent and cytologic abnormalities are often more subtle. For this reason, in order to maintain a robust sensitivity, the cutoff for an abnormal CVC interpretation is usually at the level of ASC-US.

The risk of cancer or a high grade precursor lesion of cancer in the cervix varies with the cytologic interpretation and, if performed, the risk is modified by the results of hrHPV testing.

NILM: The sensitivity of a single CVC cytology is difficult to assess due to the variation in methods used in studies to investigate sensitivity. A wide range has been reported, from a low of 50 % to as high as 94 % [88]. Repeating the CVC on an annual basis compensates for the potentially low sensitivity. When coupled with hrHPV testing (as in women over 30 years), the sensitivity increases to 100 % but specificity is somewhat diminished [89]. Most importantly, a combined NILM CVC and negative test for hrHPV has close to a 100 % negative predictive value for high grade disease.

ASC-US: This is the most common CVC abnormality in the United States, reported in about 5 % of samples. When hrHPV testing is used to triage ASC-US, biopsy-proven CIN2-3 is found in 4.3–26.7 % of women. In fact, most biopsy proven CIN2-3 is preceded by an ASC-US CVC.

ASC-H: The interpretation of ASC-H is about 10 times less common than ASC-US. However, the risk of subsequent biopsy-proven CIN2-3 is significantly higher than for ASC-US, about 40 %. Studies have suggested that testing for hrHPV may help better define the risk. However, per current guidelines, women with ASC-H should go directly to colposcopy.

LSIL: This interpretation is made in about 2.5 % of all CVC, but the incidence varies with the age group studied. Subsequent biopsy-proven CIN2-3 occurs in 12–16 % of women.

HSIL: About 0.7 % of CVC samples are interpreted as HSIL. The rate varies with the age group, being less common in older women. Subsequent biopsy-proven CIN2-3 is identified in 84–97 % of women with an HSIL CVC.

AGC: Similar to HSIL, about 0.7 % of CVC samples are interpreted as AGC (all degrees together). The interpretation of AGC can encompass both HPV-related disease and non-HPV-related disease. Many studies indicate a benefit from performing hrHPV testing to alert the practitioner to the possibility of HPV-related disease (CIN2/3 and/or adenocarcinoma in situ of the endocervix). In women with hrHPV negative AGC, noncervical glandular neoplasia remains a possibility, especially in older women.

10.2.6 Regulatory Issues and Quality Assurance

Gynecologic cytology screening is highly regulated by the Federal Government. The Clinical Laboratory Improvement Amendment of 1988 (CLIA'88) spells out in exquisite detail the regulations by which the lab must abide by (http://wwwn.cdc.gov/clia/regs/toc.aspx) [90]. 10 % of CVC samples interpreted as negative must be rescreened, cytology–histology correlation must be evaluated, following a new interpretation of HSIL all CVC samples interpreted as NILM for the prior 5 years must be reviewed.

10.2.7 Guidelines for Screening Interval and Follow-Up

In the United States, several professional organizations regularly issue updated guidelines screening for cervical cancer and for follow-up of cytological abnormalities as new data becomes available. The most recent guidelines for screening were published in 2011 by the USPSTF (www.ahrq.gov) [51] and in 2012 by a consortium of the ACS, ASCCP, and the ASCP [52]. In response to the updated guideline, the American College of Obstetrics and Gynecology (ACOG) published an updated practice bulletin with up-dated screening recommendations [91].

The recommendations by all organizations are in substantial agreement that screening be stratified according to patient age and risk factors as follows:

1. Women under 21 years should not be screened
2. Women between the ages of 21 and 29 should have cervical cytology (Pap test) alone every 3 years. They should not be tested for HPV unless as triage following an abnormal Pap test result (ASC-US).
3. Women between the ages of 30 and 65 should be screened with a Pap test and an HPV test ("co-testing") every 5 years (the preferred approach) or a Pap test alone every 3 years (acceptable).
4. Women over age 65 who have had regular screenings with normal results should not be screened for cervical cancer. Women who have been diagnosed with cervical pre-cancer (CIN2 or more severe) should continue to be screened for 20 years.
5. Women who have had a hysterectomy with the cervix removed and have no history of cervical cancer or precancer should not be screened.

6. Women who have had the HPV vaccine should be screened according to recommendations for their age group.
7. Women who are at high risk for cervical cancer may need to be screened more often or alternatively. Women at high risk might include those with a history of cervical cancer or immunocompromised (e.g., infection with human immunodeficiency virus or status-post organ transplant), or exposure in utero to the drug diethylstilbestrol (DES).

In summary, the ACS and the other organizations no longer recommend annual screening for cervical cancer, because an analysis of the benefits of screening weighed against the harm of overtreatment favored a prolongation of the screening interval [52]. The development of cervical carcinoma is generally long, as long as 10–20 years, so that even with the longer screening interval of 5 years, invasive cervical cancer is unlikely to develop.

The ASCCP previously published guidelines for the management of women with abnormal cervical cancer screening tests in 2007 [6, 74]. The ASCCP convened a conference in the fall of 2012 to discuss updated guidelines which were released in early 2013 [92]. The 2006 guidelines propose choices for management of ASC-US that include testing for hrHPV, repeat cervical cytology or colposcopy. However, when residual cells from a LBC sample are available, "reflex" hrHPV testing is preferred. Women who are hrHPV negative should have a repeat cytology in 12 months (this interval will probably be lengthened to 3 or 5 years depending on the age of the woman). Women who test positive for hrHPV have the equivalent of LSIL and should be referred for colposcopy. If no lesion is identified on the exocervix at colposcopy, blind endocervical sampling should be performed. If the colposcopy is negative, hrHPV testing should be repeated in 1 year (never less than 1 year) or cytology should be repeated at 6 and 12 months.

The recommended management of ASC-H is colposcopy. If CIN2+ is not identified, hrHPV testing should be repeated in 12 months, or cytology should be repeated at 6 and 12 months. LSIL is managed with colposcopy; if CIN2+ is not identified, hrHPV testing should be repeated at 1 year or cytology repeated at 6 and 12 months. In postmenopausal women with LSIL, "reflex" hrHPV testing may be performed or repeat cytology testing at 6 and 12 months can be done in lieu of colposcopy. If either hrHPV testing is positive or cytology is ≥ASC-US, colposcopy is recommended. Women with HSIL on cervical cytology should be referred for colposcopy. Post-excision/ablation of CIN2+, follow-up is intended to detect persistent or recurrent disease. The ASCCP recommends either cervical cytology alone or with colposcopy every 4–6 months until three negative cytologies or a single hrHPV test at 6 months.

Women with AGC need multiple tests including colposcopy, endocervical evaluation and sampling, HPV testing, and endometrial evaluation. The 2012 revised ASC-ASCCP-ASCP guidelines for cervical cancer screening also made some recommendations on management. One particularly challenging problem occurs in co-testing of women over 30 years old who have a negative cytology result but a positive test for hrHPV. Two management options were recommended:

1. Repeat co-testing in 12 months; if the co-test is positive, the woman is referred to colposcopy; if the test is negative, the woman may return to 5 year screening interval.
2. immediate, HPV genotype-specific testing for HPV 16 and/or HPV 18; women testing positive go directly to colposcopy; if negative, repeat co-testing in 12 months; if negative (that is HPV negative AND ASC-US or negative cytology), return to 5 year interval but if the co-test is positive (HPV positive OR LSIL or more severe cytology), refer to colposcopy.

Women testing hrHPV positive and cytology negative should not be referred directly to colposcopy, should not be genotyped for hrHPV other than 16 or 18, and should not be tested with other non-HPV biomarkers.

Women between 30 and 65 years with ASC-US cytology results and negative hrHPV testing should continue to be screened by either co-testing at 5 years or by cytology alone at 3 years.

Essential Changes in ASCCP 2012 Guidelines From Prior 2006 Management Guidelines [92]

- Cytology reported as negative but lacking endocervical cells can be managed without early repeat.
- CIN 1 on endocervical curettage should be managed as CIN 1, not as a positive ECC.
- Cytology reported as unsatisfactory requires repeat even if HPV negative.
- Genotyping triages HPV-positive women with HPV type 16 or type 18 to earlier colposcopy only after negative cytology; colposcopy is indicated for all women with HPV and ASC-US, regardless of genotyping result.
- For ASC-US cytology, immediate colposcopy is not an option. The serial cytology option for ASC-US incorporates cytology at 12 months, not 6 months and 12 months, and then if negative, cytology every 3 years.
- HPV-negative and ASC-US results should be followed with co-testing at 3 years rather than 5 years.
- HPV-negative and ASC-US results are insufficient to allow exit from screening at age 65 years.
- The pathway to long-term follow-up of treated and untreated CIN 2+ is more clearly defined by incorporating co-testing.
- More strategies incorporate co-testing to reduce follow-up visits. Pap-only strategies are now limited to women younger than 30 years, but co-testing is expanded even to women younger than 30 years in some circumstances. Women aged 21-24 years are managed conservatively.

CIN, cervical intraepithelial neoplasia; ECC, endocervical curettage; HPV, human papil-lomavirus; ASC-US, atypical squamous cells of undetermined significance. *Prior management guidelines were from the ''2006 Consensus Guidelines for the Management of Women With Abnormal Cervical Screening Tests'' (6). Prior guidelines not changed were retained.

10.3 Cytology of the Endometrium

10.3.1 Epidemiology of Endometrial Cancer

Endometrial adenocarcinoma (EMCa) is the most common gynecologic cancer and corresponds to approximately 6 % of all cancers in women [93]. Most cases are diagnosed at an early stage. Epidemiologic and prognostic factors suggest that there exist two forms of endometrial cancer [94]:

- Type I, estrogen-related, low grade endometrioid-type, often arising in a background of endometrial hyperplasia. Risk factors for type I include obesity, nulliparity, estrogen excess, either exogenous (tamoxifen, hormone replacement therapy) or endogenous, diabetes melitis, and hypertension. Type 1 makes up approximately 80 % of EMCa.
- Type II, unrelated to estrogen, tends to be of higher grade, of poorer prognostic type, and includes serous carcinoma and clear cell carcinoma. Type II does not arise in association with hyperplasia and the patients do not share the risk factors of type I.

Most cases of EMCa are diagnosed after menopause, usually over the age of 60. Twenty-five percent are diagnosed before menopause with only 5–10 % before 40. A hereditary form, part of the Lynch syndrome associated with hereditary non-polyposis colorectal cancer, occurs in a minority of patients [95].

Screening of the general population is not advocated. Most cases are detected without screening by the presence of abnormal uterine bleeding in 90 % of patients [96]. Even a minimal amount of blood in a postmenopausal patient is cause for exploration and while atrophy of the endometrium is the most usual case of bleeding in this age group, the further one is from menopause, the more likely is EMCa. Overall, 5–20 % of postmenopausal bleeding is related to EMCa. Abnormal uterine bleeding should be investigated by physical exam and Pipelle endometrial biopsy, a technique that can be performed in the office without anesthesia. The Pipelle biopsy sample permits examination of the cytology and architecture of the endometrium. Transvaginal ultrasound is often added as part of the diagnostic work-up.

10.3.2 Cytology of Endometrial Cells Obtained from the Endometrial Cavity

Diagnosis of endometrial lesions by cytology can be made by two methods. First, endometrial cells may be fortuitously exfoliated in cervical cytology, providing cells for evaluation even though CVC is not designed to sample the endometrium. The sensitivity of finding EMCa in CVC has been calculated to be 40–55 % on

CSs and 60–65 % on LBC [97, 98]. Despite the Pap test's unpredictability for detecting EMCa, the presence of endometrial cells may be significant. For this reason, in women 40 years old or older, when benign appearing endometrial cells are identified, they are mentioned in the cytology report under "other" [18]. The clinician should correlate with the menstrual status and determine if follow-up is warranted [99]. If the endometrial cells are cytologically atypical, they will be reported under "Epithelial cell abnormality—Glandular".

The second method, direct sampling of the endometrium for cytology, can be fortuitous or deliberate. Fortuitous abrasion of endometrial glandular and stromal cells or lower uterine segment cells occurs not infrequently with thorough sampling with an endocervical brush, especially in women who have undergone LEEP or cone biopsy of the cervix that shortens the endocervical canal [100]. Abraded, directly sampled benign appearing endometrium is not associated with increased risk of EMCa and is not reported in a Pap test report [101]. Deliberate, direct sampling of the endometrium has been advocated by cytologists for a number of years. A variety of sampling devices that brush or aspirate the endometrium have been developed, most recently the Tao brush. The sample is smeared thinly on a glass slide, stained with Papanicolaou stain, and read in a manner similar to CVC slide or the sample is suspended in alcohol [102]. The technique has not caught on as a routine test probably due to the number of inadequate smears obtained, from 8 to 20 %, the learning curve needed to skillfully read a slide and the amount of time needed to adequately screen the slide. In the end, the Pipelle biopsy is simpler to obtain and simpler to read [103].

10.3.3 Peritoneal Wash Cytology and Staging Endometrial Cancer

Surgical staging of cancer of the uterine corpus has been recommended for more than 20 years by the International Federation of Gynecology and Obstetrics (FIGO). The original staging system included peritoneal wash cytology (PWC), but FIGO revised the staging system in 2009 and eliminated PWC as a variable dictating a more advanced stage when positive [104]. The reason given was the uncertain prognostic significance of isolated positive PWC [105]. According to the committee, there is evidence that positive PWC is not an independent predictor of poor outcome in the absence of other evidence of aggressive disease. However, discovery of occult primary tumors following positive PWC have been reported [106]. The method of PWC collection entails instillation of 100 ml of sterile saline into the peritoneal cavity immediately after entry into the peritoneum and lysis of adhesions. The fluid is then aspirated and sent to cytology. Differentiation of benign mesothelial cells from malignant glandular cells is often straightforward, but pitfalls can be encountered, such as hyperplastic mesothelial cells from adhesions or cells derived from endometriosis or endosalpingiosis (Fig. 10.11).

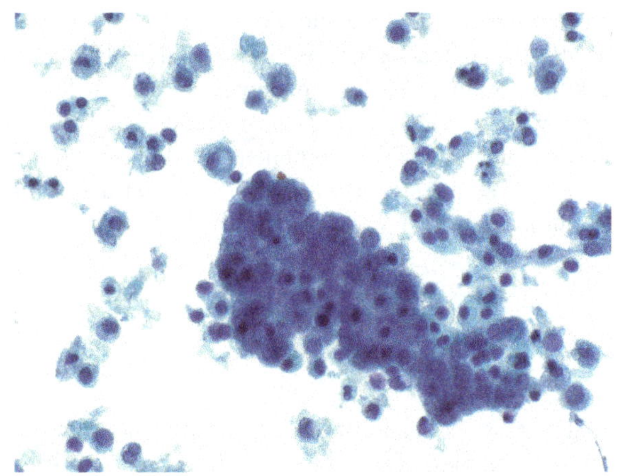

Fig. 10.11 Pelvic washing with benign, uniform mesothelial cells on the *left* contrasted with a cluster of serous adenocarcinoma on the *right*

The cytologist should correlate the PWC findings with surgical pathology findings if any question as to the origin of the cells in the sample arises [107].

10.3.4 Diagnosis of Recurrent Endometrial Adenocarcinoma in the Vaginal Cuff

The National Comprehensive Cancer Network has developed posttreatment surveillance consensus-based guidelines for EMCa that includes vaginal cytology every 6 months for 2 years, then annually (http://www.nccn.org/professionals/physician_gls/f_guidelines.asp).

However, studies indicate that the use of vaginal cuff cytology may not be cost effective [108, 109].

10.4 Cytology of the Female Adnexa

The female adnexa include the ovaries, fallopian tubes, and accompanying ligaments and soft tissues. Cysts and mass lesions in the adnexa occur at all ages and most adnexal masses arise in the ovary [110]. The lesions may be symptomatic or may be found incidentally on physical exam or imaging. The risk of malignancy depends on the several factors, being higher in prepubertal girls and in postmenopausal women. If the mass is solid or is a complex cyst with solid components, if the woman has a history of malignancy elsewhere or if ascites is present, the risk is also elevated. Besides a good history and physical exam, the most important diagnostic tool in the evaluation of an adnexal mass is pelvic ultrasound (US). Certain benign lesions (simple cyst, dermoid cyst, hemorrhagic cyst, and endometrioma) produce characteristic US features [111]. Watchful waiting is usually advocated for simple cysts less than 10 cm in premenopausal women and less than 5 cm in the postmenopausal woman. Surgical exploration, by laparoscopy or laparotomy, is advised for larger cysts or if other worrisome features are present, such as a solid component [112]. Two types of cytology samples are used as part of the diagnostic work-up of adnexal masses: Peritoneal washings and fine needle aspiration (FNA) [113].

10.4.1 Peritoneal Washings

Peritoneal washing is the technique used to sample a large surface area of the pelvis at the time of laparotomy or laparoscopic surgery. The findings compliment visualization of the pelvic and abdominal organs by the surgeon and histologic examination of the tissues by the pathologist. In case of malignant tumors of the ovary, the findings of the peritoneal washing will be taken into account in the FIGO staging. In tumors confined to the ovary, positive peritoneal washings will upstage the tumor to IC.

10.4.1.1 Collection Technique, Processing and Interpretation

The pelvic cavity can be accessed by the laparotomy incision or by the laparoscopic trocar. Sterile saline is washed over the pelvic organs prior to disruption by surgery. The saline dislodges mesothelial cells in sheets and as single cells, along with inflammatory cells, red blood cells and if present, cells extraneous to the peritoneal lining. The extraneous cells may be benign, such as cells from endometriosis, or malignant, such as serous carcinoma of the ovary. The wash fluid is aspirated into a collection container. In the cytology laboratory, the fluid is centrifuged. The cell rich pellet is used to make smears, LBC slides and if sufficiently cellular, a cell block for histology. A cell block can also be made from the residual of the LBC suspension and is particularly useful if the origin of cells is in question. The usual question is whether epithelioid-appearing cells are of mesothelial, histiocytic, or glandular origin. A panel of antibodies including pan-cytokeratin, calretinin, CD68, BerEP4, B72.3, CEA, and MOC31 can be used [107, 114, 115].

Although not a washing, aspiration of small amounts of fluid that accumulate in the pouch of Douglas by cul-de-sac during many benign or malignant processes can be obtained by culdocentesis. The fluid is processed in a manner similar to the peritoneal wash.

Correlation of the cytology sample with the histology is mandatory in order to interpret the peritoneal washing. For example, atypical cells may be found in histologically benign lesions such as torsion, acute salpingitis, or endometriosis that provoke serosal adhesions with reactive hyperplasia of the mesothelium [116]. Unless the cytology sample is compared with the histology, there is a potential for a false positive diagnosis. Another example is the case of malignant appearing cells with no histologic evidence of tumor on the serosal surface of the adnexa or uterus. In this case, comparison to the primary tumor will confirm the origin of the abnormal cells in the pelvic washing.

10.4.1.2 Diagnostic Performance

In ovarian cancer, the sensitivity of peritoneal washing when the peritoneal surface is found to be histologically involved by tumor has been found in several studies to vary from 73 to 82.9 % [117–119]. However, one more recent study found a sensitivity of only 25 % for all malignant ovarian tumors; but, the sensitivity varied with the tumor type [120]. For the five most common tumors of epithelial origin the overall sensitivity was 51 % with a specificity of 93 %. Among these five types, the PWC was most sensitive for serous type at 71 % and lowest for clear cell type at 20 %. The sensitivity for malignancy has also been found to be lower at posttreatment "second look" [117] but despite this, peritoneal washing has been deemed an important test because women are identified with tumors are more likely to recur [121].

10.4.2 Fine Needle Aspiration of Adnexal Masses

FNA has been advocated by some cytopathologists as an aid in diagnosis of adnexal masses in women. FNA is a low risk procedure that offers the possibility of avoiding surgery on the ovary [122]. The main objections to FNA of an adnexal mass include inadvertent rupture of a malignant cyst and concerns about the accuracy of an FNA diagnosis.

10.4.2.1 Procedure, Cytology Preparation and Interpretation

Aspiration of adnexal masses may be performed by the transvaginal or transrectal route or percutaneously through the abdominal wall, with or without imaging guidance [123]. An FNA can also be performed during laparotomy or laparoscopic surgery. By whatever route chosen, a 14- to 22-gauge needle is used. If a cyst is aspirated, all of the aspirated fluid should be sent to cytology for centrifugation. The cell pellet is used to make smears, liquid-based preparations or cell blocks. If a solid lesion is aspirated, the material is smeared on glass slides by the operator and the slides are either air dried for Wright-Giemsa staining (the same stain as is used for peripheral blood smears) or fixed immediately by spray or immersion in 95 % ethanol. The aspirate may also be expressed into a liquid fixative/preservative or saline for transport to the cytology laboratory for processing as a liquid-based slide.

Fig. 10.12 Follicular cells aspirated from a functional, follicular cyst of the ovary

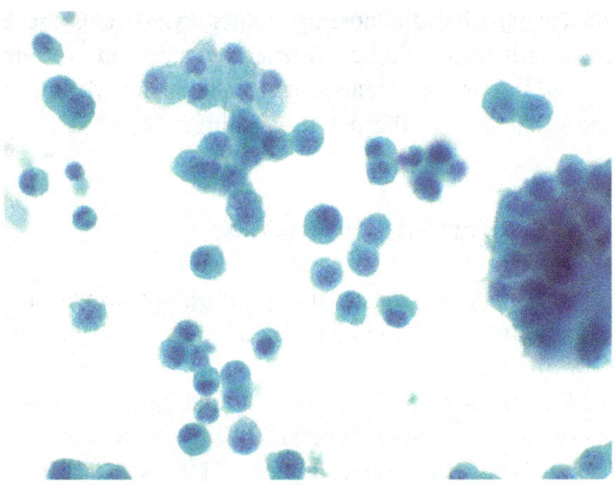

Interpretation of the FNA sample depends on the type of mass sampled. Unilocular ovarian cysts may be functional, non-neoplastic cysts such as preovulatory follicle cysts or postovulatory corpus luteum cysts (Fig. 10.12). Cysts of less than 3 cm in diameter are considered physiologic. Aspiration of functional cysts are variably cellular, from highly cellular with many diagnostic granulosa cells, to nondiagnostic paucicellular samples comprised of only macrophages. In follicle cysts, the granulosa cells can be shed singly or in clusters. The cells often have scant cytoplasm, dark round to oval, occasionally creased nuclei. Mitoses may be identified. The differential diagnosis includes unilocular cystic neoplasms including cystic granulosa cell tumor, carcinoid tumor, and serous tumors. Aspiration of a corpus luteum cyst will produce granulosa cells with abundant luteinized, foamy, eosinophilic cytoplasm.

Aspiration of an endometriotic cyst usually contains almost only hemosiderin laden macrophages and lysed blood. Benign epithelial cysts can be found in the ovary or paratubal tissue. Hydrosalpinx can appear to be a cyst. The FNA sample is usually sparsely cellular, containing mainly macrophages, but also low cuboidal epithelial cells, sometimes ciliated. The epithelial cells can appear atypical due to degenerative changes [124]. The presence of benign appearing mucinous cells may be derived from a mucinous cystadenoma.

Aspiration of complex solid and cystic lesions or entirely solid lesions of the adnexa is not usually recommended. The more common lesions, such as mature cystic teratomas, are usually diagnosed by ultrasound. If there is any clinical suspicion of malignancy, aspiration is not recommended [125].

However, the cytopathologist will be expected to recognize the cytologic appearance of metastatic ovarian tumors, some of which may be difficult. For instance, a granulosa cell tumor is a potentially malignant neoplasm that has a predilection to metastasize long after the primary tumor has been removed.

10.4.2.2 Diagnostic Performance

Most series of adnexal mass FNA considered only cysts [124–126]. And most of the cyst aspirates in these studies were done, at least for some of the cases in each series, not in vivo, but after surgical removal of cyst, creating a somewhat artificial scenario. The results of these studies were variable. In the studies that commented on the number of samples without diagnostic cells, the rate varied from 11 to 46 % [125–127]. The sensitivity for malignancy varied from 25 to 75 % [123, 125]. The false positive rate varied from 0 to 73 % and the false negative rate varied from 12 to 35 %. The problem of nondiagnostic samples and false negative cases appears to be due to the presence of only macrophages and other inflammatory cells in many cyst fluid samples. Conversely, the cells lining non-neoplastic cysts or benign cysts can become atypical when shed into the cyst fluid, leading to false positive interpretations.

Only a few studies have dealt with real time aspiration of both solid and cystic ovarian lesions. One comprehensive study from 1972 in Sweden obtained FNA samples from palpable adnexal masses using either a transvaginal or a transrectal route [128]. Categorization of 80 samples into benign or malignant categories was highly accurate with a false positive and false negative rate of 5 and 7 %, respectively. A separate group of 52 malignant ovarian tumors were reliably categorized in almost each case with an unsatisfactory rate of only 6 %.

A more recent study of 235 cystic ovarian lesions sampled by FNA under ultrasound guidance found the nondiagnostic rate to be much higher at 56 %. An elevated cyst fluid estradiol was measured to help identify follicular cysts. The sensitivity was lowest (36 %) for endometriotic cysts, presumably due to excess blood. The highest sensitivity was found for proliferating and malignant neoplasms including surface epithelial tumors, granulosa cell tumor, and an immature teratoma. Specificity for all lesions approached 100 % except for paratubal cysts (83 %) [129].

As evidenced by the cited studies, the accuracy of cytology results varies widely. Therefore, if the practitioner wishes to use cytology in the work-up and treatment of adnexal masses, communication with the cytopathologist is advised to determine their level of experience with adnexal samples. Some clinicians have employed cytology in conjunction with other parameters, such as ultrasound findings and estradiol measurement to more selectively aspirate cystic lesions [130–132]. However, when benign appearing cysts are aspirated, a recurrence rate as high as 54 % has been found [133]. A single randomized controlled study of cyst aspiration including 278 women aged 14–81 years with unilocular cysts 4–7 cm found no difference in outcome between women undergoing cyst puncture and those managed expectantly after 6 months of observation [134]. Some clinicians have used cyst aspiration in conjunction with sclerotherapy to treat benign non-neoplastic cysts [135–137].

References

1. Bosch FX, Burchell AN, Schiffman M et al (2008) Epidemiology and natural history of human papillomavirus infections and type-specific implications in cervical neoplasia. Vaccine 26(Suppl 10):K1–K16
2. Dunne EF, Unger ER, Sternberg M et al (2007) Prevalence of HPV infection among females in the United States. JAMA 297:813–819
3. Munoz N, Bosch FX, de Sanjose S et al (2003) Epidemiologic classification of human papillomavirus types associated with cervical cancer. N Engl J Med 348:518–527
4. Wright TC Jr, Schiffman M (2003) Adding a test for human papillomavirus DNA to cervical-cancer screening. N Engl J Med 348:489–490
5. Siegel R, Naishadham D, Jemal A (2012) Cancer statistics, 2012. CA Cancer J Clin 62:10–29
6. Wellings K, Collumbien M, Slaymaker E et al (2006) Sexual behaviour in context: a global perspective. Lancet 368:1706–1728
7. Sirovich BE, Welch HG (2004) The frequency of Pap smear screening in the United States. J Gen Intern Med 19:243–250
8. Diamantis A, Magiorkinis E, Androutsos G (2009) What's in a name? Evidence that Papanicolaou, not Babes, deserves credit for the PAP test. Diagn Cytopatho 138(7):473–476)
9. Janerich DT, Hadjimichael O, Schwartz PE et al (1995) The screening histories of women with invasive cervical cancer, Connecticut. Am J Public Health 85:791–794
10. Koliopoulos G, Arbyn M, Martin-Hirsch P, Kyrgiou M, Prendiville W, Paraskevaidis E (2007) Diagnostic accuracy of human papillomavirus testing in primary cervical screening: a systematic review and meta-analysis of non-randomized studies. Gynecol Oncol 104:232–246
11. Wright TC Jr (2003) Cervical cancer screening using visualization techniques. J Natl Cancer Inst Monogr 31:66–71
12. Marchand L, Mundt M, Klein G, Agarwal SC (2005) Optimal collection technique and devices for a quality pap smear. WMJ 104:51–55
13. Martin-Hirsch P, Jarvis G, Kitchener H, Lilford R (2000) Collection devices for obtaining cervical cytology samples. Cochrane Database Syst Rev 2:CD001036
14. Ferris DG, Berrey MM, Ellis KE, Petry LJ, Voxnaes J, Beatie RT (1992) The optimal technique for obtaining a Papanicolaou smear with the Cervex-Brush. J Fam Pract 34:276–280
15. Harrison DD, Hernandez E, Dunton CJ (1993) Endocervical brush versus cotton swab for obtaining cervical smears at a clinic. A cost comparison. J Reprod Med 38:285–288
16. Arbyn M, Herbert A, Schenck U et al (2007) European guidelines for quality assurance in cervical cancer screening: recommendations for collecting samples for conventional and liquid-based cytology. Cytopathology 18:133–139
17. Day SJ, O'Shaughnessy DL, O'Connor JC, Freund GG (2004) Additional collection devices used in conjunction with the SurePath Liquid-Based Pap Test broom device do not enhance diagnostic utility. BMC Womens Health 4:6
18. Solomon D, Nayar R (2004) The Bethesda System for reporting cervical cytology. Springer, New York
19. Barr Soofer S, Sidawy MK (1997) Reactive cellular change: is there an increased risk for squamous intraepithelial lesions? Cancer 81:144–147
20. Malik SN, Wilkinson EJ, Drew PA, Hardt NS (2001) Benign cellular changes in Pap smears: causes and significance. Acta Cytol 45:5–8
21. Moriarty AT, Young NA (2003) The four R's: reactive/repair, reporting, and regulations. Diagn Cytopathol 29:1–3
22. Tambouret R, Pitman MB, Bell DA (1998) Benign glandular cells in posthysterectomy vaginal smears. Acta Cytol 42:1403–1408

23. Bean SM, Connolly K, Roberson J, Eltoum I, Chhieng DC (2006) Incidence and clinical significance of morphologically benign-appearing endometrial cells in patients age 40 years or older: the impact of the 2001 Bethesda System. Cancer 108:39–44
24. Chang A, Sandweiss L, Bose S (2001) Cytologically benign endometrial cells in the papanicolaou smears of postmenopausal women. Gynecol Oncol 80:37–43
25. Gray JA, Nguyen GK (1999) Cytologic detection of endometrial pathology by Pap smears [letter]. Diagn Cytopathol 20:181–182
26. Nguyen TN, Bourdeau JL, Ferenczy A, Franco EL (1998) Clinical significance of histiocytes in the detection of endometrial adenocarcinoma and hyperplasia. Diagn Cytopathol 19:89–93
27. Tambouret R, Bell DA, Centeno BA (2001) Significance of histiocytes in cervical smears from peri/postmenopausal women. Diagn Cytopathol 24:271–275
28. Ashfaq R, Gibbons D, Vela C, Saboorian MH, Iliya F (1999) ThinPrep Pap Test: accuracy for glandular disease. Acta Cytol 43:81–85
29. Bose S, Kannan V, Kline TS (1994) Abnormal endocervical cells. Really abnormal? Really endocervical? Am J Clin Pathol 101:708–713
30. DiTomasso JP, Ramzy I, Mody DR (1996) Glandular lesions of the cervix. Validity of cytologic criteria used to differentiate reactive changes, glandular intraepithelial lesions and adenocarcinoma. Acta Cytol 40:1127–1135
31. Betsill WL Jr, Clark AH (1986) Early endocervical glandular neoplasia. I. Histomorphology and cytomorphology. Acta Cytol 30:115–126
32. Lee KR, Minter LJ, Granter SR (1997) Papanicolaou smear sensitivity for adenocarcinoma in situ of the cervix. A study of 34 cases. Am J Clin Pathol 107:30–35
33. Drijkoningen M, Meertens B, Lauweryns J (1996) High grade squamous intraepithelial lesion (CIN 3) with extension into the endocervical clefts. Difficulty of cytologic differentiation from adenocarcinoma in situ. Acta Cytol 40:889–894
34. Selvaggi SM (2002) Cytologic features of high-grade squamous intraepithelial lesions involving endocervical glands on ThinPrep cytology. Diagn Cytopathol 26:181–185
35. Gupta D, Balsara G (1999) Extrauterine malignancies. Role of Pap smears in diagnosis and management. Acta Cytol 43:806–813
36. Belsley NA, Tambouret RH, Misdraji J, Muzikansky A, Russell DK, Wilbur DC (2008) Cytologic features of endocervical glandular lesions: comparison of SurePath, ThinPrep, and conventional smear specimen preparations. Diagn Cytopathol 36:232–237
37. Hanley KZ, Tadros TS, Briones AJ, Birdsong GG, Mosunjac MB (2009) Hematologic malignancies of the female genital tract diagnosed on liquid-based Pap test: cytomorphologic features and review of differential diagnoses. Diagn Cytopathol 37:61–67
38. Pasternak S, MacIntosh R (2006) Uterine adenosarcoma detected by Papanicolaou smear: a case report. Diagn Cytopathol 34:495–498
39. McGill F, Adachi A, Karimi N et al (1990) Abnormal cervical cytology leading to the diagnosis of gastric cancer. Gynecol Oncol 36:101–105
40. McCluggage WG, Hurrell DP, Kennedy K (2010) Metastatic carcinomas in the cervix mimicking primary cervical adenocarcinoma and adenocarcinoma in situ: report of a series of cases. Am J Surg Pathol 34:735–741
41. Reid R, Greenberg MD, Lorincz A et al (1991) Should cervical cytologic testing be augmented by cervicography or human papillomavirus deoxyribonucleic acid detection? Am J Obstet Gynecol 164:14611469; discussion 9–71
42. Cox JT, Schiffman MH, Winzelberg AJ, Patterson JM (1992) An evaluation of human papillomavirus testing as part of referral to colposcopy clinics. Obstet Gynecol 80:389–395
43. Manos MM, Kinney WK, Hurley LB et al (1999) Identifying women with cervical neoplasia: using human papillomavirus DNA testing for equivocal Papanicolaou results [see comments]. JAMA 281:1605–1610
44. Human papillomavirus testing for triage of women with cytologic evidence of low-grade squamous intraepithelial lesions: baseline data from a randomized trial. The Atypical

Squamous Cells of Undetermined Significance/Low-Grade Squamous Intraepithelial Lesions Triage Study (ALTS) Group. J Natl Cancer Inst 92:397–402 (2000)

45. Wright TC, Cox JT, Massad LS, Twiggs LB, Wilkinson EJ (2002) 2001 consensus guidelines for the management of women with cervical cytological abnormalities. JAMA 287:2120–2129

46. Wright TC Jr, Massad LS, Dunton CJ, Spitzer M, Wilkinson EJ, Solomon D (2007) 2006 consensus guidelines for the management of women with abnormal cervical cancer screening tests. Am J Obstet Gynecol 197:346–355

47. Kitchener HC, Almonte M, Wheeler P et al (2006) HPV testing in routine cervical screening: cross sectional data from the ARTISTIC trial. Br J Cancer 95:56–61

48. Naucler P, Ryd W, Tornberg S et al (2007) Human papillomavirus and Papanicolaou tests to screen for cervical cancer. N Engl J Med 357:1589–1597

49. Mayrand MH, Duarte-Franco E, Rodrigues I et al (2007) Human papillomavirus DNA versus Papanicolaou screening tests for cervical cancer. N Engl J Med 357:1579–1588

50. Ronco G, Giorgi-Rossi P, Carozzi F et al (2010) Efficacy of human papillomavirus testing for the detection of invasive cervical cancers and cervical intraepithelial neoplasia: a randomised controlled trial. Lancet Oncol 11:249–257

51. Kulasingam SL, Havrilesky L, Ghebre R, Myers ER (2011) Screening for cervical cancer: a decision analysis for the U.S. Preventive Services Task Force [Internet]. Agency for Healthcare Research and Quality (US), Rockville

52. Saslow D, Solomon D, Lawson HW et al (2012) American Cancer Society, American Society for Colposcopy and Cervical Pathology, and American Society for Clinical Pathology screening guidelines for the prevention and early detection of cervical cancer. Am J Clin Pathol 137:516–542

53. Lyamichev V, Brow MA, Dahlberg JE (1993) Structure-specific endonucleolytic cleavage of nucleic acids by eubacterial DNA polymerases. Science 260:778–783

54. Hsu TM, Law SM, Duan S, Neri BP, Kwok PY (2001) Genotyping single-nucleotide polymorphisms by the invader assay with dual-color fluorescence polarization detection. Clin Chem 47:1373–1377

55. Stillman MJ, Day SP, Schutzbank TE (2009) A comparative review of laboratory-developed tests utilizing Invader HPV analyte-specific reagents for the detection of high-risk human papillomavirus. J Clin Virol 45(Suppl 1):S73–S77

56. Johnson LR, Starkey CR, Palmer J et al (2008) A comparison of two methods to determine the presence of high-risk HPV cervical infections. Am J Clin Pathol 130:401–408

57. Ginocchio CC, Barth D, Zhang F (2008) Comparison of the Third Wave Invader human papillomavirus (HPV) assay and the digene HPV hybrid capture 2 assay for detection of high-risk HPV DNA. J Clin Microbiol 46:1641–1646

58. Bartholomew DA, Luff RD, Quigley NB, Curtis M, Olson MC (2011) Analytical performance of Cervista HPV 16/18 genotyping test for cervical cytology samples. J Clin Virol 51:38–43

59. Einstein MH, Martens MG, Garcia FA et al (2010) Clinical validation of the Cervista HPV HR and 16/18 genotyping tests for use in women with ASC-US cytology. Gynecol Oncol 118:116–122

60. Cuzick J, Arbyn M, Sankaranarayanan R et al (2008) Overview of human papillomavirus-based and other novel options for cervical cancer screening in developed and developing countries. Vaccine 26(Suppl 10):K29–K41

61. Rozendaal L, Walboomers JM, van der Linden JC et al (1996) PCR-based high-risk HPV test in cervical cancer screening gives objective risk assessment of women with cytomorphologically normal cervical smears. Int J Cancer 68:766–769

62. Walboomers JM, Jacobs MV, Manos MM et al (1999) Human papillomavirus is a necessary cause of invasive cervical cancer worldwide. J Pathol 189:12–19

63. de Sanjose S, Quint WG, Alemany L et al (2010) Human papillomavirus genotype attribution in invasive cervical cancer: a retrospective cross-sectional worldwide study. Lancet Oncol 11:1048–1056

64. Castle PE, Porras C, Quint WG et al (2008) Comparison of two PCR-based human papillomavirus genotyping methods. J Clin Microbiol 46:3437–3445
65. Castle PE, Sadorra M, Lau T, Aldrich C, Garcia FA, Kornegay J (2009) Evaluation of a prototype real-time PCR assay for carcinogenic human papillomavirus (HPV) detection and simultaneous HPV genotype 16 (HPV16) and HPV18 genotyping. J Clin Microbiol 47:3344–3347
66. Heideman DA, Hesselink AT, Berkhof J et al (2011) Clinical validation of the cobas 4800 HPV test for cervical screening purposes. J Clin Microbiol 49:3983–3985
67. Lapierre SG, Sauthier P, Mayrand MH et al (2012) Human papillomavirus (HPV) DNA triage of women with atypical squamous cells of undetermined significance with cobas 4800 HPV and Hybrid Capture 2 tests for detection of high-grade lesions of the uterine cervix. J Clin Microbiol 50:1240–1244
68. Martinez SB, Palomares JC, Artura A et al (2012) Comparison of the Cobas 4800 Human Papillomavirus test against a combination of the Amplicor Human Papillomavirus and the Linear Array tests for detection of HPV types 16 and 18 in cervical samples. J Virol Methods 180:7–10
69. Lindemann ML, Dominguez MJ, de Antonio JC et al (2012) Analytical comparison of the cobas HPV Test with Hybrid Capture 2 for the detection of high-risk HPV genotypes. J Mol Diagn 14:65–70
70. Gage JC, Sadorra M, Lamere BJ et al (2012) Comparison of the cobas Human Papillomavirus (HPV) test with the hybrid capture 2 and linear array HPV DNA tests. J Clin Microbiol 50:61–65
71. Wright TC Jr, Stoler MH, Sharma A, Zhang G, Behrens C, Wright TL (2011) Evaluation of HPV-16 and HPV-18 genotyping for the triage of women with high-risk HPV+ cytology-negative results. Am J Clin Pathol 136:578–586
72. Stoler MH, Wright TC Jr, Sharma A, Apple R, Gutekunst K, Wright TL (2011) High-risk human papillomavirus testing in women with ASC-US cytology: results from the ATHENA HPV study. Am J Clin Pathol 135:468–475
73. Castle PE, Stoler MH, Wright TC Jr, Sharma A, Wright TL, Behrens CM (2011) Performance of carcinogenic human papillomavirus (HPV) testing and HPV16 or HPV18 genotyping for cervical cancer screening of women aged 25 years and older: a subanalysis of the ATHENA study. Lancet Oncol 12:880–890
74. Stoler MH, Wright TC Jr Sharma A et al (2012) The interplay of age stratification and HPV testing on the predictive value of ASC-US cytology. Results from the ATHENA HPV study. Am J Clin Pathol 137:295–303
75. Cox JT, Castle PE, Behrens CM, Sharma A, Wright TC Jr, Cuzick J (2013) Comparison of cervical cancer screening strategies incorporating different combinations of cytology, HPV testing and genotyping for HPV 16/18: results from the ATHENA HPV study. Am J Obstet Gynecol 208(3):e181–184
76. Dockter J, Schroder A, Eaton B et al (2009) Analytical characterization of the APTIMA HPV Assay. J Clin Virol 45(Suppl 1):S39–S47
77. Getman D, Aiyer A, Dockter J, Giachetti C, Zhang F, Ginocchio CC (2009) Efficiency of the APTIMA HPV Assay for detection of HPV RNA and DNA targets. J Clin Virol 45(Suppl 1):S49–S54
78. Dockter J, Schroder A, Hill C, Guzenski L, Monsonego J, Giachetti C (2009) Clinical performance of the APTIMA HPV Assay for the detection of high-risk HPV and high-grade cervical lesions. J Clin Virol 45(Suppl 1):S55–S61
79. Wu R, Belinson SE, Du H et al (2010) Human papillomavirus messenger RNA assay for cervical cancer screening: the Shenzhen Cervical Cancer Screening Trial I. Int J Gynecol Cancer 20:1411–1414
80. Monsonego J, Hudgens MG, Zerat L et al (2011) Evaluation of oncogenic human papillomavirus RNA and DNA tests with liquid-based cytology in primary cervical cancer screening: the FASE study. Int J Cancer 129:691–701

81. Clarke MA, Wentzensen N, Mirabello L et al (2012) Human Papillomavirus DNA Methylation as a Potential Biomarker for Cervical Cancer. Cancer Epidemiol Biomarkers Prev 21:12 2125–2137

82. Wentzensen N, Sherman ME, Schiffman M, Wang SS (2009) Utility of methylation markers in cervical cancer early detection: appraisal of the state-of-the-science. Gynecol Oncol 112:293–299

83. Saha B, Chaiwun B, Tsao-Wei DD et al (2007) Telomerase and markers of cellular proliferation are associated with the progression of cervical intraepithelial neoplasia lesions. Int J Gynecol Pathol 26:214–222

84. Tsoumpou I, Arbyn M, Kyrgiou M et al (2009) p16(INK4a) immunostaining in cytological and histological specimens from the uterine cervix: a systematic review and meta-analysis. Cancer Treat Rev 35:210–220

85. Schmidt D, Bergeron C, Denton KJ, Ridder R (2011) p16/ki-67 dual-stain cytology in the triage of ASCUS and LSIL papanicolaou cytology: results from the European equivocal or mildly abnormal Papanicolaou cytology study. Cancer Cytopathol 119:158–166

86. Ravarino A, Nemolato S, Macciocu E et al (2012) CINtec PLUS immunocytochemistry as a tool for the cytologic diagnosis of glandular lesions of the cervix uteri. Am J Clin Pathol 138:652–656

87. Samarawardana P, Singh M, Shroyer KR (2011) Dual stain immunohistochemical localization of p16INK4A and ki-67: a synergistic approach to identify clinically significant cervical mucosal lesions. Appl Immunohistochem Mol Morphol 19:514–518

88. Renshaw AA (2002) Measuring sensitivity in gynecologic cytology: a review. Cancer 96:210–217

89. Results of a randomized trial on the management of cytology interpretations of atypical squamous cells of undetermined significance. Am J Obstet Gynecol 188:1383–1392 (2003)

90. Cibas ES (2008) Laboratory management. In: Cibas ES, Ducatman BS (eds) Cytology, diagnostic principles and clinical correlates, 3rd edn. Saunders, Philadelphia, pp 495–522

91. American College of Obstetricians and Gynecologists (2012) Screening for Cervical Cancer. Practice Bulletin No. 131. Obstet Gynecol 120:1222–1238

92. Massad LS, Einstein MH, Huh WK et al. (2013) 2012 updated consensus guidelines for the management of abnormal cervical cancer screening tests and cancer precursor. J Low Genit Tract Dis 17(5):S1–S27

93. Jemal A, Siegel R, Ward E, Hao Y, Xu J, Thun MJ (2009) Cancer statistics, 2009. CA Cancer J Clin 59:225–249

94. Sherman ME (2000) Theories of endometrial carcinogenesis: a multidisciplinary approach. Mod Pathol 13:295–308

95. Koornstra JJ, Mourits MJ, Sijmons RH, Leliveld AM, Hollema H, Kleibeuker JH (2009) Management of extracolonic tumours in patients with Lynch syndrome. Lancet Oncol 10:400–408

96. Sonoda Y, Barakat RR (2006) Screening and the prevention of gynecologic cancer: endometrial cancer. Best Pract Res Clin Obstet Gynaecol 20:363–377

97. Guidos BJ, Selvaggi SM (2000) Detection of endometrial adenocarcinoma with the ThinPrep Pap test. Diagn Cytopathol 23:260–265

98. Schorge JO, Hossein Saboorian M, Hynan L, Ashfaq R (2002) ThinPrep detection of cervical and endometrial adenocarcinoma: a retrospective cohort study. Cancer 96:338–343

99. Greenspan DL, Cardillo M, Davey DD, Heller DS, Moriarty AT (2006) Endometrial cells in cervical cytology: review of cytological features and clinical assessment. J Low Genit Tract Dis 10:111–122

100. de Peralta-Venturino MN, Purslow MJ, Kini SR (1995) Endometrial cells of the "lower uterine segment" (LUS) in cervical smears obtained by endocervical brushings: a source of potential diagnostic pitfall. Diagn Cytopathol 12:263–268; discussion 8–71

101. Solomon D, Davey D, Kurman R et al (2002) The Bethesda System 2001: terminology for reporting the results of cervical cytology. JAMA 287:2114–2119

102. Kipp BR, Medeiros F, Campion MB et al (2008) Direct uterine sampling with the Tao brush sampler using a liquid-based preparation method for the detection of endometrial cancer and atypical hyperplasia: a feasibility study. Cancer 114:228–235

103. Dijkhuizen FP, Mol BW, Brolmann HA, Heintz AP (2000) The accuracy of endometrial sampling in the diagnosis of patients with endometrial carcinoma and hyperplasia: a meta-analysis. Cancer 89:1765–1772

104. Creasman W (2009) Revised FIGO staging for carcinoma of the endometrium. Int J Gynaecol Obstet 105:109

105. Fadare O, Mariappan MR, Hileeto D, Wang S, McAlpine JN, Rimm DL (2005) Upstaging based solely on positive peritoneal washing does not affect outcome in endometrial cancer. Mod Pathol 18:673–680

106. Jorns JM, Knoepp SM (2009) Occult fallopian tube carcinoma detected in routine pelvic washing specimens submitted for staging: another justification for pelvic washing cytology? Diagn Cytopathol 37:923–929

107. Lin O (2009) Challenges in the interpretation of peritoneal cytologic specimens. Arch Pathol Lab Med 133:739–742

108. Bristow RE, Purinton SC, Santillan A, Diaz-Montes TP, Gardner GJ, Giuntoli RL 2nd (2006) Cost-effectiveness of routine vaginal cytology for endometrial cancer surveillance. Gynecol Oncol 103:709–713

109. Cooper AL, Dornfeld-Finke JM, Banks HW, Davey DD, Modesitt SC (2006) Is cytologic screening an effective surveillance method for detection of vaginal recurrence of uterine cancer? Obstet Gynecol 107:71–76

110. Myers ER, Bastian LA, Havrilesky LJ et al (2006) Management of adnexal mass. Evid Rep Technol Assess (Full Rep) 130:1–145

111. Brown DL (2007) A practical approach to the ultrasound characterization of adnexal masses. Ultrasound Q 23:87–105

112. Gostout BS, Brewer MA (2006) Guidelines for referral of the patient with an adnexal mass. Clin Obstet Gynecol 49:448–458

113. Bibbo M, Wood MD, Fitzpatrick BT (2008) Peritoneal washings and ovary. In: Bibbo M, Wilbur DC (eds) Comprehensive cytopathology, 3rd edn. Elsevier, Amsterdam, pp 291–301

114. Davidson B, Risberg B, Kristensen G et al (1999) Detection of cancer cells in effusions from patients diagnosed with gynaecological malignancies. Evaluation of five epithelial markers. Virchows Arch 435:43–49

115. Selvaggi SM (2003) Diagnostic pitfalls of peritoneal washing cytology and the role of cell blocks in their diagnosis. Diagn Cytopathol 28:335–341

116. Zuna RE, Mitchell ML (1988) Cytologic findings in peritoneal washings associated with benign gynecologic disease. Acta Cytol 32:139–147

117. Lowe E, McKenna H (1989) Peritoneal washing cytology: a retrospective analysis of 175 gynaecological patients. Aust N Z J Obstet Gynaecol 29:55–61

118. Zuna RE, Mitchell ML, Mulick KA, Weijchert WM (1989) Cytohistologic correlation of peritoneal washing cytology in gynecologic disease. Acta Cytol 33:327–336

119. Zuna RE, Behrens A (1996) Peritoneal washing cytology in gynecologic cancers: long-term follow-up of 355 patients. J Natl Cancer Inst 88:980–987

120. Fadare O, Mariappan MR, Wang S, Hileeto D, McAlpine J, Rimm DL (2004) The histologic subtype of ovarian tumors affects the detection rate by pelvic washings. Cancer 102:150–156

121. Kudo R, Takashina T, Ito E et al (1990) Peritoneal washing cytology at second-look laparotomy in cisplatin-treated ovarian cancer patients. Acta Cytol 34:545–548

122. Zanetta G, Trio D, Lissoni A et al (1993) Early and short-term complications after US-guided puncture of gynecologic lesions: evaluation after 1,000 consecutive cases. Radiology 189:161–164

123. Ganjei P (1995) Fine-needle aspiration cytology of the ovary. Clin Lab Med 15:705–726

124. Davila RM (1993) Cytology of benign cystic uterine adnexal masses. Acta Cytol 37:385–390

125. Higgins RV, Matkins JF, Marroum MC (1999) Comparison of fine-needle aspiration cytologic findings of ovarian cysts with ovarian histologic findings. Am J Obstet Gynecol 180:550–553
126. Lu D, Davila RM, Pinto KR, Lu DW (2004) ThinPrep evaluation of fluid samples aspirated from cystic ovarian masses. Diagn Cytopathol 30:320–324
127. Wojcik EM, Selvaggi SM (1992) Diagnostic accuracy of fine-needle aspiration cytology in persistent or recurrent gynecologic malignancies. Diagn Cytopathol 8:322–326
128. Angstrom T, Kjellgren O, Bergman F (1972) The cytologic diagnosis of ovarian tumors by means of aspiration biopsy. Acta Cytol 16(4):336–341
129. Mulvany NJ (1996) Aspiration cytology of ovarian cysts and cystic neoplasms. A study of 235 aspirates. Acta Cytol 40:911–920
130. Mulvany N, Ostor A, Teng G (1995) Evaluation of estradiol in aspirated ovarian cystic lesions. Acta Cytol 39:663–668
131. Yee H, Greenebaum E, Lerner J, Heller D, Timor-Tritsch IE (1994) Transvaginal sonographic characterization combined with cytologic evaluation in the diagnosis of ovarian and adnexal cysts. Diagn Cytopathol 10:107–112
132. Allias F, Chanoz J, Blache G, Thivolet-Bejui F, Vancina S (2000) Value of ultrasound-guided fine-needle aspiration in the management of ovarian and paraovarian cysts. Diagn Cytopathol 22:70–80
133. Lipitz S, Seidman DS, Menczer J et al (1992) Recurrence rate after fluid aspiration from sonographically benign-appearing ovarian cysts. J Reprod Med 37:845–848
134. Zanetta G, Lissoni A, Torri V et al (1996) Role of puncture and aspiration in expectant management of simple ovarian cysts: a randomised study. BMJ 313:1110–1113
135. Fisch JD, Sher G (2004) Sclerotherapy with 5% tetracycline is a simple alternative to potentially complex surgical treatment of ovarian endometriomas before in vitro fertilization. Fertil Steril 82:437–441
136. Kafali H, Yurtseven S, Atmaca F, Ozardali I (2003) Management of non-neoplastic ovarian cysts with sclerotherapy. Int J Gynaecol Obstet 81:41–45
137. Mesogitis S, Daskalakis G, Pilalis A et al (2005) Management of ovarian cysts with aspiration and methotrexate injection. Radiology 235:668–673

Chapter 11
Beyond the Standard of Care: The Role of Cytopathology in Molecular Testing of Cancer

Peter Kulesza

11.1 Introduction

Cytopathology is a rather unique branch of anatomic pathology: it is defined not by the organ system affected by disease, not by patient characteristics, but by the manner of procurement of the specimen. Cytopathologists diagnose Fine Needle Aspiration (FNA) and other smears, exfoliated cellular suspensions present in body fluids, irrespective of the histologic type or anatomic origin of the specimen. Additionally, contemporary practice of solid tumor diagnostics reflects a profound dichotomy in the molecular state of the art: some specimen types, e.g., cervical smears are routinely and often reflexively evaluated using molecularly based HPV assays [1], while most other specimen types are diagnosed by morphologic means, occasionally in conjunction with immunohistochemical stains. Hematologic malignancies have been an exception to this rule, as molecular characterization by flow cytometry is the current standard of care [2]. In recent years, cytopathologists increasingly have the advantage of being the first to evaluate lesional tissue, as the progress of radiologically guided tissue procurement allows access to smaller and smaller lesions with FNA. With increasing frequency the FNA (and subsequent core biopsy) allows for a definitive diagnosis, and in some cases becoming the diagnostic standard of care [3, 4]. Consequently, any molecular assays have to be performed on the available material procured at the time, if merely to avoid the cost and morbidities of additional tissue procurement procedures. This paradigm, which is *de facto* becoming the standard of care, links the diagnosis of the malignancy with the prediction of its response to therapy.

This concept has been termed "theragnostics" and refers to simultaneous detection of a disease and tailoring of a therapeutic intervention for the individual patient [5]. To realize this concept in practice, assays which match the diagnostic

P. Kulesza (✉)
Department of Pathology, Northwestern University,
251 E. Huron St. Galter Pavilion 7-132E, Chicago, IL 60611, USA
e-mail: p-kulesza@northwestern.edu

R. Nayar (ed.), *Cytopathology in Oncology*,
Cancer Treatment and Research 160, DOI: 10.1007/978-3-642-38850-7_11,
© Springer-Verlag Berlin Heidelberg 2014

component (i.e., evaluation of lesional tissue) with the therapeutic modality (i.e., the appropriate pharmacologic agent) must be developed. Such assays utilize biomarkers defined as "an objectively measured characteristic indicative of a normal or pathogenic process, or a pharmacologic response to a therapeutic intervention" [6]. Biomarkers which define the pathogenic process (one might think of cytokeratin for carcinoma, or S-100 for melanoma) are frequently prognostic; they narrow down the probability of outcome, most frequently measured as actuarial, or progression-free survival. Biomarkers which are linked to pharmacologic or therapeutic intervention are by definition predictive and can determine the patient's response to a specific drug or treatment. Some can be "purely" predictive, i.e., their status has bearing on survival only in the case of treatment with a specific drug, however, some are not. For example, b-raf mutation prognosticates a worse outcome independently of treatment [7], while at the same time predicts lack of response to treatment with cetuximab or panitumumab [8].

The necessity of incorporating in vitro tests or biomarkers in order to define and elucidate patient-specific pathophysiology has been recognized in the context of new, "targeted" agents, and was emphasized in the "Critical Path Initiative" of the Food and Drug Administration in 2004 [9]. It therefore can be expected that new drug development, and consequently clinical trials will involve an associated biomarker assay or a "companion diagnostic".

11.2 The Dawn of Predictive Biomarkers: Chemotherapy Sensitivity-Resistance Assays (CSRA)

It has been postulated since the 1950s, that an *in vitro* assay which evaluates tumor response to drugs would be predictive of the therapeutic outcome for the individual patient although many molecular pathways and profiles have been discovered in cancers [10, 11]; ultimately all malignancies are characterized either by uncontrolled cell proliferation or enhanced cell survival. Often, both processes contribute; therefore, a quantitative assay of cell proliferation and cell death should provide necessary information regarding the effects of a particular chemotherapeutic compound on the particular tumor. While the magnitude of effects or measured rates may differ, this paradigm should hold true for all malignancies, whether carcinomas, melanomas, or lymphomas.

The central premise of CSRA is the presumed correlation of an *in vitro* result of tumor cell proliferation, viability, or death with patient outcome, defined as time to tumor progression and death [12].

Early approaches to assess tumor cell response to *in vitro* drug administration began with clonogenic assays which required tumor cells to grow in soft agar [13]. The samples were dissociated to produce single cell suspension, inoculated on agar plates, and grown with various drugs for approximately 2–3 weeks until visible colonies appeared. The drugs which reduced the colony counts the most were presumed to be most efficacious. Since many tumors cannot proliferate *in vitro* long enough to obtain meaningful colony counts, development of assays focused on techniques which required shorter time frames and smaller inocula [14]. One of the first assays to replace soft agar was Differential Staining Cytotoxicity (DiSC) [15]. This assay evaluated the *ex vivo* drug response of human tumor cells by determining their structural state. The principle was that only cells with intact membranes are viable. Tumor cells were plated, exposed to drug for 3–4 days, and then membrane integrity of cells scored by microscopic examination. The scoring is very labor intensive, and the assay has not been commonly used [16].

Another assay type that has gained popularity due to ease of application and quantitation is the MTT and more recently, the MTS assay [17]. These are colorimetric assays which measure the activity of enzymes that reduce MTT or MTS. In living cells, these reactions take place only when reductases, particularly mitochondrial succinate dehydrogenase are active. Thus, the color conversion is, therefore, a measure of cell viability. While the scoring of the assay is free of observer error and fully quantitative, the assays cannot distinguish between inhibition of proliferation, inhibition of metabolic activity, and induction of cell death. In this sense, any change in metabolic activity can suggest large changes in viability by MTT (or MTS) while the number of viable cells in fact remains unchanged. A similar in vitro approach is the determination of ATP content as a marker of cell viability [18]. This assay (Adenosine Triphosphate Luminescence Assay) in a single step ruptures cells, releases ATP, and through the addition of recombinant luciferase generates a luminescence which is detected and quantified. The assay is based on the principle that light-emission is proportionally dependent on amount of ATP and, thus, number of viable cells.

The cell viability assays discussed above are methodologically very different, but the correlation of results between them appears reasonable. While there is no data comparing all the assays in the context of a clinical trial, Wiesenthal determined correlation coefficients of 0.84, 0.81, and 0.83 ($p < 0.0001$ for each) for MTT/DiSC, ATP/DiSC, and ATP/MTT, respectively, in a comparison of 20 drugs in five adenocarcinomas [19]. Thus, it may not be important which specific assay is used if any of the assay results can be translated to clinical benefit.

Rather than focusing on tumor cell sensitivity to a drug, many argue that the main application of CSRA in the current standard of care is the detection of resistance, since historically the accuracy of detection of resistance is higher. A pure proliferation assay which has been used for determination of drug resistance is the Extreme Drug Resistance (EDR) assay [20], which is based on *in vitro* incorporation of radioactive thymidine into tumor cells in the presence of suprapharmacologic drug concentrations. While this assay does require tumor growth, it is very sensitive, and the results are objectively quantitative. The EDR-thymidine assay gained for a time commercial popularity; however, the company which performed the assay (Oncotech, Inc.) has discontinued operations as of June 2010.

11.3 Translation of CSRA into Standard of Care

So, are the CSRA, such as the ones described above, clinically useful? This most important issue was addressed by the American Society of Clinical Oncology (ASCO) working group in special articles [21, 22]. Although to date, no prospective, randomized trials of CSRA-guided therapy had been conducted, the reviewed data suggested that CSRA may have been of benefit by improving tumor response rates in cohorts where assay-guided therapy was implemented. In small-cell lung cancer patients, tumor response to drug was 25 % for DiSC–guided therapy versus 7 % for empiric therapy [23]; in metastatic breast cancer, use of the MTT assay correlated with 77 % response rate in contrast to 39 % response with empiric therapy [24]. In recurrent ovarian cancer, ATP assay-guided therapy resulted in a 65 % response rate, while empiric therapy showed a 35 % response rate [25]. In a similar patient population, the EDR assay resulted in a 56 %, and empiric therapy in 28 %, response rate [26]. In addition, 2 of the 11 studies showed prolonged survival in the assay-guided group.

Reviewing these results, the ASCO working group concluded that the use of CSRA was *not* recommended outside of clinical trial settings. This conclusion was based on the numerous problems which have confounded the analysis, such as lack of randomization, failure to account for baseline patient characteristics, and insufficient numbers of patients to draw comparisons between assay-guided and empiric arms, particularly given the heterogeneity of lesions and assays [22]. Despite this, CSRA have continued to be utilized, particularly in ovarian malignancies which has been recognized in the most recent NCCN clinical practice guidelines in oncology [27]. Even in this setting the data is conflicting: while the EDR assay showed no association with survival outcomes, a simpler type of assay did show association to progression-free interval [28, 29]. The latter assay (ChemoFX) uses less cells per data point, establishes a broader dose-response curve, and relies on scoring live cells only, which may explain the findings. No study to date, however, proved the effectiveness of the CSRA-guided therapy in a prospective manner.

11.4 Targeted Therapies: Molecular Specificity

More recently, the CSRA has been placed in a new context by the increased use of targeted therapeutics, i.e., the utilization of drugs designed to effect a single molecule, placed at a point critical to the "well-being" of the malignancy. Detailed understanding of the molecular mechanism of drug action can theoretically permit the development of specific *in vitro* or *ex vivo* assays reflective of the biological activity of the drug and serving, at a minimum, as pharmacodynamic marker assays; in practice, this has been remarkably difficult to accomplish [30, 31].

Almost exclusively, the assay design has been focused not on live tumor material but on fixed tissue. This was mainly due to the "target enrichment" strategies which equated the presence, or overexpression of a molecule with the putative therapeutic effect of the drug targeting that molecule. Thus, it was proposed that only the patients whose lesions express the target molecule will receive, and benefit from the therapy. In some cases, this has been remarkably successful, as evidenced in the case of Gastrointestinal Stromal Tumors, c-kit, and imatinib [32].

One of the earliest targeted cancer drugs was tamoxifen, an estrogen receptor antagonist which was developed for use in estrogen receptor-expressing breast cancer [33]. It is used in the context of estrogen receptor identification by immunohistochemistry (IHC). There is no molecular assay in living cancer cells that can be used to predict tumor response, or resistance, to tamoxifen and other estrogen blockers. A similar situation exists for a newer drug-target pair, trastuzumab and erbB2. Trastuzumab is used only in patients whose cancers overexpress erbB2, IHC for erbB2 was implemented as companion test, and was part of the FDA approval process for trastuzumab [34]. Despite the regulatory scrutiny, the performance of IHC in clinical practice has been problematic. Results were affected by subjective interpretation and specimen processing [35]. The former has been addressed by the development of specific criteria, such as identification of membranous staining, and stratification of results based on fraction of positive cells (HercepTest, Dako) [36]. Addressing specimen processing has been particularly challenging, leading the ASCO to issue a set of restrictive fixation guidelines (10 % neutral-buffered formalin; not less than 6, and not more than 48 h) [37]. The effect on cytopathology which uses alcohol-based fixatives (a source of false positive results) has been minimal, most likely because the vast majority of breast cancer samples are core biopsies which are processed by surgical histopathology labs where alcohol-based fixatives are not used [38]. IHC has also been approved for detection of Epidermal Growth Factor Receptor (EGFR, erbB1) in formalin-fixed samples (EGFR PharmDx), but has proven even more problematic than HercepTest [39]. Furthermore, while this test utilized a priori similar scoring criteria as HercepTest, its utility is questionable, and in some cases has been proven to be of no value at all [40]. Thus, colon cancer patients had been treated empirically on the basis of large phase III studies. The subsequent discovery of the resistance to cetuximab and panitumumab despite EGFR overexpression in cancers bearing k-ras mutations resulted in abandonment of "target-enrichment" strategy for EGFR [41].

Assays for k-ras mutations and activating EGFR mutations have been utilized as very successful predictive biomarkers to exclude cetuximab-resistant patients in the former, and to offer gefitinib and erlotinib as therapy in the latter [42, 43]. Due to chemical stability and ability to amplify DNA, the specimen requirements are less stringent than for IHC-based tests: a typical FNA contains sufficient amount of material for IHC as well as nucleic acid-based tests [44]. Since almost all FNA smear slides are alcohol-fixed, the rare but real false positives induced by formalin are avoided [45]. In all mutation-detection testing the issue of specimen purity is critical, i.e., the proportion of lesional material to the "contaminating" benign, or nonlesional cells. Typical dye-terminator sequencing utilized in the majority of labs requires a minimum of 25 % of lesional tissue in the sample, since neither the PCR amplification step, nor the DNA extension reaction favors mutant template over wild type [46]. This limitation can be circumvented by implementing "single strand" sequencing analyses such as Solexa (now Illumina) or SOLiD, in which a single DNA template is clonally expanded and each individual sequence read by a high resolution camera [47, 48]. The other approach is to use methods which "ignore" the wild type sequence and preferentially amplify, (TheraScreen KRAS and EGFR29, DxS, Ltd) [49] or preferentially extend the abnormal sequence (k-ras Mutector, TrimGen [50]). Commercial laboratories (Genzyme Genetics, Quest) do accept cytologic specimens such as aspirates and fluids. While such applications rarely have been validated in published studies [51], they are increasingly utilized given that FNA samples are often the only diagnostic samples available.

11.5 Slow Progress in Biomarker-Guided Therapeutics

It is sobering to realize that despite thousands of scientific papers describing the molecular basis of malignancy and mechanisms of action of chemotherapeutic agents, no live tumor CSRAs which address a defined molecular end-point are yet available. While live tumor assays may not be the only answer, the current approach of random assignment of patients in clinical trials may not be optimal and it certainly does not produce benefits proportional to the amount of clinical, cognitive, and financial resources devoted to the task [52]. It has been estimated that approximately 5 % of applications for new drugs in oncology submitted to the FDA move beyond investigational stage [53]. This clearly is not sustainable, and requires new drug development strategies. The FDA Critical Pathway initiative provides for an Exploratory Investigational Drug Application (xIND) which uti-lizes a Phase 0 clinical trial approach [9, 54]. The central premise of Phase 0 is the realization that the pharmacodynamic measurements, i.e., the effect of drug on biomarker(s) is the essential step in transfer of any targeted drug from preclinical (typically murine xenograft) to clinical realm. The consequences of this approach, however, extend beyond Phase 0 into the entire drug development process, and change the design of Phase I through Phase III. Aside from statistical conse-quences which on average decrease the number of patients compared to "classic" Phase I through III system, the main change is in the tissue procurement. In the "new" schema, all patients undergo protocol biopsies at baseline, and at multiple points during therapy: this is to follow the biomarker changes. Irrespective of the specific end-point assays, whether performed on live or fixed material, the para-digm of multiple tissue procurement must have minimal morbidities to be feasible, thus requiring either FNA or core biopsies.

11.6 Cytopathology as an Indispensible Component of Oncologic Drug Development

Typical practices in cytopathology make it ideal for the development of theragnostic approaches, particularly for live cell, predictive CSRA. First, the source of material in cytopathology is uniquely suitable: fine needle aspirates consist of dissociated cells and cell clusters, and effusions are both dispersed and usually voluminous. This avoids the need for digestion of specimens with elastases and collagenases, and does not require any mechanical specimen manipulation beyond pipetting. These specimens are routinely obtained and maintained without fixation, allowing for adequate preservation of live cells. Second, specimens can be used for CSRA without interfering with the standard of care, since most of the specimens are collected by clinical colleagues as part of routine care of cancer patients. Third, cytopathologists and cytotechnologists are trained to recognize malignant or lesional cells in small specimens. This provides for easily available and qualified expertise, useful at a minimum in validation of quantitative assays to assure that preanalytical variables are stringently controlled for. Fourth, the costs associated with adaptation of the CSRA technology are minimal compared to the overall sums expended on cancer therapeutics [55]. The staining and microscopy personnel and infrastructure already exists in all cytopathology laboratories, and most laboratories can adapt existing structures to provide a biosafety cabinet suitable for tissue culture and humidified CO_2 incubators. Fifth, since cytopathology has been the heaviest-regulated subspecialty in anatomic pathology, it can claim the advantage of superior quality control and quality assurance. The standard of care practices in cytopathology includes "chain of custody" process, with individuals signing off on the specimen processing and diagnosis (beginning with the preparation technicians, through cytotechnologists, and then attending pathologists). Such a system is well-suited for the FDA registration process with minimal changes. Sixth, most of the chemotherapeutic compounds used in the clinic are easily available in their pure (or active) form from hospital pharmacies or from independent vendors. Thus, the adoption of *ex vivo* live tumor assays even without material transfer agreements is feasible. Given the above, it is easy to envision the increasing use of cytopathologic techniques in the context of drug development and clinical trials. The main challenge is in the effective, and evidence-based communication of these unique advantages to the treating physicians.

References

1. Kinney W, Stoler MH, Castle PE (2010) Special commentary: patient safety and the next generation of HPV DNA tests. Am J Clin Pathol 134(2):193–199
2. Craig FE, Foon KA (2008) Flow cytometric immunophenotyping for hematologic neoplasms. Blood 111(8):3941–3967

3. Hawes RH (2010) The evolution of endoscopic ultrasound: improved imaging, higher accuracy for fine needle aspiration and the reality of endoscopic ultrasound-guided interventions. Curr Opin Gastroenterol 26(5):436–444

4. Baloch ZW, Cibas ES, Clark DP et al (2008) The national cancer institute thyroid fine needle aspiration state of the science conference: a summation. Cytojournal 5:6

5. Pene F, Courtine E, Cariou A, Mira JP (2009) Toward theragnostics. Crit Care Med 37(1 Suppl):S50–S58

6. Downing GJ (2000) Biomarkers and surrogate endpoints: clinical research and applications. Elsevier Scientific, Amsterdam

7. Roth AD, Tejpar S, Delorenzi M et al (2010) Prognostic role of KRAS and BRAF in stage II and III resected colon cancer: results of the translational study on the PETACC-3, EORTC 40993, SAKK 60–00 trial. J Clin Oncol 28(3):466–474

8. Di Nicolantonio F, Martini M, Molinari F et al (2008) Wild-type BRAF is required for response to panitumumab or cetuximab in metastatic colorectal cancer. J Clin Oncol 26(35):5705–5712

9. FDA (2004) Challenges and opportunities report. Introduction or stagnation: challenge and opportunity on the critical path to new medical products

10. Von Hoff DD (1990) He's not going to talk about in vitro predictive assays again, is he? J Natl Cancer Inst 82(2):96–101

11. Brown E, Markman M (1996) Tumor chemosensitivity and chemoresistance assays. Cancer 77(6):1020–1025

12. Kern DH (1997) Tumor chemosensitivity and chemoresistance assays. Cancer 79(7):1447–1450

13. Hamburger AW, Salmon SE (1977) Primary bioassay of human tumor stem cells. Science 197(4302):461–463

14. Furukawa T, Kubota T, Hoffman RM (1995) Clinical applications of the histoculture drug response assay. Clin Cancer Res 1(3):305–311

15. Hoy CA, Salazar EP, Thompson LH (1984) Rapid detection of DNA-damaging agents using repair-deficient CHO cells. Mutat Res 130(5):321–332

16. Mason JM, Drummond MF, Bosanquet AG, Sheldon TA (1999) The DiSC assay. A cost-effective guide to treatment for chronic lymphocytic leukemia? Int J Technol Assess Health Care 15(1):173–184 (Winter)

17. Cory AH, Owen TC, Barltrop JA, Cory JG (1991) Use of an aqueous soluble tetrazolium/formazan assay for cell growth assays in culture. Cancer Commun 3(7):207–212

18. Bradbury DA, Simmons TD, Slater KJ, Crouch SP (2000) Measurement of the ADP: ATP ratio in human leukaemic cell lines can be used as an indicator of cell viability, necrosis and apoptosis. J Immunol Methods 240(1–2):79–92

19. Weisenthal LM, Dill PL, Kurnick NB, Lippman ME (1983) Comparison of dye exclusion assays with a clonogenic assay in the determination of drug-induced cytotoxicity. Cancer Res 43(1):258–264

20. Kern DH, Weisenthal LM (1990) Highly specific prediction of antineoplastic drug resistance with an in vitro assay using suprapharmacologic drug exposures. J Natl Cancer Inst 82(7):582–588

21. Schrag D, Garewal HS, Burstein HJ, Samson DJ, Von Hoff DD, Somerfield MR (2004) American society of clinical oncology technology assessment: chemotherapy sensitivity and resistance assays. J Clin Oncol 22(17):3631–3638

22. Samson DJ, Seidenfeld J, Ziegler K, Aronson N (2004) Chemotherapy sensitivity and resistance assays: a systematic review. J Clin Oncol 22(17):3618–3630

23. Gazdar AF, Steinberg SM, Russell EK et al (1990) Correlation of in vitro drug-sensitivity testing results with response to chemotherapy and survival in extensive-stage small cell lung cancer: a prospective clinical trial. J Natl Cancer Inst 82(2):117–124

24. Xu JM, Song ST, Tang ZM et al (1999) Predictive chemotherapy of advanced breast cancer directed by MTT assay in vitro. Breast Cancer Res Treat 53(1):77–85

25. Kurbacher CM, Cree IA, Bruckner HW et al (1998) Use of an ex vivo ATP luminescence assay to direct chemotherapy for recurrent ovarian cancer. Anticancer Drugs 9(1):51–57
26. Loizzi V, Chan JK, Osann K, Cappuccini F, DiSaia PJ, Berman ML (2003) Survival outcomes in patients with recurrent ovarian cancer who were treated with chemoresistance assay-guided chemotherapy. Am J Obstet Gynecol 189(5):1301–1307
27. NCCN Guidelines™ (2010) http://www.nccn.org/professionals/physician_gls/f_guidelines.asp
28. Gallion H, Christopherson WA, Coleman RL et al (2006) Progression-free interval in ovarian cancer and predictive value of an ex vivo chemoresponse assay. Int J Gynecol Cancer 16(1):194–201
29. Matsuo K, Eno ML, Im DD, Rosenshein NB, Sood AK (2010) Clinical relevance of extent of extreme drug resistance in epithelial ovarian carcinoma. Gynecol Oncol 116(1):61–65
30. Kaiser J (2004) Cancer research…and NCI hears a pitch for biomarker studies. Science 306(5699):1119
31. Sawyers CL (2008) The cancer biomarker problem. Nature 452(7187):548–552
32. Dagher R, Cohen M, Williams G et al (2002) Approval summary: imatinib mesylate in the treatment of metastatic and/or unresectable malignant gastrointestinal stromal tumors. Clin Cancer Res 8(10):3034–3038
33. Ward HW (1973) Anti-oestrogen therapy for breast cancer: a trial of tamoxifen at two dose levels. Br Med J 1(5844):13–14
34. Cobleigh MA, Vogel CL, Tripathy D et al (1999) Multinational study of the efficacy and safety of humanized anti-HER2 monoclonal antibody in women who have HER2-overexpressing metastatic breast cancer that has progressed after chemotherapy for metastatic disease. J Clin Oncol 17(9):2639–2648
35. Perez EA, Suman VJ, Davidson NE et al (2006) HER2 testing by local, central, and reference laboratories in specimens from the North Central Cancer Treatment Group N9831 intergroup adjuvant trial. J Clin Oncol 24(19):3032–3038
36. Dako. HercepTest Interpretation Manual (2009) http://www.dako.com/us/index/knowledgecenter/kc_publications/kc_publications_interpret.htm
37. Wolf AM, Wender RC, Etzioni RB et al (2010) American cancer society guideline for the early detection of prostate cancer: update 2010. CA Cancer J Clin 60(2):70–98
38. Bilous M, Dowsett M, Hanna W et al (2003) Current perspectives on HER2 testing: a review of national testing guidelines. Mod Pathol 16(2):173–182
39. Derecskei K, Moldvay J, Bogos K, Timar J (2006) Protocol modifications influence the result of EGF receptor immunodetection by EGFR pharmDx in paraffin-embedded cancer tissues. Pathol Oncol Res 12(4):243–246
40. Hecht JR, Mitchell E, Neubauer MA et al (2010) Lack of correlation between epidermal growth factor receptor status and response to Panitumumab monotherapy in metastatic colorectal cancer. Clin Cancer Res 16(7):2205–2213
41. Allegra CJ, Jessup JM, Somerfield MR et al (2009) American society of clinical oncology provisional clinical opinion: testing for KRAS gene mutations in patients with metastatic colorectal carcinoma to predict response to anti-epidermal growth factor receptor monoclonal antibody therapy. J Clin Oncol 27(12):2091–2096
42. Lievre A, Bachet JB, Le Corre D et al (2006) KRAS mutation status is predictive of response to cetuximab therapy in colorectal cancer. Cancer Res 66(8):3992–3995
43. Lynch TJ, Bell DW, Sordella R et al (2004) Activating mutations in the epidermal growth factor receptor underlying responsiveness of non-small-cell lung cancer to gefitinib. N Engl J Med 350(21):2129–2139
44. Centeno BA, Enkemann SA, Coppola D, Huntsman S, Bloom G, Yeatman TJ (2005) Classification of human tumors using gene expression profiles obtained after microarray analysis of fine-needle aspiration biopsy samples. Cancer 105(2):101–109
45. Williams C, Ponten F, Moberg C et al (1999) A high frequency of sequence alterations is due to formalin fixation of archival specimens. Am J Pathol 155(5):1467–1471
46. Smith LM, Sanders JZ, Kaiser RJ et al (1986) Fluorescence detection in automated DNA sequence analysis. Nature 321(6071):674–679

47. Schuster SC (2008) Next-generation sequencing transforms today's biology. Nat Methods 5(1):16–18
48. Mardis ER (2008) Next-generation DNA sequencing methods. Annu Rev Genomics Hum Genet 9:387–402
49. Angulo B, Garcia–Garcia E, Martinez R et al (2010) A commercial real-time PCR kit provides greater sensitivity than direct sequencing to detect KRAS mutations: a morphology-based approach in colorectal carcinoma. J Mol Diagn 12(3):292–299
50. Shackelford W, Deng S, Murayama K, Wang J (2004) A new technology for mutation detection. Ann N Y Acad Sci 1022:257–262
51. Franklin WA, Haney J, Sugita M, Bemis L, Jimeno A, Messersmith WA (2010) KRAS mutation: comparison of testing methods and tissue sampling techniques in colon cancer. J Mol Diagn 12(1):43–50
52. Peppercorn JM, Weeks JC, Cook EF, Joffe S (2004) Comparison of outcomes in cancer patients treated within and outside clinical trials: conceptual framework and structured review. Lancet 363(9405):263–270
53. Gutman S, Kessler LG (2006) The US food and drug administration perspective on cancer biomarker development. Nat Rev Cancer 6(7):565–571
54. Kummar S, Kinders R, Rubinstein L et al (2007) Compressing drug development timelines in oncology using phase '0' trials. Nat Rev Cancer 7(2):131–139
55. Rimm DL, Stastny JF, Rimm EB, Ayer S, Frable WJ (1997) Comparison of the costs of fine-needle aspiration and open surgical biopsy as methods for obtaining a pathologic diagnosis. Cancer 81(1):51–56